# ADVANCES IN DRUG RESEARCH
## VOLUME 27

# ANTIDIABETIC AGENTS

Recent Advances in their Molecular
and Clinical Pharmacology

# ADVANCES IN DRUG RESEARCH
## VOLUME 27

Edited by

BERNARD TESTA

*School of Pharmacy, University of Lausanne*
*Lausanne, Switzerland*

and

URS A. MEYER

*Institute of Pharmacology*
*University of Basel, Basel*
*Switzerland*

# ANTIDIABETIC AGENTS

Recent Advances in their Molecular
and Clinical Pharmacology

by

## H. P. T. Ammon, H. U. Häring,
## M. Kellerer, H. Laube, L. Mosthaf,
## E. J. Verspohl and M. A. Wahl

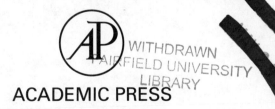

ACADEMIC PRESS

*Harcourt Brace & Company, Publishers*

LONDON   SAN DIEGO   NEW YORK   BOSTON
SYDNEY   TOKYO   TORONTO

ACADEMIC PRESS LIMITED
24–28 Oval Road
LONDON NW1 7DX


*U.S. Edition Published by*
ACADEMIC PRESS INC.
San Diego, CA 92101


This book is printed on acid-free paper

A catalogue record for this book is available from the British Library


ISBN 0-12-013327-X

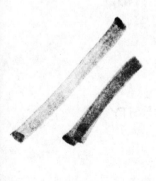

Typeset by Keyset Composition, Colchester, Essex
Printed in Great Britain by Hartnolls Ltd, Bodmin, Cornwall

# CONTENTS

### Regulation of Glucose Homoeostasis

### Clinical Aspects of Diabetes Mellitus

### Mechanisms of Insulin Action

### Therapeutic Use of Insulin

The Secretory Machinery of Insulin Release

Compounds Acting on Insulin Secretion: Sulphonylureas

Compounds Acting on Glucose Uptake: Biguanides

Compounds Acting on Glucose Absorption

Aldose Reductase Inhibitors as New Antidiabetic Drugs

# CONTRIBUTORS

H. P. T. Ammon, *Lehrstuhl Pharmakologie, Pharmazeutisches Institut, Universität Tübingen, Auf der Morgenstelle 8, D–72076 Tübingen, Germany*

H. U. Häring, *Institut für Diabetes-Forschung, Krankenhaus Schwabing, Kölner Platz 1, D–80804 München, Germany*

M. Kellerer, *Institut für Diabetes-Forschung, Krankenhaus Schwabing, Kölner Platz 1, D–80804 München, Germany*

H. Laube, *Medizinische Klinik der Universität Gießen, Rodthohl 6, D–35392 Gießen, Germany*

L. Mosthaf, *Institut für Diabetes-Forschung, Krankenhaus Schwabing, Kölner Platz 1, D–80804 München, Germany*

E. J. Verspohl, *Institut für Pharmazeutische Chemie, Hittorfstrasse 58–62, D–48149 Münster, Germany*

M. A. Wahl, *Lehrstuhl Pharmakologie, Pharmazeutisches Institut, Universität Tübingen, Auf der Morgenstelle 8, D–72076 Tübingen, Germany*

# FOREWORD

When Professor Ammon accepted to write a chapter on antidiabetics for *Advances in Drug Research*, he set himself to the task with great enthusiasm and dedication. His first priority was to enlist the help of a few distinguished colleagues whose fields of competence were complementary to his own. However, Ammon and his co-authors soon realized that what they had in mind would not fit into a single chapter, even a very large one.

The present volume is the result of the writers' ambition towards comprehensiveness and timeliness. In one chapter after the other, they examine such facets as glucose homeostasis, clinical aspects of diabetes, mechanisms of insulin action, therapeutic use of insulin, insulin release and drugs that act on its secretion, agents that influence glucose uptake or absorption, and some novel drugs. The coverage is impressive in its breadth and depth, ranging from molecular physiology and pharmacology to pathology and therapy.

For *Advances in Drug Research*, a monograph such as this one is a novelty. Whether and how much it will remain an exception will depend on a number of factors including the readers' response.

BERNARD TESTA
URS A. MEYER

# PREFACE:
## ANTIDIABETIC AGENTS: RECENT ADVANCES IN THEIR MOLECULAR AND CLINICAL PHARMACOLOGY

This book tries to give an overview on present knowledge about pharmacological and clinical aspects of antidiabetic drugs. In this connection it was found to be important to include chapters on the regulation of glucose homoeostasis and pathophysiology of Type-I and Type-II diabetes mellitus. Since diabetes mellitus is a disease of inadequate insulin secretion and inadequate action of insulin, especially in Type-II diabetes mellitus, special emphasis has been put on the molecular basis of insulin secretion and insulin actions. Several experts have contributed different topics. The clinical part was written by H. Laube, and insulin action by H. U. Häring, M. Kellerer and L. Mosthaf. The secretory machinery and mechanisms of sulphonylurea actions were contributed by H. P. T. Ammon. The author of pharmacodynamics of other antidiabetic drugs, side effects and drug interactions is E. J. Verspohl and finally M. A. Wahl added the pharmacokinetic properties of antidiabetic agents. Only antidiabetic drugs on the market have been included.

By discussing the pathophysiology of diabetes mellitus, the regulation of glucose homoeostasis and the molecular aspects of insulin action and secretion, this book aims to stimulate future considerations on possible concepts in the development of new antidiabetic drugs.

H. P. T. Ammon
H. U. Häring
M. Kellerer
H. Laube
L. Mosthaf
E. J. Verspohl
and M. A. Wahl

# ABBREVIATIONS

| | |
|---|---|
| Acetyl-CoA | Acetyl-coenzyme A |
| ACTH | Adrenocorticotrophic hormone |
| ADA | American Diabetes Association |
| ADH | Alcohol dehydrogenase |
| ADP | Adenosine diphosphate |
| AEP | Artifical endocrine pancreas |
| AVP | Arginine-vasopressin |
| BCH | 2-Aminobicyclo[2.2.1]heptane-2-carboxylic acid |
| BB rats | Bio-Breeding rats (a model for Type-I diabetes) |
| BCNU | 1,3-bis-(2-chloroethyl)-1-nitrosourea |
| BSA | Bovine serum albumin |
| BSO | Buthionine-sulphoximine |
| $C_{max}$ | Peak plasma concentration |
| cAMP | Cyclic adenosine monophosphate |
| $[Ca^{2+}]_i$ | Cytosolic calcium concentration |
| CaCaMK | Calcium–calmodulin-dependent protein kinase |
| CCK | Cholecystokinin |
| $CCK_4$ | Cholecystokinin analogue: 4 amino acids |
| $CCK_8$ | Cholecystokinin analogue: 8 amino acids |
| cDNA | Complementary desoxyribonucleic acid |
| CGRP | Calcitonin-gene-related peptide |
| CPAF | Chloropropamide–alcohol flushing |
| C-peptide | Connecting peptide |
| CRF | Corticotrophin-releasing hormone |
| CSF | Colony-stimulating factor |
| CSII | Continuous subcutaneous insulin infusion |
| DAG | Diacylglycerol |
| db-cAMP | Dibutyryl cyclic adenosine monophosphate |
| diamide | Diazenedicarboxylic acid bis-($NN$-dimethylamide) |
| DIP | Diazenedicarboxylic acid bis-($N'$-methylpiperazide) |
| EGF | Epidermal growth factor |
| ERKs | Extracellular-signal-regulated kinases |
| F-2,6-$P_2$ | Fructose-2,6-bisphosphate |
| FDA | Food and Drug Administration |
| FFA | Free fatty acids |
| $G_i$ | Inhibitory G-protein |
| $G_s$ | Stimulatory G-protein |
| GABA | $\gamma$-Aminobutyric acid |
| GAP | GTPase-activating protein |

| | |
|---|---|
| GDP | Guanosine diphosphate |
| GH | Growth hormone |
| GHRH | Growth hormone-releasing hormone |
| GIP | Glucose-dependent-insulinotropic polypeptide = Gastric inhibitory peptide |
| GLP | Glucagon-like peptide |
| GLP-1$_{(7-36)}$ | Glugacon-like peptide analogue: 7–36 amino acids |
| GLUT-1 | Glucose transporter 1 |
| GLUT-2 | Glucose transporter 2 |
| GLUT-3 | Glucose transporter 3 |
| GLUT-4 | Glucose transporter 4 |
| GLUT-5 | Glucose transporter 5 |
| G-protein | GTP-binding protein |
| Grb2 | Growth factor receptor-bound protein 2 |
| GRP | Gastrin-releasing peptide |
| GSH | Glutathione – reduced |
| GSSG | Glutathione – oxidized |
| GTP | Guanosine triphosphate |
| HbA$_1$ | Adult haemoglobin |
| HDL | High-density lipoprotein |
| HIR-A | Human insulin receptor-A |
| HIR-B | Human insulin receptor-B |
| HIT cells | Hamster insulin tumour cells |
| HLA | Human leucocyte antigen |
| HMG-CoA | Hydroxymethylglutaryl-coenzyme A |
| HM-insulin | Human insulin |
| HGP | Hepatic glucose production |
| IAA | Insulin autoantibodies |
| IAB | Insulin antibodies |
| IAPP | Islet amyloid polypeptide |
| ICA | Islet cell antibodies |
| ICIT | Intensified conventional insulin therapy |
| ICT | Intensified conventional therapy |
| IDDM | Insulin-dependent diabetes mellitus |
| IDL | Intermediate-density lipoprotein |
| IFN | Interferon |
| IgE | Immunoglobulin E |
| IGF-I | Insulin-like growth factor I |
| IgG | Immunoglobulin G |
| IL-1 | Interleukin-1 |
| Ins(1,4,5)$P_3$ | Inositol (1,4,5)-trisphosphate |
| IP$_3$ | Inositol (1,4,5)-trisphosphate |
| IPO | Inositol phospho-oligosaccharide |
| IR-GIP | Immunoreactive glucose-induced polypeptide |

| | |
|---|---|
| IRS-1 | Insulin receptor substrate-1 |
| $K_m$ | Michaelis constant |
| $K_d$ | Dissociation constant |
| LDL | Low-density lipoprotein |
| LDL-cholesterol | Low-density lipoprotein-cholesterol |
| LH | Luteinizing hormone |
| L-PIA | L-Phenylisopropyl adenosine |
| MAPK | Mitogen-activated protein kinase |
| MAPKK | Mitogen-activated protein kinase kinase |
| MAPKKK | Mitogen-activated protein kinase kinase kinase |
| MC-insulin | Monocomponent-insulin |
| MDI | Multiple daily injections |
| MI | Multiple injections |
| MODY | Maturity-onset diabetes of the young |
| MW | Molecular weight |
| Na/K-ATPase | Sodium-potassium pump |
| NEFA | Non-esterified fatty acids |
| NIDDM | Non-insulin-dependent diabetes mellitus |
| NPH | Neutral protamine Hagedorn insulin |
| NPY | Neuropeptide Y |
| PDGF | Platelet-derived growth factor |
| $PGE_2$ | Prostaglandin $E_2$ |
| PHI | Peptide histidine-isoleucinamide |
| PI 3-kinase | Phosphatidylinositol 3-kinase |
| PKA | Protein kinase A |
| PKC | Protein kinase C |
| $PLA_2$ | Phospholipase $A_2$ |
| PLC | Phospholipase C |
| PP-1 | Protein phosphatase 1 |
| PPS | Pentose phosphate shunt |
| $R_i$ | Inhibitory receptor |
| $^{86}Rb^+$ | $^{86}$Rubidium |
| RIN | Rat insulinoma |
| RINm5F | Rat insulinoma tumour cell line m5F |
| SDS-PAGE | Sodium dodecyl sulphate–polyacrylamide gel electrophoresis |
| $t_{1/2}$ | Elimination half-life |
| $t_{max}$ | Time of peak plasma concentration following drug intake |
| t-BHP | *tert*-butyl hydroperoxide |
| TMG | Tetramethyleneglutaric acid |
| t-PA | Tissue plasminogen activator |
| UGDP | University Group Diabetes Program |
| UK-P.D.S. | United Kingdom-Prospective Diabetes Study |

| | |
|---|---|
| u + n regimen | Background (u) and soluble (n) insulin |
| $V_d$ | Volume of distribution |
| VIP | Vasoactive intestinal peptide |
| VLDL | Very-low-density lipoprotein |
| W-7 | $N$-(6-aminohexyl)-5-chloro-1-naphthalenesulphonamide |

# Introduction

Diabetes is a life-threatening disease which can be found in all population groups and countries all over the world. Recent advances in the chemistry and molecular pharmacology of antidiabetic drugs have considerably improved the therapeutic situation and have increased chances to treat diabetic patients with "near normoglycaemia". Nevertheless, morbidity and mortality in diabetic patients have clearly not decreased and are now not much better than they were years ago. The diagnosis of diabetes mellitus still means a considerable reduction of life expectancy (30%) for the average untrained patient. This suggests that our basic knowledge of glucose homoeostasis and the advances in understanding of the pathophysiology of diabetes mellitus are still not sufficiently great or transformed into clinical practice to the benefit of our patients and therefore should be further improved.

# Regulation of Glucose Homoeostasis

## 1 Introduction

The glucose regulatory system is one of the most important homoeostatic systems in physiology. Glucose homoeostasis is the sum of various processes that regulate the production and metabolism of glucose *in vivo*. In healthy individuals, fuel homoeostasis and blood glucose levels are remarkably well maintained. The fundamental mechanism underlying the regulation of glucose homoeostasis, however, is rather complex. The maintenance of glucose homoeostasis depends on substrate supply, primarily glucose ingestion and glucose uptake (peripheral and splanchnic), insulin secretion, hormonal counter-regulation and hepatic glucose efflux (gluconeogenesis and glycogenolysis). These processes are simultaneously ongoing and are coordinated physiologically to avoid hypo- and hyper-glycaemic states. In the postabsorptive state, normal blood glucose levels are maintained by hepatic glucose production from gluconeogenesis and glycolysis. Extrahepatic tissues utilize glucose, and corresponding amounts of glucose are provided by the liver, thus keeping glucose homoeostasis in balance.

**Glycogenolysis** in the liver is the major source of rapid release of glucose in the fasting state (Fig. 1). Glucagon, catecholamines and the sympathetic nervous system stimulate glycogenolysis, with insulin having the opposite action. Glucose *per se* suppresses glycogenolysis directly. The main substrates for gluconeogenesis are glycogenic amino acids, mainly alanine and glutamine from muscle protein, and lactate and pyruvate derived initially from triglycerides.

**Gluconeogenesis** is stimulated by glucagon and supported by catecholamines. Gluconeogenesis is also stimulated by high fatty acid concentrations, and inhibited by insulin. The ratio of insulin to glucagon,

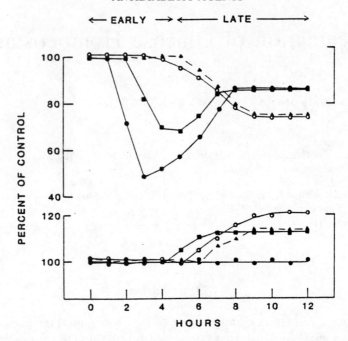

FIG. 1. Effects of lack of glucagon (●), catecholamine (■), growth hormone (▲), and cortisol (○) responses on counter-regulatory changes in glucose production (top) and glucose utilization (bottom) in non-diabetic volunteers. (Source: Gerich, 1988.)

however, is more important than the absolute concentration of either hormone alone. Insulin physiologically released in a pulsatile fashion – the pulses lasting from 8 to 30 min (Hansen et al., 1982; Waldahäusl et al., 1984) – is the key regulatory factor of glucose homoeostasis. Conversely, the major regulator of insulin secretion is plasma glucose concentration. Insulin suppresses glucose output of the liver and stimulates glucose uptake by extrahepatic peripheral tissues, primarily muscle and adipose tissue.

In the fasting state, glucose homoeostasis is maintained at the expense of other fuel sources, mainly free fatty acids (FFA). Lipolysis is initiated in adipose tissue, and triglycerides are hydrolysed to FFA and glycerol. Ketogenesis is increased. Ketones are synthesized in the liver from fatty acids and utilized progressively during prolonged starvation. An increased rate of fatty acid oxidation is stimulated through an increase in intrahepatic citrate and acetyl-CoA concentrations. Free fatty acids cause a decrease in glucose uptake and metabolism and subsequently a decrease in glucose utilization (glucose–fatty acid cycle; Fig. 2).

The major stimuli to lipolysis are insulin deficiency and catecholamines. Lipolysis is also stimulated by the sympathetic nervous system through both

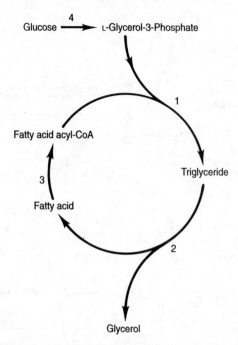

FIG. 2. Metabolic interrelationships between free fatty acid and glucose metabolism. (Source: Randle *et al.*, 1963.)

$\alpha$- and $\beta$-adrenergic actions. Muscle and liver as sites of $\beta$-oxidation are the major consumers of circulating fatty acids.

Following glucose ingestion a rapid rise in arterial glucose concentration, as well as splanchnic output, is seen as the result of glucose absorbed from the gut and passing through the liver. This is accompanied by a mean 50% suppression of endogenous glucose production. Normally 30% of the glucose load is retained by the liver and the remainder is translocated and available to peripheral tissues, with insulin-supported uptake into muscle and adipose tissue. Plasma glucose is the major regulator of insulin secretion.

Our understanding of the fundamental mechanism underlying the complex regulation of glucose homoeostasis has been dramatically transformed recently by the realization that glucose transport in mammalian tissues is mediated by a family of structurally related, but genetically distinct, glucose transporter proteins. This, however, will be discussed in detail later.

After ingestion of food, a small rise in serum insulin suppresses effectively fatty acid mobilization from adipose tissue but has little effect on glucose transport. A single intravenous injection of insulin does not decrease serum triglycerides. However, small amounts of insulin infused for a number of hours result in significant reduction, leading finally to an increase in insulin

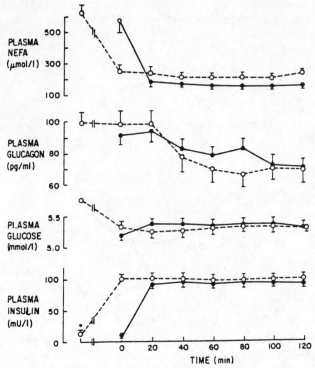

FIG. 3. Time-related changes in plasma glucose, non-esterified (or free) fatty acids (NEFA), insulin and glucagon concentrations in controls (—●—) and normal-weight NIDDM patients (—○—) during insulin clamp. *P < 0.01. (Source: Golay et al., 1988.)

sensitivity. The inhibitory effect of insulin on FFA mobilization has to persist for a certain period of time, until the influx of lipoproteins from the liver can be demonstrated. Significant lowering of blood sugar will only be achieved at serum insulin levels of at least $30–40 \, \text{mU} \, \text{l}^{-1}$.

Insulin has long been thought to play a role in the general regulation of protein biosynthesis. It inhibits urea production and markedly suppresses the release of amino acids from the liver of non-fasting mammalians. Insulin has a direct effect in regulation of circulating amino acid levels. It lowers concentrations of valine, leucine, isoleucine, threonine, phenylalanine and tyrosine. It augments protein synthesis and participates in gluconeogenesis to maintain glucose homoeostasis (Fig. 3). Glucose homoeostasis is also influenced by physical training. The beneficial effect on glucose tolerance is mainly based on enhanced insulin sensitivity.

Glucose homoeostasis is also influenced by the central nervous system. The hypothalamo-autonomic nervous system coordinates visceral activities and modulates hormonal secretion, both through production of hypothalamic-releasing and -inhibiting hormones and by sending neural signals to the endocrine organs (Shimazu, 1981). Sympathetic denervation influences glucose homoeostasis. The effect of neural activation upon islet function has been explained by adrenergic and cholinergic neural inputs (Ahrén et al., 1986). The role of the adrenergic system appears to be predominantly directed at the insulin response to acute stress. In contrast, during chronic stress where increased delivery of substrate is desired, the catecholamines play a minor role. Stress is characterized by an increase in fuel delivery to insulin-sensitive tissues. In this situation insulin secretion may be only mildly impaired and glucose uptake maximized (Ahrén et al., 1986).

## 2 Effect of Insulin Deficiency

### 2.1 GLUCOSE

The most dramatic manifestation of acute insulin deficiency is the effect on carbohydrate metabolism. Absolute or relative deficiency of insulin results in hyperglycaemia with an early increase in hepatic glucose output, which is evident within 1 h of insulin withdrawal and is due to stimulated glycogenolysis and gluconeogenesis from glycerol, lactate and amino acids. This results in an increased concentration of extracellular glucose and excessive loss of glucose in the urine. At the same time, glucose uptake by extrahepatic tissues, primarily muscle and adipose tissue, is decreased (Fig. 4). A diminished translocation of glucose in muscle and fat and lower oxidation and glycogen synthesis are prevalent.

In the state of prolonged insulin deficiency, the metabolic situation is further aggravated by stress hormones and sympathetic nerve reaction. An increase in cortisol, catecholamines and growth hormone (GH) stimulates glycogenolysis and gluconeogenesis further (Bratusch-Marrain, 1983). Whereas in insulin deficiency hepatic glucose output is primarily increased, in insulin resistance it may be normal, and only peripheral glucose utilization may be decreased initially. This may be primarily due to a loss of insulin-stimulated glucose uptake and secondarily due to the glucose–fatty acid cycle (Randle et al., 1963).

In diabetes mellitus, blood glucose homoeostasis and rate of lipolysis in adipose tissue appear to be associated. This relationship is most apparent in an insulin-deficient state, where glucose homoeostasis is maintained at the expense of other fuel sources, mainly FFA. Insulin deficiency initiates lipolysis. The increase in fatty acid oxidation further favours hepatic gluconeogenesis.

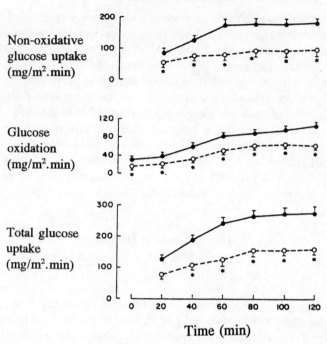

Non-oxidative glucose uptake (mg/m².min)

Glucose oxidation (mg/m².min)

Total glucose uptake (mg/m².min)

Time (min)

FIG. 4. Time-related change in total glucose uptake in controls (—●—) and in normal weight NIDDM patients (—O—) during insulin clamp. *P < 0.01. (Source: Golay et al., 1988.)

## 2.2 LIPIDS

In insulin deficiency, basal plasma FFA levels and lipid oxidation are elevated and fail to decrease normally (DeFronzo, 1988). Fatty acid production rates are increased up to threefold. This reflects the deficiency of insulin in the presence of normal sympathetic nervous system activity and normal level of circulating catecholamines.

With loss of insulin action and an excess of catabolic hormones, hydrolysis of triglycerides is markedly increased, glycerol supply rises and triglyceride turnover in plasma increases with a concomitant increase in ketoacid derived from hepatic oxidation of FFA. Fatty acids are partly oxidized to ketonic compounds. Ketone synthesis increases more than threefold in the state of insulin deficiency as the result of a low insulin/glucagon ratio and a high FFA supply to the liver. At low insulin levels, ketone uptake and utilization of peripheral tissue is also significantly reduced.

In diabetic ketoacidosis, plasma ketone concentrations are often raised to 200–300 times the normal fasting values because of additional impaired renal elimination. An excessive mobilization of FFA is due to an augmented breakdown of triglycerides and to a reduced rate of utilization of FFA for esterification in adipose tissue. The increase in fatty acid oxidation favours hepatic gluconeogenesis.

There is a diminished capacity of peripheral tissue to take up triglycerides in diabetes with insulin deficiency or in an insulin-resistant state. FFA and ketones depress glucose uptake and oxidation in muscle, contributing to hyperglycaemia and, as first noted by Randle et al. (1963), FFA inhibit pyruvate oxidation, glycolysis and possibly glucose transport. There is a reciprocal relationship between the metabolism of glucose and that of FFA, known as the glucose–fatty acid cycle.

### 2.3 PROTEINS

It was noted as early as 1889 that removal of the pancreas resulted, quite apart from the effects on carbohydrate metabolism, in an increase in amino acid release from muscles (v. Mering and Minkowski, 1889), with consequent increased loss of nitrogen in the urine and wasting of body tissues. Treatment with insulin prevents this excessive loss of protein (Chaikoff and Forker, 1950). During insulin deficiency, muscle proteolysis provides gluconeogenic substrates for fuel for those tissues metabolizing glucose. Insulin deficiency is the signal for this process and its time constant is measurable in hours (slow insulin effect), thus avoiding hypoglycaemic reactions.

Insulin stimulates protein biosynthesis by a mechanism which is not directly dependent upon its action in stimulating the uptake and accumulation of amino acids by the cells. Insulin increases the incorporation of amino acids into the protein of a number of tissues, an effect which is dependent on the presence of glucose.

## 3 Regulation of Glucose Homoeostasis in Type-I Diabetes Mellitus (IDDM)

### 3.1 HORMONES AND CYTOKININS

In patients taking insulin, especially those with Type-I diabetes, an impaired glucose homoeostasis is common (Gerich, 1988). This is due to the independence of plasma glucose concentration and the availability of insulin and varies with dose, site of insulin injection, subcutaneous blood flow, insulin–antibody binding, insulin catabolism, diet and physical activity.

More importantly, IDDM patients have a defective glucose counter-regulation. As Bolli and Perriello (1990) pointed out, counter-regulatory mechanisms in IDMM, compared with controls, are intact only in the first months after onset of diabetes. Thereafter, impaired insulin kinetics (due to

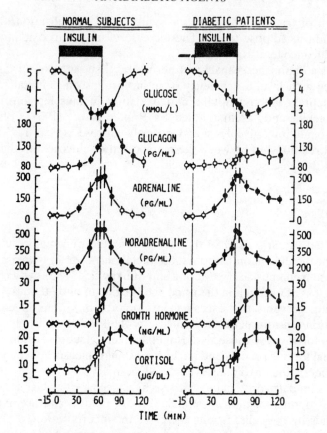

Fɪɢ. 5. Blood glucose and plasma counter-regulatory hormone levels before, during and after a constant intravenous insulin infusion. ● = $P \leqslant 0.05$ versus basal; ○ = n.s. versus basal. (Source: Bolli et al., 1984c.)

antibodies) and reduced counter-regulatory hormone response lead to a delay in recovery from hypoglycaemia.

The most important counter-regulatory hormone defect is a reduced glucagon response which is almost universally present after approximately 5 years of diabetes and is selective, because the secretory response to other stimuli is normal or even exaggerated (Gerich et al., 1973; Bratusch-Marrain, 1983) (Fig. 5). Glucagon secretion is increased over basal levels leading to a decline in the insulin/glucagon ratio. The mechanism for this deficient response is not known. It is not due to autonomic neuropathy or changes in the β-cell function (Gerich, 1988). Sustained hyperglucagonaemia has an effect on glucose homoeostasis for at least 2 hours after the initiation of a continuous infusion (Clarke et al., 1983) with higher blood glucose concentrations and higher insulin requirements. As a consequence it is not the glucagon-mediated compensatory increase in glucose production but the suppression of glucose utilization that reverses insulin-induced hypoglycaemia in IDDM and, less severely, in NIDDM (Shilo et al., 1990).

After 5–10 years of diabetes, glucose counter-regulation in IDDM becomes further impaired when adrenaline secretion also becomes deficient. This, however, can be attributed to diabetic autonomic neuropathy, because it is usually accompanied by reduced pancreatic polypeptide response (Cryer, 1983; White et al., 1985a; Gerich, 1988).

Plasma GH and cortisol response appear to be appropriate in most IDDM patients. During prolonged insulin deficiency, however, there is an increased secretion of glucocorticoids and stress hormones (Johnston and Alberti, 1982). With long-standing diabetes, impaired secretory responses have also been noted (Boden et al., 1981; Bolli et al., 1984a).

The diabetogenic action of GH is not mediated by its effect on glucagon secretion, and GH is of little importance in the acute counter-regulation of insulin-induced changes in glucose homoeostasis (Adamson, 1981). A reduction in counter-regulatory hormone response in IDDM through successful intensive therapy, however, is still a controversial approach (Bergenstal et al., 1983; Bolli et al., 1984b; Simonson et al., 1984; Amiel et al., 1987).

Prostaglandins also seem to participate in glucose homoeostasis. Despite some controversy, the weight of evidence appears to favour an inhibitory role of prostaglandins when all in vivo and in vitro data are considered. The in vitro observation that prostaglandins has stimulatory effects on $\beta$-cell function at normal glucose concentration, but inhibitory effects at high glucose concentration, may be an important clue for the ultimate resolution of this problem (Robertson, 1981).

An interesting possible explanation for the abnormalities in glucose homoeostasis in viral and bacterial infections was offered by Shimizu et al. (1985), who observed a decrease in the production of insulin after administration of interferon (IFN), suggesting that viral and bacterial infections with induced production of IFN may be responsible for abnormalities in carbohydrate metabolism.

Interleukin (IL-1), a cytokinin mainly produced by monocytes–macrophages, may also affect glucose homoeostasis (Gerich, 1988). Its hypoglycaemic effect was first observed in an insulin-resistant state, and this constitutes an example of the biological relevance of immune–neuroendocrine interaction in glucose homoeostasis (Besedovsky and Del Rey, 1989).

IL-1$\beta$ has a potentiating effect on insulin secretion, suggesting a priming effect on B-cell function and also a paracrine effect on A + B-cell function. IL-1$\beta$ should be considered to be a physiological modulator of insulin and glucagon secretion, e.g. during the acute phase response, but also as pathogenic factor in Type-I diabetes mellitus (Wogensen *et al.*, 1990).

## 3.2 PHYSICAL EXERCISE

Fuel homoeostasis and blood glucose levels are remarkably well maintaine during physical exercise in healthy individuals. A decline in plasma insuli and an increase in glucagon are known to occur during intense and/o prolonged exercise. In diabetics, physical training improves glucose homoeo stasis. In IDDM, however, the very basis for fuel homoeostasis adjustments i.e. normal insulin production, is absent. Recent studies have pointed ou that in trained diabetics, increased circulating insulin levels are present an may also contribute to the improvement in glucose homoeostasis (Rousseau Migneron *et al.*, 1988).

The glucose homoeostatic response to exercise in IDDM, in contrast t healthy controls, is critically dependent on the adrenergic system (Simonso *et al.*, 1984). Thus, exercise in hyperinsulinaemic patients may result i hypoglycaemic reactions and, in hypoinsulinaemic diabetics, in increasec blood glucose levels. There are many adjustments to the therapeutic regimen which an individual with IDDM can make in order to avoid changes ir glucose homoeostasis during or after exercise. Thus, individualized recom mendations for exact treatment modification in association with exercise arc necessary.

Exercise-induced glycogen depletion, with an increase in glucose storagc and insulin-stimulated glucose disposal, both of which may add to post exercise hypoglycaemia in Type-I diabetes, is associated with increasec peripheral sensitivity to insulin. The finding, however, that exercise will have a long-term effect on the metabolic control of diabetes or prevent the development of complications of diabetes remains to be firmly established (Zinman and Vranic, 1985).

Changes in glucose homoeostasis with an increase in blood glucose concentration, primarily in the early morning (dawn phenomenon), is a secondary phenomenon (Waldhäusl, 1986) which reflects the state of insulin sensitivity, the size of the hepatic glycogen pool, lack of insulin and the availability of glycogenolytic and/or gluconeogenic counter-regulatory hor mones. It is more frequent in Type-I diabetics, with an intake the preceding day of a hypercaloric diet, than in fasting patients. The dawn phenomenon is defined as an early-morning increase in plasma glucose concentration, without antecedent hypoglycaemia, in patients with IDDM or NIDDM (Somogyi, 1959).

A rebound hyperglycaemia, caused by counter-regulatory hormones provoked by insulin-induced hypoglycaemia, is called the Somogyi phenomenon (Gerich, 1988). Attvall *et al.* (1987) have shown that prolonged insulin resistance occurs after hypoglycaemia in IDDM patients. Increase in cortisol, GH and catecholamines play a role in causing the prolonged post-hypoglycaemic insulin resistance.

While GH is essential in this respect, the diabetogenic effect of cortisol is evident only in conjunction with GH (Kollind *et al.*, 1987). Insulin resistance occurs for at least 12 hours after hypoglycaemic episodes in patients with IDDM. Adrenaline causes immediate insulin resistance, whereas GH exerts a sustained resistance only after a lag period of about 4 hours (Kollind, 1988).

It is important to prevent nocturnal hypoglycaemia, not only to protect brain function, but also to prevent insulin resistance. This may easily result in exaggerated hyperglycaemia and initiate the vicious circle – hypoglycaemia, hyperglycaemia, increase in insulin dose and risk of subsequent hypoglycaemia (Bolli and Perriello, 1990). The mechanism, frequency and even the existence of the Somogyi phenomenon, however, are all still controversial.

## 4   Regulation of Glucose Homoeostasis in Type-II Diabetes Mellitus (NIDDM)

### 4.1   CHARACTERISTICS OF NIDDM

NIDDM is a heterogeneous disorder that may be initiated by a defect in insulin action. A reduction in glucose clearance is one of the earliest abnormalities. At that time, the early phase of insulin secretion tends to be reduced, priming the insulin target tissues, primarily the liver, that are responsible for the maintenance of glucose homoeostasis. As the first phase of insulin secretion is impaired, the resulting postprandial hyperglycaemia initiates a hyperinsulinaemia, returning blood glucose to normal. In NIDDM, with a fasting glucose concentration up to 120 mg/100 ml, insulin secretion is increased to twice normal with a fasting glucose concentration of 80 mg/100 ml.

As the pancreatic exhaustion continues, insulin response becomes insufficient and the absolute amount of insulin decreases. Basal blood glucose begins to rise. Once the fasting blood glucose concentration exceeds 120 mg/100 ml there is a further progressive decline in reactive insulin release in response to glucose. Basal insulin, however, still remains elevated. Finally, the early and late phases of insulin secretion disappear, and a decrease in the absolute amount of insulin is noted.

At a glucose level of 150–160 mg/100 ml the amount of insulin secreted is similar to that of a normal non-diabetic individual. With a further increase in glucose to more than 160 mg/100 ml the insulin response becomes insulinopenic, and markedly reduced when basal glucose exceeds 200–220 mg/100 ml.

## 4.2 INSULIN SENSITIVITY

Insulin controls glucose homoeostasis through three coordinated mechanisms, i.e. suppression of hepatic glucose production (HGP), stimulation of splanchnic (hepatic) glucose uptake and peripheral uptake. The tissues responsible for the insulin resistance in the basal state are quite different from those responsible for the insulin resistance in the insulin-stimulated (hyperinsulinaemic) state.

Glucose, which is released by the liver, can be derived from either glycogenolysis or gluconeogenesis. However, while no defect in hepatic glucose uptake is demonstrable, the effects on HGP depend on insulin and glucose levels.

At low glucose (hyperinsulinaemic) levels (120 mg/100 ml) a normal suppressive action of insulin on HGP is noted (Gerich et al., 1973). A normal rate of HGP, however, in the presence of fasting hyperglycaemia, and a plasma insulin concentration nearly twofold greater, demonstrates that a latent hepatic resistance to the suppressive action of insulin is already present early in the course of NIDDM. HGP still remains within normal range because of the suppressive effect of hyperglycaemia. Tissue glucose uptake, however, is markedly reduced. In diabetic subjects, the glucose uptake of muscle tissue is delayed and retarded. While in control subjects muscle glucose uptake accounts for 75% of the total glucose uptake, normal-weight NIDDM patients have a 50% reduction in insulin-mediated peripheral glucose uptake. Thus in the early stages of NIDDM, the site of insulin resistance is not at the level of the liver. The principal defect causing the elevated postprandial glucose is a defect in muscle glucose uptake (Fig. 6).

The suppression of hepatic glucose uptake is very sensitive to small increments in plasma glucose. With more severe fasting hyperglycaemia, an augmented rate of HGP causes the progressive rise in plasma glucose concentration.

If fasting glucose levels exceed 200–220 mg/100 ml and an insulinopenic state is present (basal state), an impairment of the ability of insulin to suppress HGP is noted (Gerich et al., 1979). In that state, the liver now represents the major site of insulin resistance, leading finally to high fasting blood glucose concentrations. Chronic hyperglycaemia leads to insulin resistance through interference with the regulation of the glucose-transport system and desensitizes the $\beta$-cell to acute glycaemic stimuli. Glucose oxidation (Berger et al., 1986) and glycogen formation (Gerich, 1985) are impaired and an excessive amount of glucose is converted to lactate, which

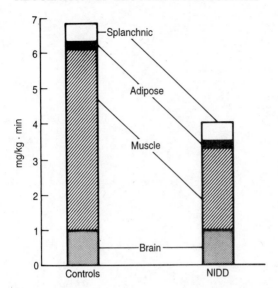

F<small>IG</small>. 6. Summary of glucose metabolism during euglycaemic insulin-clamp studies in NIDDM subjects and controls. (Source: DeFronzo, 1988.)

is subsequently released and can serve as a substrate to drive gluconeogenesis by the liver.

### 4.3 LIPIDS

The increased fat mass in obese individuals, associated with enhanced lipolysis in insulin-resistant NIDDM, leads to elevated plasma FFA and stimulates lipid oxidation by peripheral tissues. In non-insulin-dependent diabetics, ketone formation, however, is not increased because sufficient insulin is available to restrain hepatic production and stimulate peripheral utilization.

Elevated FFA oxidation restricts glucose oxidation in muscle and accounts for the defect in glucose oxidation and glucose storage in NIDDM. Lipid and glucose oxidation have been found to be inversely related to each other. These results suggest that elevated rates of lipid oxidation contribute to the defect in glucose oxidation and, to a lesser extent, glucose storage in insulin-resistant diabetics. In normal-weight NIDDM patients, however, lipid oxidation is not significantly increased.

The treatment of obese NIDDM patients should primarily aim at a reduction in insulin resistance by hypocaloric diet (reducing hyperglycaemia), weight reduction (reducing hyperinsulinaemia) and a reduction in hyper-lipidaemia (with interruption of the fatty acid cycle).

# Clinical Aspects of Diabetes Mellitus

## 1 Type-I Diabetes Mellitus

### 1.1 AETIOLOGY

Type-I diabetes is the result of an immunologically mediated genetically programmed destruction of the B-cells. This process may require many years and can be documented by several humoral and cellular immunological abnormalities preceding the clinical onset of the disease. Islet cell surface antibodies (ICA) and insulin autoantibodies (IAA) are often detected years before overt clinical symptoms start. A florid insulitis, however, has mainly been observed only close to the time of diagnosis (Bottazzo et al., 1985).

There is also strong evidence of a genetic component in the aetiology of Type-I diabetes, with a close human leucocyte antigen (HLA)-DR association. The relative risk of becoming diabetic is six times higher for HLA-DR4 and 14 times higher for HLA-DR3 + 4 but only 0.2 for HLA-DR2. At least one of the diabetic risk antigens is found in more than 80% of patients with Type-I diabetes but in only 30% of the general population. However, there is also evidence that HLA genes alone do not determine the disease and we are probably dealing with a multistage aetiology. Among monozygotic twins, there is a concordance value of only 30–50% for Type-I diabetes, pointing to a strong environmental factor.

The incidence of Type-I diabetes rises from birth to 12 years of age and is most frequent around puberty. The pattern of age of onset, however, may vary widely and Type-I diabetes may also start in the 6th or even 7th decade of life (Jarret, 1991).

The onset of the disease shows a striking seasonal variation with a high incidence rate in autumn and winter, suggesting a prominent role for environmental trigger factors in the genesis of Type-I diabetes. However, attempts to relate the occurrence of the disease to common viral infections have failed (Yoon and Ray, 1985).

New working hypotheses should take into account slow viruses as precipitating agents that are tropic for B-cells, acting close to the time of diagnosis (Bottazzo et al., 1985).

The incidence of Type-I diabetes (insulitis) varies considerably in its geographic distribution among countries and has increased dramatically, up to 3 times during the past 3 decades in Finland. The highest rates of occurrence are found predominantly in the northern hemisphere. Finland has a leading position with 28 cases/100 000 per year. In contrast, there is a very low national incidence in France and Japan (0.8/100 000). This again suggests a predominant effect of environmental factors in the genesis of Type-I diabetes.

The incidence rate of Type-I diabetes may also vary considerably over a narrow geographic range. In Israel, the Ashkenazi Jews are affected with 6.8 new cases of Type-I diabetes per 100 000 per year while Arabs in Israel suffer only in 1.2/100 000, pointing to an effect of different genetic background.


1.2   CLINICAL SYMPTOMS

The onset of the autoimmune disease Type-I diabetes has a protracted prodromal period. Overt symptoms such as hyperglycaemia occur only months and years after initial metabolic and immunological abnormalities such as impaired glucose tolerance, ICA and IAA are noted.

Chances of detecting early symptomatic Type-I diabetic patients therefore depend on glucose studies of relatives and monitoring of a combination of immunological serum parameters and assessment of insulin secretion in persons who are at high risk. Clinical symptoms in Type-I diabetes usually start when more than 90% of vital B-cells are destroyed. Patients present acute with symptoms of hyperglycaemia such as polyuria, polydipsia, weight loss and tiredness (Table 1). Minor symptoms may include cramps, skin infections and blurred vision. The duration of these symptoms is usually very short and may last for only 1–2 weeks (Gill, 1991).

The most dangerous acute symptom of Type-I diabetes is the ketoacidotic coma, which is noted as a first sign in 10% of newly diagnosed patients.

The acute clinical symptoms in Type-I diabetes can only be treated with exogenous insulin. The metabolic situation will improve rapidly after the start of the treatment. Hyperglycaemia, ketonaemia, hypertriglyceridaemia and other metabolic complications, however, may continue in view of a still imperfect unphysiological insulin-application regimen.

Next to the insulin pump, intensified conventional insulin therapy is the most effective way of imitating the homoeostatic regulation of blood glucose levels by means of several daily injections of clear insulin before meals and basal insulin to suppress gluconeogenesis during the night.

TABLE 1[a]
Symptoms of insulin-dependent diabetes

| Major symptoms | Minor symptoms | Features of ketoacidosis |
|---|---|---|
| Thirst | Cramps | Nausea |
| Polyuria | Constipation | Vomiting |
| Weight loss | Blurred vision | Drowsiness |
| Fatigue | Candidiasis | Abdominal pain |
| | Skin sepsis | |

[a]Source: Gill (1991).

A spontaneous temporary improvement in B-cell function can be observed during the "honeymoon period", which may last for a few weeks or months. But as the autoimmune destruction of the B-cells continues, insulin requirements increase again. Some patients may retain a few functioning B-cells with some endogenous insulin production in the long term, thus having better blood glucose control and being less prone to diabetic complications.

## 1.3  NATURAL HISTORY AND PROGNOSIS

The natural history of the disease is determined by the onset and extent of chronic diabetic complications. Microangiopathic changes are diabetes-specific, causing retinopathy, nephropathy and alterations in the peripheral and autonomous nervous system. Macroangiopathy, which is more typical for Type-II diabetes, leads predominantly to cardiovascular complications with coronary heart disease, myocardial infarction and peripheral vascular occlusion.

For diabetic patients overall, the mortality risk is about twice that in the age-matched non-diabetic population. For Type-I, the overall life expectancy is reduced by about 30%. The most frequent cause of mortality in Type-I diabetes is **nephropathy** (Palmberg et al., 1981): 35% of Type-I diabetics die from renal failure, 15% from coronary heart disease and 15% from infectious disease. Type-I diabetics whose disease appears before puberty have a still higher risk of developing nephropathy, associated with premature death.

After 5 years of diabetes, the risk of nephropathy rises rapidly. However, only a subset of patients are susceptible and only a small proportion develop total renal failure, predominantly those with a familial clustering and parents with hypertensive disease.

Nephropathy is initially manifested as a persistent urinary excretion of albumin, a decreasing glomerular filtration rate and increasing blood pressure. Once proteinuria occurs, patients have a poor prognosis. The median survival is about 10 years, which is determined by diastolic blood pressure, dietary protein intake and the severity of diabetes exposure. A family history of longevity, however, may be helpful and also regular clinical contact.

The complication risk in Type-I diabetes is related not only to duration of the disease but also to the degree of glycaemic control, blood pressure and genetic susceptibility (Hanssen, 1991). The most frequent chronic complication in Type-I diabetes is diabetic background **retinopathy**, with a near-100% occurrence rate after 15 years diabetes duration. Manifestations of diabetes, however, can be found in all ocular structures (Table 1).

The lesions of diabetic retinopathy can be divided into two major groups: background retinopathy and proliferative retinopathy. Microaneurysms are the hallmark of diabetic retinopathy. Once microaneurysms are present, multiple haemorrhages indicate increasing severity of diabetic retinopathy. Proliferative diabetic retinopathy carries a poor prognosis for vision and is the commonest sight-threatening lesion in IDDM. Diabetic retinopathy is now the leading cause of blindness in persons 25–74 years of age. Regular screening of patients is therefore crucial.

**Diabetic neuropathy** is grouped into various types (Ward, 1991):

(1) chronic insidious sensory neuropathy;
(2) acute painful neuropathy;
(3) proximal motor neuropathy;
(4) diffuse motor neuropathy;
(5) focal vascular neuropathy.

The most common syndrome is sensory neuropathy with clinical signs of tingling, burning, cramps and pains, mainly in the legs and feet.

Autonomic neuropathy presents clinically as damage to the cardiovascular, genitourinary and gastrointestinal tracts. The mortality rate appears to be high (50% in 3 years) resulting from renal failure and "sudden unexpected death".

Despite the potential problems of Type-I diabetes, some patients do remarkably well and may survive 50 years or more without major complications. Again, a family history of longevity and good metabolic control are important factors in achieving this goal.

1.4 PROGNOSIS OF TYPE-I DIABETES MELLITUS

The introduction of insulin by Banting and Best and colleagues (1922) dramatically improved the prognosis of Type-I diabetes. However, life expectancy is still considerably lower than in non-diabetics. As shown by Green *et al.* (1985) relative mortality in insulin-dependent diabetes decreases with increasing age at diagnosis and increases with increased duration of diabetes to a maximum at 15–25 years, after which it declines. Up to the age of 20 years, acute hypo- and hyper-glycaemic complications lead the diabetes-related death rates in Type-I diabetes. Between 20 and 40 years of age, renal failure (microangiopathy) and then coronary heart disease (macroangiopathy) are the most frequent causes of death.

Acute complication rates increase with low glycaemia, but decrease rapidly with intensified training programmes. Micro- and macro-vascular complication rates can also be significantly reduced by improved metabolic control and low levels of glycosylated haemoglobin. As shown in the DCC Trial (1993), intensive therapy slows the progression of retinopathy by more than 50%, reduces microalbuminuria by 39–54% and neuropathy by 60%. Severe hypoglycaemia, however, increases two- to three-fold.

The prognosis of Type-I diabetes can be greatly improved by lowering glycaemia by intensive therapy. The risk of severe hypoglycaemic reactions, however, means that close blood-sugar monitoring is required.

## 2  Type-II Diabetes Mellitus

### 2.1  AETIOLOGY

Type-II diabetes mellitus is defined and classified as non-insulin-dependent, although many patients receive insulin to improve their glycaemic control; there is a relative deficit in insulin-secretory capacity. Maturity-onset diabetes of the young (MODY) and gestational diabetes are both variants of Type-II diabetes mellitus. There are two subgroups of Type-II: normal-weight type IIa and obese-type IIb.

The prevalence of Type-II diabetes shows a large variation among populations, depending on ethnic, racial and social factors, age and genetic determinants. Pima-Indians have a rate of 50%, Eskimos far below 1% (Bennett, 1990) and Chinese and Africans less than 0.1%, which increases with urbanization and living standard.

In Europe, two-thirds of all Type-II patients are overweight. Obesity and age are regarded as being the most important external risk factors. The average age of Type-II diabetics is 67 years, 70% of the patients being over 70. The disease is characterized by reduced insulin-secretory capacity as the major defect in normal-weight (Type-IIa) patients and an additional insulin resistance in obese (Type-IIb) patients (O'Rahilly *et al.*, 1986). Monozygotic twin studies where one twin already had Type-II diabetes revealed that 91% of the co-twins also developed Type-II diabetes. A strong genetic factor is demonstrated by some 40% of the patients having a first-degree relative with

NIDDM (Pyke and Nelson, 1976). In dizygotic co-twins only 7% more than the expected number in the general population were diabetic.

There is a strong familial component of the susceptibility to Type-II diabetes, with nearly complete concordance in identical twins (Pyke, 1979).

Type-II diabetes may remain undetected for many years. In Europe and North America the ratio of undiagnosed to diagnosed cases may be as high as 1:1. Specific criteria have been adopted by WHO (1985a) for the diagnosis of Type-II diabetes mellitus.

Concordance rates among monozygotic twins range from 55% to 100% compared with 17% in dizygotic twins. Type-II diabetes predisposition is best described as dependent on the inheritance of a single major gene in a co-dominant manner. Type-II diabetes is often associated with normal or high levels of circulating insulin, the absence of distinct HLA, insulin antibodies (IAB) and spontaneous ketoacidosis.

It is now recognized that the development of Type-II diabetes requires a genetic component which predisposes to the disease, an abnormality in pancreatic B-cell function and the presence of insulin resistance in skeletal muscle, adipose tissue and the liver. Obesity is the most common condition associated with Type-II diabetes by hyperinsulinaemia and insulin resistance.

## 2.2 CLINICAL SYMPTOMS

The classic symptoms of metabolic disturbance are rare in Type-II diabetes and more insidious than in Type-I. Hyperglycaemia, thirst, polyuria and fatigue are the classic symptoms, but weight loss is infrequent and diagnosis is often made after intercurrent infections or as an incidental finding (Table 2).

## 2.3 NATURAL HISTORY

The natural history of Type-II diabetes mellitus is characterized by a progression of B-cell dysfunction. Many patients are initially well controlled by diet but, as the years go by, they need oral hypoglycaemic agents and eventually insulin for satisfactory glycaemic control. Some 17% of all Type-II diabetics are treated with insulin, and 5% of Type-II diabetics are switched to insulin each year (Marble and Camerini-Davalos, 1961). The point at which a patient should be put on a insulin regimen, however, is not always easy to assess and may be determined by life expectancy, morbidity and compliance of the patient.

TABLE 2[a]

Modes of detection of NIDDM

| Mode of detection | Percentage detected |
|---|---|
| Diabetic symptoms | 53 |
| Incidental finding (usually glycosuria) | 29 |
| Infections (e.g. candidiasis) | 16 |
| Complications (e.g. retinopathy) detected by an optician | 2 |

[a]Source: UK Prospective Diabetes Study (1988).

2.4 PROGNOSIS OF TYPE-II DIABETES MELLITUS

Morbidity and mortality in Type-II diabetes is characterized mainly by problems related to **macroangiopathy**. This, however, is not specific for Type-II, but for the age at which Type-II diabetes mainly appears.

Type-II diabetes is frequently accompanied by other macroangiopathic risk factors. Arterial hypertension can be found in 65%, hypertriglyceridaemia in 60% and hypercholesterolaemia in 35% of patients. The multimetabolic syndrome caused by insulin resistance and hyperinsulinaemia leads to increased macrovascular risk the endpoint of which is death from coronary heart disease.

Life expectancy is reduced by 5–10 years in Type-II diabetes compared with the non-diabetic population. The mortality risk, however, is not related to the duration of the disease (Nathan *et al.*, 1986) but to the additional presence of other risk factors. In patients over the age of 75 at the time of diagnosis, mortality from diabetes is similar to that of age-matched non-diabetics. Coronary heart disease is the main cause of death in 58% of all Type-II diabetics (WHO, 1985b), followed by cerebrovascular accidents in 12%. Nephropathy is the cause of death in only 3%.

**Microvascular** complications are far less prominent in Type-II than in Type-I diabetes mellitus. Retinopathy is present in only 17%, and cataracts in 14% of patients.

The prevalence of diabetic neuropathy rises from 7.5% at the time of diagnosis to 50% after 25 years and seems to be directly related to the duration of diabetes. The commonest type is a symmetric sensory and autonomic polyneuropathy. Once symptomatic autonomic neuropathy is present the prognosis for survival is substantially diminished. The clinically silent phase of diabetic **nephropathy** in Type-II diabetes may last 5–10 years. It is characterized by rising urinary albumin excretion caused by a capillary lesion in the glomerulus. Microalbuminuria varies and can be found in 15–60% of all Type-II diabetics; it is defined by an excretion rate between

15 and $250\,\mu g\,min^{-1}$. In patients with microalbuminuria, coronary heart disease and proliferative retinopathy increase severalfold; without special care about 50% of the patients with persistent proteinuria will die within 7 years from uraemia, myocardial infarction or cerebral vascular accidents. Antihypertensive therapy, however, can slow down progressive renal failure. Early identification of endangered patients and appropriate therapy is therefore essential for a good prognosis.

# Mechanisms of Insulin Action

## 1 Insulin Actions

Insulin action is initiated by binding of the hormone to its specific receptor at the plasma membrane. This induces a broad spectrum of distinct effects at a number of different target cells, predominantly in muscle, liver and fat. These cellular insulin effects can be divided into four categories:

(1) stimulation of membrane transport processes (ions, glucose, amino acids); (2) anabolic effects including the stimulation of glycogen synthesis, lipogenesis and protein synthesis; (3) anticatabolic effects such as the inhibition of lipolysis, proteolysis and glycogenolysis; (4) growth-promoting effects in certain cell types, i.e. stimulation of RNA and DNA synthesis in concert with the other above-described anabolic effects. Insulin action involves rapid events (seconds to minutes) such as the stimulation of ion and glucose transport, stimulation of phospholipid turnover, generation of mediators and enzyme regulation including glycogen synthase, pyruvate dehydrogenase, triacylglycerol lipase and phosphorylase among others. Insulin also stimulates slow events (minutes to hours) such as the activation of amino acid transport, protein and lipid synthesis or stimulation of RNA and DNA synthesis. It is believed that all these different effects are initiated by binding of insulin to a single type of receptor, whereas a branching of signal transduction occurs at a post-binding or even post-receptor level. The existence of a specific insulin receptor was postulated over 25 years ago in the original studies of Cuatrecasas (1971), Freychet et al. (1971) and Kono and Barham (1971) who demonstrated specific saturable binding of $^{125}$I-labelled insulin to cell surfaces. Since then a large number of studies have been performed to characterize the structure and function of the insulin receptor.

## 2 Insulin Receptor

### 2.1 STRUCTURE

The insulin receptor is a transmembrane glycoprotein of approximately 400 kDa and comprises two $\alpha$-subunits of molecular mass 135 kDa each (Goldfine, 1987) and two 95 kDa $\beta$-subunits (Jacobs and Cuatrecasas, 1981). The two $\alpha$- and $\beta$-subunits form a heterotetrameric protein complex which is linked by disulphide bonds (Fig. 7). The $\alpha$-subunit of the insulin receptor consists of 719 or 731 amino acids (Ebina et al., 1985; Ullrich et al., 1985), it is entirely extracellular and contains the insulin-binding site. Both $\alpha$-subunits are covalently linked via disulphide bonds. The $\beta$-subunit is a transmembrane protein with a 194-amino acid extracellular domain that is glycosylated, a 23-amino acid transmembrane domain, a 403-amino acid cytoplasmic sequence (Fig. 7), which contains a well-preserved tyrosine kinase domain similar to that found in several oncogenes (ros, src, DrBB2) (Anderson et al., 1985; Semba et al., 1985; Matsushime et al., 1986), and a unique C-terminal tail. Both the $\alpha$- and the $\beta$-subunits are glycosylated at their N-terminal region (Hedo et al., 1981; Deutsch et al., 1983; Ronnet et al., 1984; Ullrich et al., 1985).

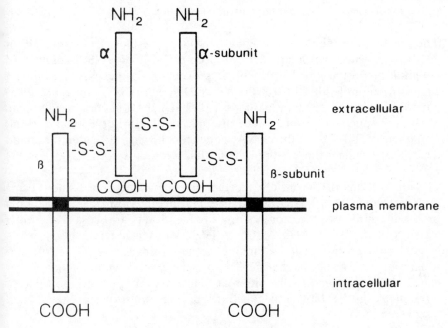

FIG. 7. Model of the insulin receptor protein.

## 2.2 THE INSULIN RECEPTOR GENE AND INSULIN RECEPTOR PROCESSING

The cDNA of the human insulin receptor was isolated by Ebina *et al.* (1985) and Ullrich *et al.* (1985). The gene spans more than 150 kb and contains 22 exons on chromosome 19, 11 coding for the α-subunit and 11 for the β-subunit. Seino *et al.* (1989) suggested that exon 1 encodes the signal peptide, exon 2 the binding region and exon 3 the so-called cysteine-rich region. Exon 11 contains the site for alternative splicing which gives rise to two preproreceptor isoforms, exon 12 contains the proreceptor processing site, exon 15 the transmembrane region, exons 17–21 encode the tyrosine kinase domain and exon 22 encodes the *C*-terminal tail (Yang-Feng *et al.*, 1985).

The insulin receptor is synthesized as a preproreceptor of 1370 amino acids. The proreceptor (molecular mass 190 kDa on SDS–PAGE) is glycosylated (Kahn, 1985) in the Golgi region, proteolytically cleaved into mature α- and β-subunits, and inserted in the plasma membrane (Fehlmann *et al.*, 1982) or degraded. The half-life of the insulin receptor was determined to be 7–12 hours (Kahn, 1985).

2.3   ISOFORMS OF THE INSULIN RECEPTOR

The α-subunit of the insulin receptor exists in two isoforms of either 719 or 731 amino acids, which are derived from a 1370- or a 1382-amino acid common preproreceptor by proteolytic processing. Two cDNAs encoding a preproreceptor of either 1370 (Ullrich et al., 1985) or 1382 (Ebina et al., 1985) amino acids were originally described. The length difference results from alternative splicing of exon 11. The presence or absence of a 36 bp segment (amino acids 718–729) in the cDNA sequence following the codon for amino acid 717 determines the length of the insulin receptor isoform A (−exon 11) or isoform B (+exon 11).

Both isoforms of the insulin receptor are expressed in a tissue-specific pattern (Moller et al., 1989; Mosthaf et al., 1990). Most of the functional properties of the two receptor isoforms are identical (Carrascosa et al., 1991; Kellerer et al., 1991a, 1992; McClain, 1991; Yamaguchi et al., 1991), while some characteristics such as binding affinity (Mosthaf et al., 1990), internalization (Yamaguchi et al., 1991), recycling and down-regulation (Vogt et al., 1991a) appear to be different. However, at present, no specific differences in the biological functions of the two isoforms have been discovered.

The tissue-specific expression patterns of the isoforms were studied in NIDDM and severe insulin resistance. Conflicting results have been reported. While we and others found evidence at both the protein and mRNA levels for an altered isoform pattern (Mosthaf et al., 1991; Kellerer et al., 1993a), this finding was not confirmed by other investigators (Benecke et al., 1992; Hansen et al., 1992). The reason for the discordant results is unclear. Although the biological significance of an altered insulin receptor isoform expression in NIDDM cannot be interpreted at present, it is interesting to note that in a prediabetic population the altered expression of the receptor isoforms in the skeletal muscle was associated with skeletal muscle insulin resistance (Mosthaf et al., 1993). This suggests that altered splicing of mRNA for the proreceptor might be associated with development of skeletal muscle insulin resistance.

2.4   HOMOLOGY OF INSULIN- AND INSULIN-LIKE GROWTH FACTOR I (IGF-I)
      RECEPTOR

The insulin and IGF-I receptors are similar in their structure, both being heterotetrameric glycoproteins (α-ββ-α) (Massague and Czech, 1982). They show high sequence homology particularly in the domain that encodes the tyrosine kinase of the β-subunit (approx. 80%) (Ullrich et al., 1986). Their specific ligands, insulin and IGF-I, also show significant homology of approximately 50% (Rinderknecht and Humbel, 1978). IGF-I binds to the insulin receptor with 10–100-fold lower affinity than to its own receptor. The same was observed with insulin which also binds with 50–100-fold lower affinity to the IGF-I receptor (Czech, 1985). Insulin binding to the IGF-I receptor stimulates the tyrosine kinase of this receptor and parallel results have been found after binding of IGF-I to the insulin receptor (Czech, 1985). The IGF-I receptor also exists in at least two different isoforms as the result of alternative splicing of RNA (Abbott et al., 1992).

As a consequence of structural similarities, the insulin and IGF-I receptors are immunologically related (Soos and Siddle, 1989). The two receptors seem to share common signalling elements (White et al., 1985b,c; Kadowaki et al., 1987; Shemer et al., 1987). Although the insulin receptor predominantly induces metabolic effects, it also induces growth-promoting effects in specific cell types (King and Kahn, 1984). Conversely, the IGF-I receptor primarily elicits growth-promoting effects although it is able to induce metabolic effects such as, for example, stimulation of glucose uptake and muscle glycogen synthesis (Meuli and Froesch, 1977; Poggi et al., 1979). However, these effects can only be measured at much higher IGF-I concentrations than would be necessary for the respective insulin effects (Froesch and Zapf, 1985; Jacob et al., 1989; Rosetti et al., 1991).

Furthermore, the insulin and IGF-I receptors form hybrid heterotetrameric receptors. The hybrid receptor consists of an insulin receptor heterodimer $(\alpha,\beta)$ and an IGF-I heterodimer $(\alpha,\beta)$ which are connected via disulphide bonds (Soos et al., 1990; Moxham and Jacobs, 1992). Such hybrid receptors are not only formed in vitro, but also occur naturally in intact cells and bind insulin and IGF-I with high affinity (Moxham et al., 1989; Soos and Siddle, 1989). Studies with different cell models suggested that low concentrations of IGF-I and insulin are able to stimulate both $\beta$-subunits of an insulin/IGF-I receptor hybrid (Moxham et al., 1989). These naturally occurring hybrid receptors could give new insights into the specific forms of insulin resistance. This is suggested by studies with hybrid receptors that consist of mutated kinase-inactive $\alpha,\beta$-insulin receptor dimers or IGF-I receptor dimers. A transdominant inhibition of the kinase-inactive $\alpha,\beta$ dimer to the kinase-active wild-type $\alpha,\beta$ dimer was observed (Frattali et al., 1992). Furthermore, studies with chimeric insulin receptors in which residues 191–290 of the IGF-I receptor replaced the corresponding domain of the insulin receptor gave interesting results, conferring on insulin and IGF-I ligand specificity and affinity. The creation of such a chimeric receptor results in a markedly increased affinity for insulin and IGF-I compared with the wild-type insulin receptor (Schäffer et al., 1993). Thus, the existence of such chimeric insulin receptors might imply new possibilities for alteration of ligand specificity and affinity (Schäffer et al., 1993).

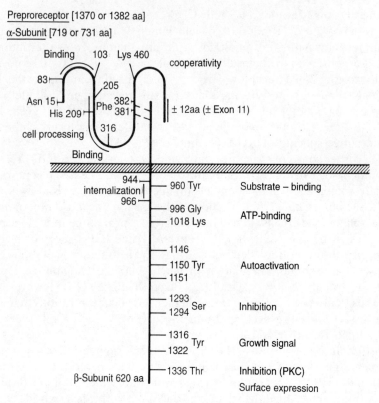

FIG. 8. Functional domains of the insulin receptor.

## 2.5 FUNCTIONAL DOMAINS OF THE INSULIN RECEPTOR

### 2.5.1 Functional Domains of the α-Subunit

Insulin binds with high affinity to the α-subunit of its receptor. The exact binding site has, however, not been defined. Syndromes of extreme insulin resistance have revealed several important domains for ligand binding (Fig. 8).

It was suggested that the binding domain is located between amino acids 83 and 103 (DeMeyts *et al.*, 1988, 1989). Furthermore the so-called cysteine-rich region, a 23 kDa fragment spanning amino acids 205–316 (Yip *et al.*, 1988) which is encoded by exon 3, was implicated in insulin binding (Rafaeloff *et al.*, 1989) and specificity for ligand binding. The lysine at position 460 appears to be involved in positive and negative cooperativity of insulin–receptor interaction (Kadowaki *et al.*, 1989).

The 12 amino acids at the C-terminus of the α-subunit also appear to play a role in insulin binding, since the presence of these amino acids (insulin receptor isoform B) results in a decrease in insulin affinity.

The coupling of the α-subunit to the extracellular part of the β-subunit occurs through disulphide bonds. There is some evidence from tryptic cleavage experiments (Frias and Waugh, 1989) that the amino acids involved in the disulphide coupling are located in positions 435, 468 or 524 in the α-chain.

### 2.5.2 Functional Domains of the β-Subunit

In 1982 it was first shown that the β-subunit of the insulin receptor contains an intrinsic tyrosine-specific kinase (Kasuga et al., 1982a). Binding of insulin to intact hepatoma cells (Kasuga et al., 1982b), IM9 lymphocytes (Kasuga et al., 1982a), adipocytes (Häring et al., 1982b) and liver cells (Van Obberghen and Kowalski, 1982) leads to phosphorylation of the β-subunit of the insulin receptor. In the intact cell the phosphorylation occurs at tyrosine and serine residues (Kasuga et al., 1982b; Häring et al., 1984). The mechanism for insulin signal transduction through the receptor is not fully understood, but many studies with mutated or truncated insulin receptors have provided indirect evidence for functional properties of distinct regions of the insulin receptor (Fig. 8).

The transmembrane domain of the β-subunit seems to be involved in regulation of the catalytic domain, since substitution or mutation of this region constitutively stimulates the insulin receptor tyrosine kinase (Yamada et al., 1992). The juxtamembrane domain of the β-subunit is located between the transmembrane region and the ATP-binding domain. It is encoded by exon 16 and spans the 23 amino acids 944–966, which shows a high degree of homology with an analogous region of the low-density lipoprotein (LDL) receptor (Seino et al., 1989). It includes two potential tyrosine-phosphorylation sites at amino acids 953 and 960. Tyr-960 which is weakly phosphorylated (Tavare and Denton, 1988; Tavare et al., 1988) appears to be important for substrate binding (White et al., 1988a); it is, however, not necessary for autophosphorylation of the receptor β-subunit. Moreover, the juxtamembrane region seems to be required to allow the internalization of the insulin receptor (Backer et al., 1991a).

The ATP-binding region of the receptor is located around Lys-1018 (Ebina et al., 1987) and Gly-996 (Odawara et al., 1989). The cytoplasmic sequence of the insulin receptor contains 13 tyrosine residues and it is believed that at least six of these tyrosines become phosphorylated (White et al., 1984, 1985c, 1988a; Tornqvist et al., 1987, 1988; Tavare and Denton, 1988; Tavare et al., 1988; Tornqvist and Avruch, 1988) after insulin stimulation. The triplet of tyrosines at 1146, 1150 and 1151 in the preserved tyrosine kinase region, which contains 50–60% of the phosphate after insulin stimulation (Tornqvist et al., 1988; White et al., 1988b), are crucial for autoactivation (Ellis et al., 1986).

The function of Tyr-1316 and -1322 at the *C*-terminus, which contains 20–30% of the phosphate (Tornqvist *et al.*, 1988; White *et al.*, 1988b), is not known. They are obviously not important for kinase activity, but may be related to growth signals (Debant *et al.*, 1988). Moreover studies with proteolytically truncated receptor at the *C*-terminus suggest a role for this region in the specificity for signal transmission of the insulin receptor. Related receptors such as the IGF-I receptor and the "insulin receptor-related receptor" lack some of these tyrosine-phosphorylation sites at the *C*-terminus.

The removal of the *C*-terminal tail does not alter kinase activity, endocytosis, degradation or binding properties (Goren *et al.*, 1987; Herrera *et al.*, 1988; Maegawa *et al.*, 1988; McClain *et al.*, 1988). It might, however, be the site of serine phosphorylation at amino acids 1293 and 1294 (Lewis *et al.*, 1989) and threonine phosphorylation at 1336, which may inhibit kinase activity through a conformational change. Thr-1336 seems to be a major site for phosphorylation by protein kinase C (PKC), and is probably important for regulation of receptor cell surface expression and turnover (Czech, 1985).

## 3  Signal Transduction

### 3.1  BASIC CHARACTERISTICS OF TRANSMEMBRANE SIGNALLING THROUGH THE INSULIN RECEPTOR KINASE

The model of the insulin receptor kinase as a signal transducer across the plasma membrane is based on a great number of studies which were initiated by the original finding of Kasuga *et al.* (1982a), who showed that insulin stimulation of intact cells leads to phosphorylation of the β-subunit of the insulin receptor. It is believed that further signal transduction then occurs through phosphorylation of other cellular proteins at tyrosine residues which could transmit the insulin signal to the effector systems of the target cell (White *et al.*, 1985b,c). In addition, it is speculated that the autophosphorylated receptor β-subunit may interact directly with regulatory proteins or with enzymes that could be modulated in a non-covalent way, for example by complex formation and conformational changes (Riedel *et al.*, 1986; Schlessinger, 1988).

### 3.2  AUTOACTIVATION OF THE RECEPTOR KINASE BY TYROSINE PHOSPHORYLATION: THE AUTOPHOSPHORYLATION CASCADE

It appears that after kinase activation a signal amplification occurs through autophosphorylation. Several tyrosine residues in the β-subunit are involved in the autophosphorylation reaction including Tyr-1146, -1150 and -1151 in the regulatory region and Tyr-1316 and -1322 at the *C*-terminus (Tornqvist *et al.*, 1987, 1988; Tavare *et al.*, 1988; White *et al.*, 1988b). Autophosphorylation proceeds through a sequential mechanism in which Tyr-1146 and either

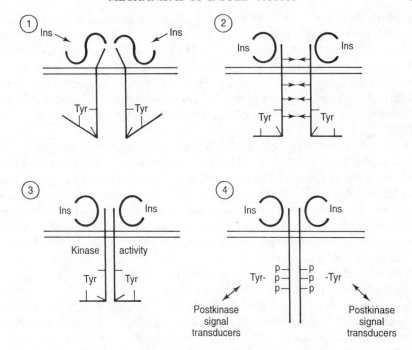

FIG. 9. Model of the signal flow through the insulin receptor.

Tyr-1150 or Tyr-1151 are phosphorylated first, generating a diphosphotyrosyl region. However, this partial autophosphorylation does not activate the phosphotransferase, and complete autophosphorylation of all three tyrosine residues in the regulatory region forming a triphosphotyrosine domain is required for full activation (White *et al.*, 1988b; Flores-Riveros *et al.*, 1989; Wilden *et al.*, 1990).

Phosphorylation of the *C*-terminus does not activate the intrinsic tyrosine kinase. Moreover, diphosphorylation of the regulatory region is poorly associated with activation of the kinase. In contrast, triphosphorylation of the regulatory region is closely associated with kinase activation, representing full activation (White *et al.*, 1988b) and probably reflecting a further allosteric change (Fig. 9). The original idea of the autophosphorylation cascade has been confirmed more recently in several cell systems (Ellis *et al.*, 1986; White *et al.*, 1988b). Furthermore, it is now clear that transphosphorylation of receptor β-subunits can also occur (Schlessinger, 1988).

3.3 SIGNAL TRANSFER FROM THE α- TO THE β-SUBUNIT

Interactions between insulin and its receptor probably occur, as outlined above, at amino acids 83–103 and 205–316. It is speculated that binding of insulin to its receptor induces dimerization and a conformational change in the receptor $\alpha$-subunit (Kahn, 1985; Sweet *et al.*, 1987; Johnson *et al.*, 1988; O'Hare and Pilch, 1988; Debant *et al.*, 1989), resulting in autophosphorylation of the intracellular insulin receptor $\beta$-subunit (Fig. 9). Very similar structural changes in the receptor molecule can be induced by certain insulin-mimetic antibodies which are able to stimulate the insulin receptor tyrosine kinase as well (Brindle *et al.*, 1990; Steele-Perkins and Roth, 1990).

There is increasing evidence that the conformational change in the $\alpha$-subunit is transduced to the $\beta$-subunit and modulates the tyrosine kinase activity of the $\beta$-subunit. The coupling of the $\alpha$-subunit to the extracellular part of the $\beta$-subunit occurs through disulphide bonds. Following the idea that the unoccupied $\alpha$-subunit functions as an inhibitor of the $\beta$-subunit (Herrera *et al.*, 1988; Shoelson *et al.*, 1988), it seems possible that the insulin-binding-induced conformational change in the $\alpha$-subunit is transduced to the $\beta$-subunit and releases the catalytic domain from inhibition.

Several findings support this interpretation. (1) Antibodies against specific regions of the $\alpha$-subunit are able to alter the kinase activity in the $\beta$-subunit. (2) Antibodies against the extracellular domain of the $\beta$-subunit can stimulate (Prigent *et al.*, 1990) or inhibit (Gherzi *et al.*, 1989) the tyrosine kinase, pointing towards a role for the extracellular domain as a transducer element. (3) The possible functional importance of conformational changes is further underlined by the observation that ATP binding to the $\beta$-subunit also causes a conformational change (Maddux and Goldfine, 1990). (4) Removal of the insulin-receptor-binding domain by proteolytic cleavage activates the insulin receptor tyrosine kinase as does insulin (Shoelson *et al.*, 1988). We have recently obtained further support for such kinase modulation through the $\alpha$-subunit structure by comparing the two receptor types human insulin receptor (HIR)-A and HIR-B which differ only in the $C$-terminal sequence of the $\alpha$-subunit (Kellerer *et al.*, 1992). We found that HIR-B exhibits higher autophosphorylation and substrate phosphorylation activities *in vitro*, suggesting that the $\alpha$-subunit of HIR-A is a more efficient inhibitor of basal and insulin-stimulated kinase activity (Kellerer *et al.*, 1992). Similarly, it was shown that a mutation at Phe-382 in the $\alpha$-subunit reduces the kinase activity of the $\beta$-subunit suggesting that in this case a conformational change in the $\alpha$-subunit also occurs which increases its inhibitory function (Taylor *et al.*, 1990).

## 3.4    POST-KINASE SIGNAL TRANSDUCTION: TYROSINE-PHOSPHORYLATED PROTEINS

### 3.4.1    The Search for Tyrosine-phosphorylated Proteins

For a long time the search for tyrosine-phosphorylated proteins which might serve as a substrate for the insulin receptor kinase was unsuccessful. White *et al.* (1985b) were the first to use a phosphotyrosine-specific antibody to identify tyrosine-phosphorylated proteins in the intact cell. They found a 185 kDa protein in hepatoma cells which was rapidly phosphorylated on tyrosine residues after insulin stimulation of the cell (White *et al.*, 1985b). Using the same experimental approach, a number of different proteins (Rees-Jones and Taylor, 1985; Sedoul *et al.*, 1985; Bernier *et al.*, 1987; Häring *et al.*, 1987; Izumi *et al.*, 1987; Machicao *et al.*, 1987; Hoffmann *et al.*, 1988; Madoff *et al.*, 1988; Margolis *et al.*, 1988; Momomura *et al.*, 1988) were identified which fulfil the criteria of putative signal-transmitting substrate proteins, i.e. rapid phosphorylation in the intact cell upon stimulation by physiological insulin concentrations.

We found 46 (Häring *et al.*, 1987) and 180 kDa proteins (Machicao *et al.*, 1987) in the plasma membrane, both with unknown function. In the cytosol a number of bands were found. The originally described 185 kDa protein was, meanwhile, found in many cells. Furthermore, a 115–120 kDa protein is seen in many cell and membrane systems (Rees-Jones and Taylor, 1985; Sedoul *et al.*, 1985; Machicao *et al.*, 1987). There is a 120 kDa protein in hepatocytes (Sedoul *et al.*, 1985), which appears to be involved in bile duct function (Margolis *et al.*, 1988). In fat cells (Häring *et al.*, 1987), hepatoma cells and transfected cells, we found a 60 kDa protein which is particularly interesting as it might function as a serine kinase (Obermaier-Kusser *et al.*, 1988a). Furthermore, there is a 15 kDa protein (Bernier *et al.*, 1987), which was identified as an abundant cell protein of the cytoskeleton (Hoffmann *et al.*, 1988). In addition, calmodulin, which is an *in vitro* substrate of the insulin receptor kinase (Häring *et al.*, 1985; Laurino *et al.*, 1988; Nong *et al.*, 1988), becomes phosphorylated in the intact cell. So far, signal transduction with respect to specific insulin effects, has not been demonstrated through any of these proteins except for the 185 kDa protein. This protein was sequenced and cloned (Rothenberg *et al.*, 1991; Sun *et al.*, 1991) and demonstrated to function as a docking protein which links the insulin receptor to other signal-transducing elements in the cell.

### 3.4.2 *Insulin Receptor Substrate-1 (IRS-1) in Post-kinase Signalling*

The first evidence of a cellular substrate of the insulin receptor kinase came from White *et al.* (1985b) who described a 185 kDa phosphoprotein in Fao hepatoma cells which was rapidly phosphorylated upon insulin stimulation. pp185, recently renamed IRS-1, is a cytosolic protein with at least 30 potential serine/threonine- and 10 potential tyrosine-phosphorylation sites (Sun *et al.*, 1991). Six of these tyrosine-phosphorylation sites lie in the amino acid sequence motif Tyr-Met-Xaa-Met which is recognized in its phosphorylated form by the SH2 (*src* homology 2) domain of the phosphatidylinositol 3-kinase (PI 3-kinase) (Sun *et al.*, 1991).

IRS-1 is highly phosphorylated on serine residues in the basal state; insulin stimulation leads to additional tyrosine phosphorylation and an increase in serine phosphorylation (Sun et al., 1991, 1992). Mutated kinase-negative insulin receptors that cannot be autophosphorylated after ligand binding are completely unable to phosphorylate IRS-1 (Chou et al., 1987). Thus phosphorylation of the insulin receptor kinase seems to be a prerequisite for IRS-1 phosphorylation at tyrosine residues (White et al., 1988a; Wilden et al., 1990; Backer et al., 1991b). After insulin stimulation, IRS-1 is rapidly tyrosine phosphorylated and thereby associated with PI 3-kinase (Backer et al., 1991b). It is believed that this association leads to activation of PI 3-kinase which results in phosphorylation of phosphatidylinositol molecules (Cantley et al., 1991).

Several studies suggest that PI 3-kinase activation and lipid phosphorylation play a role in cell growth (Cantley et al., 1991; Myers et al., 1993). Although some functional properties of IRS-1 have been defined, we can presume that not all of the functions of IRS-1 have been discovered. The role of IRS-1 is probably not restricted to its function as a docking protein for PI 3-kinase; it might rather play a multifunctional role as a signalling element for growth-promoting and metabolic effects. IRS-1 is a substrate for the insulin receptor as well as for the structure- and sequence-related IGF-I (Izumi et al., 1987; Kadowaki et al., 1987; Myers et al., 1993); in contrast, it appears not to be a substrate for the platelet-derived growth factor (PDGF) and epidermal growth factor (EGF) receptors (Kadowaki et al., 1987; Escobedo et al., 1991). IRS-1 has been identified in many different cell types (Kahn et al., 1993), animal tissues (Momomura et al., 1988; Tobe et al., 1990) and in human muscle (Kellerer et al., 1993b) as a major target for insulin. This might also suggest its general role as a signalling element in different cell types.

### 3.4.3 IRS-1 Couples the Insulin Receptor to Phospholipid Kinases

The existence of a phospholipid kinase activity associated with the insulin receptor (Machicao and Wieland, 1984; Sale et al., 1986; Carrascosa et al., 1988) has proved controversial in the past. In the meantime, activation of a PI 3-kinase by the insulin, IGF-I, EGF and PDGF receptors could be demonstrated among other growth factor receptors (Kaplan et al., 1987; Auger et al., 1989; Varticovski et al., 1989; Endemann et al., 1990; Ruderman et al., 1990).

PI 3-kinase is composed of an 85 kDa regulatory subunit and a 110 kDa catalytic subunit. Two isoforms of the 85 kDa regulatory subunit have been identified which are both able to bind phosphorylated proteins via their SH2 domains (Augustine et al., 1990; Backer et al., 1992). Activation of PI 3-kinase results in phosphorylation of phosphatidylinositol molecules. PI

3-kinase has been found to be activated by the insulin receptor as well as by several growth factor receptors such as those of IGF-I, EGF, colony-stimulating factor (CSF) and PDGF, suggesting a role in signal transduction for all of these receptors (Kaplan et al., 1987; Auger et al., 1989; Varticovski et al., 1989; Endemann et al., 1990; Ruderman et al., 1990). Several studies indicate that PI 3-kinase activation is involved in cell growth (Cantley et al., 1991; Myers et al., 1993). We have recently shown that both receptor isoforms HIR-A and HIR-B are able to stimulate PI 3-kinase (Carrascosa et al., 1991). It appears possible that insulin-stimulated phospholipid phosphorylation plays a role in a signal-transmitting system that involves the activation of a phospholipase and subsequently the release of second-messenger products cleaved from membrane phospholipids. The characterization of IRS-1 has finally provided a basis for understanding the mechanism of insulin receptor interactions with phospholipid kinases.

### 3.4.4 IRS-1 Couples the Insulin Receptor Tyrosine Kinase to a Ras-activated Signalling Cascade of Serine Kinases

It has been known for a long time that a number of enzymes are regulated by insulin through phosphorylation and dephosphorylation at serine residues (Kahn, 1985). Therefore, a signal transduction from the tyrosine-specific insulin receptor kinase to a serine-specific kinase must occur. The serine kinase that might fulfil both functions in the insulin signal-transduction chain has not yet been identified; however, there are several possible candidates for these so called "switch kinases" (Fig. 10).

Recent studies suggest that Ras might function as a switch between tyrosine and serine kinases (for a review see Satoh et al., 1992). Ras is a GTP-binding protein which is able to interact with and to activate a serine kinase cascade in different cell types (Skolnik et al., 1993a,b; Vojtek et al., 1993). It appears to be involved in mitogenic signal transduction and possibly also other signalling pathways, such as the regulation of glycogen synthesis. This serine kinase cascade includes the so-called mitogen-activated protein kinases (MAPKKK, MAPKK and MAPK), also recently called extracellular-signal-regulated kinases (ERKS), (receptor-activated kinases) (Satoh et al., 1992; Vojtek et al., 1993).

Studies in Caenorhabditis elegans, Drosophila and different mammalian cell systems have demonstrated that receptor tyrosine kinases (Let-23 in C. elegans, Sevenless in Drosophila and different growth hormone receptors such as the EGF receptor and PDGF receptor in mammalian cells) couple to adaptor proteins which contain SH2 and SH3 domains (Sem-5 in C. elegans, Drk in Drosophila, Grb2 in mammalian cells) (Egan et al., 1993; Li et al., 1993). The SH2 domains of these coupling proteins recognize phosphotyrosine-containing domains in the tyrosine kinase receptors. These

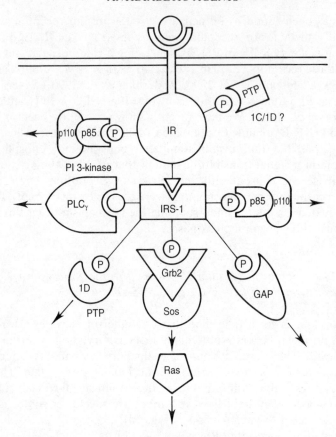

FIG. 10. Downstream elements of insulin receptor signalling. PTP, phosphotyrosine phosphatase; 1C, phosphatase 1C; 1D, phosphatase I1D.

adaptor proteins are able to form complexes with GDP–GTP exchanger proteins (Sos in *Drosophila* and mSos 1,2 in mammalian cells). These proteins catalyse the exchange of GDP for GTP in Ras which at the same time activates Ras function. GTP–Ras is then able to activate serine kinases such as Raf. Ras contains an endogenous GTPase activity which inactivates the complex to Ras–GDP. This endogenous GTPase activity is again modulated by other proteins like GTPase-activating protein (GAP) or NF1.

Recently, it was demonstrated that the insulin receptor tyrosine kinase uses IRS-1 to interact with these adaptor and GTP-exchanger proteins (Baltensperger *et al.*, 1993; Skolnik *et al.*, 1993b). It appears that in insulin-responsive cells the insulin receptor interacts with a complex formed by IRS-1, Grb2 and Sos leading to activation of Ras (Skolnik *et al.*, 1993a). It is at present unclear whether this pathway is only involved in the generation of mitogenic signals by the insulin receptor or whether this coupling to a serine kinase cascade is also involved in modulation of key enzymes of cell metabolism such as glycogen synthase.

### 3.4.5  Phosphatases

After insulin binding, protein phosphorylation and dephosphorylation appear to play a pivotal role in further signal transmission from the insulin receptor to the effector systems (Goldstein, 1992). Since at the post-kinase level tyrosine phosphorylation of substrate proteins is involved in insulin signalling, an important role for tyrosine phosphatases in the regulation of post-kinase signalling mechanisms has to be assumed (Goldstein, 1992).

Tyrosine-specific phosphatases must be involved in the regulation of the autophosphorylation status of the insulin receptor controlling its signalling activity. The same mechanism is likely to be relevant for IRS-1 and other tyrosine-phosphorylated signal-transduction elements. The tyrosine phosphatase that specifically controls the insulin receptor and IRS-1 has, however, not so far been identified. It is believed that the insulin signal-transmission mechanism switches at some point in the signalling chain from tyrosine phosphorylation to serine phosphorylation (Lewis et al., 1990; Goldstein, 1992). At this level of the signal-transduction chain, serine phosphatases play an important role. A previously characterized enzyme in this context is protein phosphatase 1 (PP-1). Insulin stimulates a serine/threonine kinase which activates this protein phosphatase by serine phosphorylation (Goldstein, 1992). Subsequently, PP-1 is able to dephosphorylate glycogen synthase and thereby activates this enzyme (see also section 4.1). Thus insulin is able to promote increased as well as decreased phosphorylation of signalling proteins which are probably involved in regulation of distinct biological effects of insulin (Ballou and Fisher, 1986; Baltensperger et al., 1992; Goldstein, 1992).

The above may be of pathophysiological relevance as a decreased basal and insulin-stimulated glycogen phosphatase activity and phosphorylase phosphatase activity (Type-1 protein phosphatase, PP-1) in the skeletal muscle of insulin-resistant individuals has been found (Freymond et al., 1988; Kida et al., 1990, 1992; Damsbo et al., 1991). Other studies suggest increased phosphotyrosine phosphatase activity in patients with NIDDM who show decreased autoactivation of the insulin receptor kinase (McGuire et al., 1991).

### 3.4.6  Serine Kinases Modulating the Insulin Receptor Functions

It is believed that the insulin receptor kinase might activate other serine-specific kinases which have a dual function, i.e. further transduction of the insulin signal to other effector systems and, in a feedback mechanism, inhibition of the first steps of insulin signalling at the level of the insulin receptor. Current opinions on the role of serine kinases in "downstream signalling" are discussed above. The role of serine kinases as "feedback inhibitors" of the insulin receptor will be discussed in the following section. We and others have shown that serine phosphorylation, in particular by PKC and cAMP kinase, counteracts the effects of tyrosine phosphorylation at the level of the receptor kinase (Jacobs et al., 1983; Takayama et al., 1984, 1988; Häring et al., 1986a,b; Obermaier et al., 1987) and at a post-kinase level (Kellerer et al., 1990). The physiological significance of the serine phosphorylation might therefore be termination of the insulin signal or a mechanism to rapidly modulate the sensitivity of cells toward insulin signals.

In this context interest is focused on PKC, which plays a key role in mediating signals generated by hormones, growth factors and neurotransmitters (Nishizuka, 1988). Several isoforms of PKC have been described which show distinct sensitivity to $Ca^{2+}$ and phospholipid-degradation products (Nishizuka, 1988). Their specific function, however, is not defined. It has been demonstrated previously that phorbol esters are potent activators of PKC and induce inhibition of the catalytic domain of the insulin receptor probably via serine phosphorylation of the insulin receptor $\beta$-subunit (Müller et al., 1991).

Insulin-dependent activation of PKC has also been demonstrated in several studies. The following mechanism was suggested for transduction of the insulin signal to PKC isoforms: insulin stimulates at the post-kinase level a specific GTP-binding protein (G-protein) and subsequently a phospholipase C (PLC) (Exton et al., 1991). This results in hydrolysis of phosphatidylinositol which generates diacylglycerol. The second messenger, diacylglycerol, is a potent activator of PKC (Housley, 1991). We recently demonstrated that hyperglycaemia reduces insulin receptor kinase activity in vitro and in vivo (Müller et al., 1991; Berti et al., 1994). Indirect evidence was obtained that this effect might be mediated by PKC. Insulin, as well as high glucose levels, is able to induce translocation of four PKC isoforms in rat-1 fibroblasts overexpressing the insulin receptor (Berti et al., 1994). Moreover our recent results suggest a direct association of PKC with the insulin receptor upon insulin stimulation (Berti et al., 1994). All these data together strongly suggest a regulatory role for PKC for insulin signal transduction.

### 3.4.7 GTP-binding Proteins

The role of the G-protein Ras in insulin signalling has already been discussed. Besides Ras, the family of heterotrimeric G-proteins might also be relevant in insulin action. These G-proteins are composed of a $\alpha$-, $\beta$- and $\gamma$-subunits. The $\alpha$-subunit has a high-affinity binding site for GDP or GTP. GTP binding to the $\alpha$-subunit induces its dissociation from the $\beta$- and $\gamma$-subunits. The $\alpha$-subunit can thereby gain regulatory functions for signalling proteins (Taylor, 1990a). The role of heterotrimeric G-proteins in post-kinase signal transduction has long been a topic for discussion. The evidence suggesting a role for these G-proteins in insulin signalling consists of the following: (1) an effect of insulin on ADP-ribosylation has been demonstrated (Heyworth and Houslay, 1983; Heyworth et al., 1985; Rothenberg and Kahn, 1988); (2) G-protein expression was altered in streptozotocin-induced diabetes (Gawler et al., 1987); (3) G-proteins serve in vitro as substrates for the insulin receptor kinase (Zick et al., 1986; O'Brian et al., 1987; Krupinski et al., 1988; Rothenberg and Kahn, 1988); (4) G-proteins are able to modulate insulin receptor kinase activity (O'Brian et al., 1987; Rothenberg and Kahn, 1988; Kellerer et al., 1991b).

We have shown that stimulation of G-proteins produces insulin-like effects (Obermaier-Kusser et al., 1988b), and have identified a 40 kDa G-proteins in adipocytes with characteristics distinct from $G_i\alpha$ and $G_S$-$\alpha$ that is activated by the insulin receptor (Kellerer et al., 1991b). Jo et al. (1990) also described a G-protein of a similar size which co-purifies with the insulin receptor. The molecular mass of this G-protein is also around 40 kDa, but a different susceptibility to cholera toxin and pertussis toxin was found. It is still unclear which effector systems might be activated by these G-proteins even though PLC is a good candidate. It is, however, interesting to note that these insulin-receptor-associated G-proteins are able to inhibit the binding and kinase function of the insulin receptor, possibly in a negative feedback manner (Kellerer et al., 1991b).

### 3.4.8 Phospholipases and Release of Chemical Mediators from Membrane Glycolipids

The action of insulin on PLC has caused long-standing controversy. However, earlier reports on the stimulatory effects of insulin on PLC (Koepfer-Hobelsberger and Wieland, 1984; Fox et al., 1987) have more recently been confirmed by others (Egan et al., 1990; Yoshimoto et al., 1990; Cooper et al., 1990a). We could show that this putative insulin-activated PLC is also under the negative control of PKC (Kellerer et al., 1990) and may be activated by both receptor (HIR-A and HIR-B) isoforms. It is believed that the substrates of these phospholipases are membrane glycolipids. On activation of PLC, inositol phospho-oligosaccharides (IPOs) might be released from the plasma membrane. Despite the many different effects of these IPOs on isolated cells and enzymes (Kelly et al., 1986, 1987; Saltiel and Cuatrecasas, 1986; Saltiel et al., 1986; Alemany et al., 1987; Mato et al., 1987; Saltiel, 1987; Standaert et al., 1988; Mato, 1989; Kellerer et al., 1993c), their physiological role is still being discussed.

We recently demonstrated that IPOs released from rat-1 fibroblasts overexpressing the human insulin receptor are able to stimulate glucose transport and lipogenesis (Kellerer et al., 1993c). As most of these glycolipids are located on the outside of the cell (Mato, 1989), this system might not be involved in intracellular signalling but might be important for cell–cell signalling. Unfortunately, precise structural data on these putative insulin second messengers is lacking. However, evidence was recently presented that several isoforms of these molecules exist which are differentially regulated (Gaulton, 1991).

## 4 Effector Systems of Insulin Signals: A Limited Selection

### 4.1 GLUCOSE UPTAKE AND METABOLISM: GLYCOGEN SYNTHASE

Despite our increasing knowledge about the post-kinase signalling systems described above, the exact mechanism linking the insulin receptor to particular effector systems remains obscure. Among the most important and intensively studied effector systems of the metabolic insulin signal are the glucose-transport system and the key enzyme of glycogen synthesis, glycogen synthase. These two effector systems have also been extensively studied in the context of the pathogenesis of NIDDM.

Glycogen synthase activity is regulated by phosphorylation and dephosphorylation. A number of serine-specific kinases phosphorylate glycogen synthase at different residues (Dent et al., 1990; Lavoinne et al., 1991), and at least two phosphatases regulate the dephosphorylation. Dephosphorylation converts the enzyme from a glucose-6-phosphate-dependent form to a glucose-6-phosphate-independent form. Insulin activates the enzyme by activating glycogen synthase phosphatase and inhibiting the cAMP-dependent kinase, one of the glycogen synthase kinases (Larner, 1983). The inhibition of cAMP-dependent kinase appears to lower the phosphorylation of glycogen synthase phosphatase-inhibitor-I leading to activation of glycogen synthase phosphatase (Larner, 1983). Although there is no experimental proof, it is speculated that the MAPK cascade might also be involved in insulin signalling to glycogen synthases.

It is generally found that the insulin effect on glycogen synthase from skeletal muscle of NIDDM patients is reduced (Bogardus et al., 1984; Mandarino et al., 1987; Freymond et al., 1988; Wright et al., 1988; Eriksson et al., 1989; Gerich et al., 1990; Nyomba et al., 1990). Conversely, it has been reported that the activation of the dependent enzyme form by glucose 6-phosphate is normal (Damsbo et al., 1991), suggesting that no defect of the enzyme itself exists in NIDDM. It has been shown by nuclear magnetic resonance technology that the decreased effect of insulin on the enzyme is indeed relevant *in vivo*, causing a decreased rate of glycogen synthesis (Shulman *et al.*, 1990).

## 4.2 THE GLUCOSE TRANSPORTER

### 4.2.1 Structure

From the work of Garcia de Herreros and Birnbaum (1989), Mueckler (1990), Fukumoto *et al.* (1988) and others, it is clear that five different isoforms of the glucose-transporter protein exist. This family of five structurally related glucose-transporter proteins have been named GLUT-1 to GLUT-5. They show tissue-specific expression (Table 3) which presumably adapts to tissue-specific demands for glucose utilization (Mueckler *et al.*, 1985; Birnbaum *et al.*, 1986; Kayano *et al.*, 1988; Thorens *et al.*, 1988; Birnbaum, 1989; Charron *et al.*, 1989; Fukumoto *et al.*, 1989; James *et al.*, 1989; Kaestner *et al.*, 1989). Of these glucose-transporter isoforms GLUT-4 and to a lesser extent GLUT-1 are insulin-sensitive glucose transporters and are expressed abundantly in skeletal muscle and fat which are major insulin target tissues (Charron *et al.*, 1989; Fukumoto *et al.*, 1989; James *et al.*, 1989; Kaestner *et al.*, 1989).

Most tissues express more than one isoform (Table 3). The different glucose transporters have distinct $K_m$ values for glucose (Table 3). This might reflect the tissue-specific demand. For example, GLUT-1 and GLUT-3 with relatively low $K_m$ values for glucose may mediate basal glucose uptake (Birnbaum *et al.*, 1986; Kayano *et al.*, 1988). In contrast, GLUT-2 with a high $K_m$ for glucose is expressed primarily in liver which is exposed to relatively high glucose levels (Fukumoto *et al.*, 1988; Thorens *et al.*, 1988). Therefore tissue-specific isoform expression of GLUT presumably allows a cell-specific response to glucose uptake and metabolism.

A model of the glucose-transporter protein structure in the plasma membrane was created as described by Mueckler *et al.* (1985). This two-dimensional structure model in Fig. 11 shows 12 membrane-spanning regions with the *N*- and *C*-terminal regions located inside the plasma membrane. The molecular structure reveals two big loops, one in the extracellular region between transmembrane regions 1 and 2, the other in the intracellular part between transmembrane regions 6 and 7. Highest homology was found between the membrane-spanning segments whereas the homology in the big intracellular loop and the *N*- and *C*-terminal regions was rather low between the different glucose-transporter isoforms (Bell *et al.*, 1990). It was speculated that the segments with high homology between all five glucose-transporter isoforms have a common general function, for example the formation of a pore for the transport of glucose from the extracellular to the intracellular pool (Kasanicki and Pilch, 1990). However, the domain for glucose binding has not been identified.

TABLE 3

Distribution and properties of glucose transporters

| Glucose transporter | Tissue | Number of amino acids | Chromosomal location | Homology to GLUT-4 (%) | Appropriate $K_m$ for glucose (mM) |
|---|---|---|---|---|---|
| GLUT-1 | Erythrocyte, placenta, brain | 492 | 1p35-31.3 | 76 | 2–20 |
| GLUT-2 | Liver, kidney | 524 | 3q26 | 67 | 20–40 |
| GLUT-3 | Brain, placenta, kidney | 496 | 12p13 | 69 | ? |
| GLUT-4 | Muscle, fat | 509 | 17p13 | | 2–10 |
| GLUT-5 | Small intestine | 501 | 1p31 | 41 | ? |

## 4.2.2   Glucose-transporter Function and Regulation

The transport and utilization of glucose is one of the most important sources of energy in organisms. Defects in this transport system can give rise to diseases such as diabetes mellitus (Friedman *et al.*, 1991; Rothmann *et al.*, 1992; Vogt *et al.*, 1992). Although the glucose-transport mechanism is being studied extensively, there are still many unanswered questions concerning the molecular mechanisms of signal transmission to the glucose-transporter proteins and their activation.

Insulin stimulates glucose transport in typical target tissues such as muscle and adipose tissue. Muscle and fat express predominantly the insulin sensitive GLUT-4 (Fukumoto *et al.*, 1989). Insulin stimulation induces recruitment of GLUT-4 from the intracellular pool to the plasma membrane (Wardzala *et al.*, 1978; Cushman and Wardzala, 1980; Suzuki and Kono, 1980; Kono *et al.*, 1981).

Recently, increasing evidence for a possible glucose-transport-mediating function for small G-proteins has been produced. Such G-proteins are identified in low-density microsomes (Cormont *et al.*, 1991) where most of the GLUT-4 protein is located before stimulation with insulin.

## 4.2.3   The Fat Cell Model

A classic cell model widely used to study the signal flow from the receptor to the glucose-transport system is the isolated adipocyte where activation and

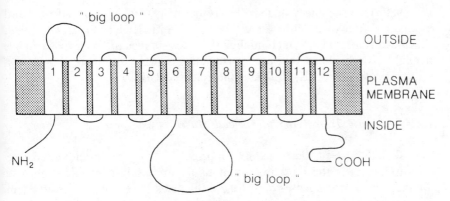

FIG. 11. Model of the glucose-transporter protein integrated into the plasma membrane.

deactivation of the glucose-transport system can be easily studied (Häring et al., 1981, 1982a). More than 10 years ago it was shown in this cell model by Cushman and Wardzala (1980) and Kono et al. (1981) that insulin induces translocation of glucose carriers from intracellular membranes to the plasma membrane. It seems to be accepted that autophosphorylation of the insulin receptor is essential for stimulation of GLUT-4. Insulin induces an acute 20–40-fold stimulation of glucose uptake rate in muscle and fat (Martz et al., 1986; Toyoda et al., 1987; Joost et al., 1988). However, data from many different groups, including our own, suggest that a simple translocation model is not sufficient to explain the effect of insulin on GLUT-4 (Joost et al., 1986; Kahn and Cushman, 1987; Karnieli et al., 1987; Matthaei et al., 1987; Mühlbacher et al., 1988; Obermaier-Kusser et al., 1989). A combined model involving translocation and activation of the glucose carriers where separate signalling chains activate the two steps (Obermaier-Kusser et al., 1989) has been suggested.

Several pharmacological substances that act like insulin have been valuable tools for testing which post-kinase signal transducers are involved in the insulin signal from the receptor to the translocation step or the activation step. We have found that the effect of insulin on glucose translocation can be mimicked by phorbol esters (Mühlbacher et al., 1988; Vogt et al., 1990, 1991b). As phorbol esters activate PKC, it is very likely that this enzyme is somehow involved in the signal between the receptor and the translocation process. The phorbol ester effect is restricted to the translocation of GLUT-4 (Vogt et al., 1990), not GLUT-1, suggesting distinct translocation mechanisms for the two carrier types (Vogt et al., 1991b). We used other pharmacological tools to investigate which signal-transducing elements are involved in the second signal-transmitting chain leading from the insulin receptor to carrier activation. As aluminium chloride (Obermaier-Kusser et *al.*, 1988b), exogenously added PLC (Obermaier-Kusser *et al.*, 1988b) and a mixture of exogenously added IPOs (Obermaier-Kusser *et al.*, 1989; Machicao *et al.*, 1990) can all mimic the effect of insulin on carrier activity, it might be speculated that carrier-activating signal transmission involves a sequence of G-proteins, PLC and the release of IPOs.

### 4.2.4 Glucose Transporter in Skeletal Muscle

The skeletal muscle accounts for approx. 85% of postprandial glucose utilization and is the most important tissue for insulin-dependent glucose uptake. However, glucose-transport mechanisms have not been studied in skeletal muscle as extensively as in fat cells, because of difficulties in measuring insulin-stimulated glucose transport in this tissue type. In skeletal muscle two glucose-transporter isoforms (GLUT-1 and GLUT-4) are expressed (Charron *et al.*, 1989; Fukumoto *et al.*, 1989; James *et al.*, 1989; Kaestner *et al.*, 1989). In the basal state GLUT-1 is found predominantly in the plasma membrane and its amount increases in the plasma membrane in response to insulin (James *et al.*, 1988). In contrast, GLUT-4 is identified primarily in intracellular vesicles in the basal state and increases dramatically in the plasma membrane after insulin stimulation (Klip *et al.*, 1987; James *et al.*, 1988). It has been proposed that GLUT-1 is primarily responsible for basal glucose transport whereas GLUT-4 is responsible for postprandial insulin-stimulated glucose uptake in skeletal muscle (James *et al.*, 1988).

Another unique feature of the skeletal muscle glucose transporter (GLUT-4) is its response to acute exercise. Several studies have demonstrated that electric stimulation of muscle as well as physical exercise results in increased glucose uptake in skeletal muscle (Ivy and Holloszy, 1981; Holloszy *et al.*, 1986). This increase in glucose uptake is parallelled by an increasing number of GLUT-4 molecules in the plasma membrane. Other studies suggest not only an increase in glucose transporters in the plasma membrane after exercise but also an increase in intrinsic carrier activity.

### 4.2.5 Alterations of the Insulin-signalling Cascade in Type-II Diabetes Mellitus

Insulin resistance, in particular in skeletal muscle, plays a pivotal role in the pathogenesis of NIDDM. Several abnormalities of the insulin-signalling chain have been found. At the receptor level a decreased tyrosine kinase activity has been described which appears to be due to a regulatory event (reviewed by Häring, 1991). Relevant mutations of the insulin receptor were not found (reviewed by Häring and Mehnert, 1993). Abnormalities at the level of glycogen synthase were observed as discussed above. There is also some evidence for irregularity of glucose transport in skeletal muscle. Nuclear magnetic resonance studies suggest that in muscle of NIDDM subjects glucose transport is decreased (Rothmann *et al.*, 1992).

The molecular mechanism has not been elucidated. The question of whether an abnormality of the glucose-transport system contributes to the insulin resistance in NIDDM patients was first addressed in adipocytes. In these studies both a decreased expression of the relevant glucose-transporter isoform (GLUT-4) and a decreased translocation to the plasma membrane and activation of glucose carriers was found (Garvey *et al.*, 1988). A number of studies have since addressed the question of whether alterations in GLUT-4 expression can be detected at the level of the skeletal muscle. The majority of the data suggest that the expression of GLUT-4 in skeletal muscle is not significantly decreased (reviewed by Häring and Mehnert, 1993).

The functional properties of the glucose transporters are not known as no studies on translocation or activation of GLUT-4 from NIDDM patients have been published. In skeletal muscle biopsies from musculus vastus lateralis, normal expression of GLUT-4 both at the mRNA and protein level was described (Handberg *et al.*, 1990; Pedersen *et al.*, 1990). In contrast, our data obtained from musculus gastrocnemius suggested a decreased level of GLUT-4 (Vogt *et al.*, 1992).

Ultimately, it will be important to know whether GLUT-4 levels in plasma membranes and transverse tubules after insulin stimulation are altered. In the basal state, at least, we observed an altered subcellular distribution of GLUT-4 in gastrocnemius muscle. The discrepancy between results might be a consequence of the different muscle types studied or, more likely, different patient characteristics. In our study patients were clearly older and had a longer duration of NIDDM than in the other studies where no abnormality was detected. This suggests that changes in GLUT-4 expression might be a very late phenomenon in the development of skeletal muscle insulin resistance and may not be considered as a primary defect in the development of NIDDM. Furthermore no mutation of the glucose-transporter gene could be detected in patients with NIDDM (O'Rahilly *et al.*, 1991). Thus, it seems that the impaired glucose uptake in NIDDM is due to unknown modulatory factors of the glucose transporter. Overall insulin resistance in NIDDM is probably due to a synergistic effect of impaired receptor signalling together with regulatory events of the glucose transporter and the signalling chain to glycogen synthase.

# Therapeutic Use of Insulin

Insulin is used for the treatment of Type-I and for Type-II diabetes mellitus, when other therapeutic measures, i.e. appropriate diet and oral antidiabetics, are not sufficient to produce normoglycaemia. The physiological actions of insulin including recent advances in our knowledge on signal transduction have been discussed above (chapter 4). Since treatment of diabetes with insulin attempts only to supplement inadequate insulin secretion, this chapter will concentrate on pharmacokinetics, unwanted effects and clinical applications of insulin and its pharmaceutical preparations.

## 1  Chemistry

The insulin molecule consists of two chains, the A-chain with 21 amino acids and the B-chain with 30 amino acids (Fig. 12). They are interconnected by two intermolecular disulphide bridges between amino acids A7 and B7 and A20 and B19. A third disulphide bridge connects amino acids 6 and 11 on chain A, giving an intramolecular loop. It is synthesized as a single-chain precursor, preproinsulin, which is converted to proinsulin after the molecule has been translocated to the endoplasmic reticulum. There, the C-peptide, which connects the A- and B-chains, is cut away forming the active insulin (Briggs and Gierasch, 1986; Bailyes et al., 1993). The most often used insulins in therapeutics (Fig. 12), bovine, porcine and human insulin, exhibit differences in their amino acid sequences; bovine insulin contains Ala instead of Thr in position 8 and Val instead of Ile in position 10 of the A-chain, and both bovine and porcine insulin differ from human insulin by an Ala instead of Thr in position 30 of the B-chain.

The positions of the three bridges, the N- and C-terminal sequences on the A-chain and the hydrophobic residues in the C-terminal region of the B-chain are invariant with respect to other species.

The insulin molecule contains six amino acid residues that can carry a positive charge and 10 that can carry a negative charge. The net charge is zero at pH 5.5 (Brange, 1987). The solubility of insulin is dependent on the pH of the solvent, being practically insoluble in water at pH 5.4 but easily soluble at pH less than 4. In alkaline media, solubility is dependent on the concentration of zinc ions and the species of insulin origin (Schlichtkrull, 1958).

Insulin is able to form at least six different crystalline modifications, either zinc-free or with two or four zinc ions per hexamer. The addition of protamine and phenol also affects the structure of the crystal (for a review see Brange, 1987).

## 2  Preparations

The preparations marketed can be divided into three types: (1) the short-acting or rapid-acting insulins, (2) the intermediate-acting insulins and

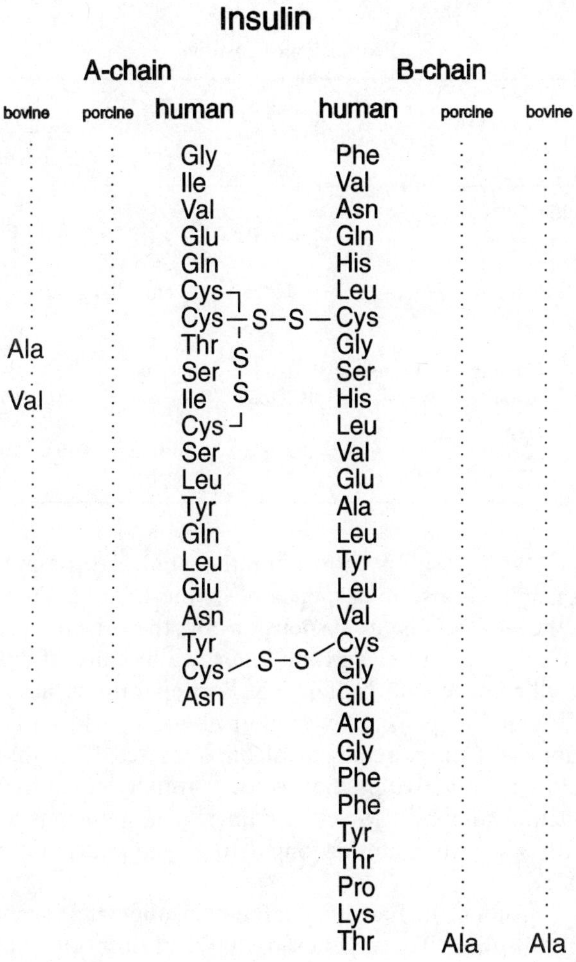

## Insulin

| A-chain | | | B-chain | | |
|---|---|---|---|---|---|
| bovine | porcine | human | human | porcine | bovine |

```
                    Gly          Phe
                    Ile          Val
                    Val          Asn
                    Glu          Gln
                    Gln          His
                    Cys┐         Leu
                    Cys┼S–S─Cys
        Ala         Thr  S       Gly
                    Ser  |       Ser
        Val         Ile  S       His
                    Cys┘         Leu
                    Ser          Val
                    Leu          Glu
                    Tyr          Ala
                    Gln          Leu
                    Leu          Tyr
                    Glu          Leu
                    Asn          Val
                    Tyr        ⸝Cys
                    Cys╱S–S╲Gly
                    Asn          Glu
                                 Arg
                                 Gly
                                 Phe
                                 Phe
                                 Tyr
                                 Thr
                                 Pro
                                 Lys
                    Thr    Ala   Ala
```

FIG. 12. Differences in the amino acid sequence of bovine, porcine and human insulin.

(3) the slow-acting or long-lasting insulins. To obtain special preparations, short- and intermediate-acting insulins may be mixed together.

The short-acting insulins are the soluble forms, which have an onset of action after about 30 min to 1 h, a peak activity at about 2–5 h, and a duration of about 6–8 h. Generally, they are of the regular crystalline zinc insulin-type and dissolved in neutral buffer. Apart from use for acute control of blood glucose levels, they are used in combination with intermediate-acting insulins and in subcutaneous insulin pump systems. Although the absorption of the Semilente insulin (a prompt-acting insulin zinc suspension) is similar to that of regular insulin, its duration of action is longer (Table 4).

TABLE 4

Properties of insulins

| | Protein | Zinc | Buffer | Action (h) | | |
|---|---|---|---|---|---|---|
| | | (mg per 100 U) | | Onset | Peak | Duration |
| Rapid-acting insulin | | | | | | |
| Regular (crystalline) | Clear | – | 0.01–0.04 | – | 0.3–0.7 | 2–4 | 5–8 |
| Semilente | Cloudy | – | 0.2–0.25 | Acetate | 0.5–1.0 | 2–8 | 12–16 |
| Intermediate-acting insulin | | | | | | |
| Isophane | Cloudy | Protein | 0.01–0.04 | Phosphate | 1–2 | 6–12 | 18–24 |
| Lente | Cloudy | – | 0.2–0.25 | Acetate | 1–2 | 6–12 | 18–24 |
| Slow-acting insulin | | | | | | |
| Ultralente | Cloudy | – | 0.2–0.25 | Acetate | 4–6 | 16–18 | 20–36 |
| Protamine | Cloudy | Protein | 0.2–0.25 | Phosphate | 4–6 | 14–20 | 24–36 |

Intermediate-acting insulins are either the neutral protamine Hagedorn insulin (NPH isophane insulin suspension) or the Lente insulin (insulin zinc suspension); the former is a suspension of the insulin–protamine–zinc complex in a phosphate buffer and the latter is a mixture of crystallized and amorphous insulin in acetate buffer. These preparations have an onset of action within about 2 h, peak activity after about 4–12 h, and a duration of up to 24 h (Table 4). Commercially available mixtures of soluble insulins and isophane insulins have activities that would normally place them within the intermediate-acting category. Mixed insulin–zinc suspensions are sometimes classified as either intermediate- or long-acting as the duration of action may be up to 30 h.

Long-acting insulins include crystalline insulin–zinc suspensions and protamine–zinc–insulins. These generally have an onset after about 4 h and a duration of up to 36 h.

## 3 Application of Insulins

The particular insulin employed, such as human or animal, the type of formulation, the route of administration, and the frequency of administration must be chosen to suit the needs of the individual patient. The dose must also be determined for each patient, and, although a precise dose range cannot be given, a total dose in excess of about 80 units daily would be unusual and may indicate the presence of a form of insulin resistance (Martindale, 1989).

The short-acting insulins are usually injected between 30 and 45 min before meals. The intermediate-acting insulins should be given once a day before breakfast or twice a day, the long-lasting insulins are given three times on the first day as a loading dose and then as one or two injections per day, the dosage being adapted as required to maintain near normoglycaemic blood glucose levels (Kahn and Schechter, 1990).

## 4 Pharmacokinetics

### 4.1 INTRODUCTION

Although the pharmacokinetical parameters of exogenously administered insulin resemble those of physiological insulin, it differs from physiological secretion of insulin in at least two major ways: the kinetics of absorption of subcutaneously or intramuscularly administered insulins are relatively slow and thus do not mimic the normal rapid increase and decline in insulin secretion in response to ingestion of nutrients; the insulin diffuses into the peripheral circulation instead of being released into the portal circulation (Kahn and Schechter, 1990). This may account for the differences in the action between physiological secretion and therapeutic administration of insulin.

### 4.2 ABSORPTION

Absorption of insulin is mainly dependent on the preparation used (see Section 2). Insulin is fairly rapidly absorbed from subcutaneous tissues and although its half-life in blood is very short (see below), the duration of action of most preparations is considerably longer because of their formulation (see Section 2). The rate of absorption from different anatomical sites may be different and may also be increased by exercise. The absorption of insulin after intramuscular administration is more rapid than that after subcutaneous administration (Martindale, 1989). Apart from the fact that absorption depends on the site of injection, it is most rapid from the subcutaneous fat tissue in the abdominal region rather than from the leg or the arm. It can be modified by massage of the tissue or by heat, both inducing an increase in subcutaneous blood flow (Berger et al., 1982).

The absorption of subcutaneously injected regular human insulin is significantly accelerated when compared with porcine or bovine insulin (Bottermann et al., 1981; Federlin et al., 1981; Cüppers et al., 1982; Sonnenberg et al., 1983; Owens et al., 1986) independent of its origin (semisynthetic or biosynthetic) (Sonnenberg et al., 1983), but the clinical relevance appears doubtful (Kemmer et al., 1983; Sonnenberg et al., 1983). A possible explanation is that human insulin is more hydrophilic than porcine insulin or it has a lesser tendency to associate into stable hexamers than porcine insulin (Brange, 1987).

Recent development of insulin analogues has altered the rates of absorption. Insulin with aspartate and glutamate substituted at positions B9 and B27 respectively crystallizes poorly and has been termed "monomeric insulin" (Vora et al., 1988). This insulin is absorbed more rapidly from subcutaneous depots and thus may be useful in meeting postprandial demands. In contrast, other insulin analogues tend to crystallize at the site of injection and are absorbed more slowly (Markussen et al., 1988). Insulins with enhanced biological potency have been produced by substitution of aspartate for histidine at position B10 and by modification of the C-terminal residues of the B-chain (Schwartz et al., 1989).

After intramuscular injection, the onset of action of all insulins is generally more rapid and the duration of action shorter (Martindale, 1989).

## 4.3 PLASMA LEVELS

For the rapid-acting insulins, the peak plasma levels are reached about 90–150 min after injection (Vora and Owens, 1991), for the intermediate-acting insulins after about 6–12 h and for the long-lasting insulins after about 7–30 h (Rang and Dale, 1991).

## 4.4 DISTRIBUTION

The volume of distribution approximates the volume of the extracellular fluid (Kahn and Schechter, 1990). Normally, insulin is not bound to plasma proteins, but this is altered in the presence of insulin antibodies (Poulsen and Deckert, 1976).

## 4.5 HALF-LIFE

The half-life of insulin in the plasma of healthy subjects is about 5–6 min. To obtain a longer duration of the therapy, the rate of absorption of insulin must be modulated. The following are useful ways of controlling the absorption of insulin.

(1) Addition of cationic organic compounds (surfen, globin) to acidic solutions of insulin. This produces poorly soluble complexes in the tissue fluids.
(2) Combination of basic proteins with neutral suspensions of insulin (protamine–zinc–insulin).
(3) Complexes of insulin in neutral suspensions with zinc ions.
(4) Alteration of the physical state and size of the insulin–zinc particles (amorphous versus crystalline).

(5) Species of origin: the duration of action of the porcine variety is somewhat shorter than that of the bovine.
(6) Coupling of the insulin molecule with phenylisocyanate or heat treatment leading to prolonged action.

## 4.6 METABOLISM AND INACTIVATION

Degradation of insulin takes place in liver, muscles and kidney. In the liver, about 50% of the insulin is extracted, therefore insulin undergoes a strong "first-pass effect" when released from the pancreas. The capacity of hepatic degradation is maximal under normal conditions but may be reduced after oral administration of glucose, possibly because of the effect of gastrointestinal hormones (Kahn and Schechter, 1990). In the kidney, insulin is filtered via the glomerula and reabsorbed in the tubules, which also degrade it.

In addition to the normal metabolic and elimination systems, circulating antibodies against insulin have important effects on its pharmacokinetic properties. Such antibodies may delay the exit of insulin from the vascular space to the extracellular interstitial space, where it exerts its actions. The insulin–antibody complex may also be cleared by the reticuloendothelial system, leading to an increased requirement of insulin. In general, insulin antibodies delay the onset of action of rapidly acting insulin and increase the duration of action of all insulins.

## 5 Toxic Effects

Extreme caution is necessary in the measurement of dosage; inadvertent overdose may lead to an irreversible insulin shock. Serious consequences may result if insulin is not used under constant medical supervision; if an overdose is untreated, hypoglycaemia may lead to convulsions and coma which should not be confused with hyperglycaemic coma.

In acute, usually suicidal, overdoses of insulin, successful management has included excision of the injection site.

## 6 Side Effects

### 6.1 HYPOGLYCAEMIA

#### 6.1.1 Symptoms

The most frequent complication of insulin therapy is hypoglycaemia, the speed of onset and duration of which may vary according to the type of preparation and the route of administration used. It is often associated with an excessive dosage of insulin, the omission of a meal by the patient, or increased physical activity, and has sometimes been reported in patients changing from bovine to other insulins (Tattersall, 1992).

Symptoms of hypoglycaemia resulting from increased sympathetic activity include hunger, pallor, sweating, palpitations, anxiety and tremulousness. Other symptoms include headache, visual disturbances such as blurred or double vision, slurred speech, paraesthesia of the mouth, alterations in behaviour, and impaired mental or intellectual ability (Anonymous, 1985). Some patients, especially the elderly or those with long-standing diabetes, may not experience the typical early warning symptoms of a hypoglycaemic attack.

The results of a 1-year study of adult patients with severe hypoglycaemia are summarized here (Potter et al., 1982; Moses et al., 1985). Of 204 episodes, one occurred in a patient with insulinoma, three in elderly diabetic patients receiving sulphonylureas, and 200 in 130 insulin-treated patients. A survey of diabetic clinics, identifying all insulin-treated adults, revealed that 9% had episodes of hypoglycaemia severe enough to warrant admission to casualty. Precipitating causes were often difficult to assess and no definite cause could be found in over one-third of patients. Comparison of patients with only one attack with those who suffered multiple attacks showed that missed or delayed meals accounted for 30 and 19% respectively, a recent increase in insulin dose for 14 and 13%, loss of warning symptoms for 4 and 11%, and exercise for 6 and 7%; other causes included carelessness, pregnancy and intake of alcohol.

During hypoglycaemia, subjects had to indicate the severity of the symptoms and their current mood. Differences between the effects of the insulins were consistently apparent after 20 min of hypoglycaemia, indicating a short-term action of these hormones on specified central nervous system functions (Kern et al., 1990). These differences, occurring during early hypoglycaemia, could contribute to the differential awareness of hypoglycaemic warning symptoms during human insulin (HI)- and porcine insulin (PI)-induced hypoglycaemia in diabetic patients.

The heart rate increases in response to hypoglycaemia; this increase is accompanied by a significant increase in systolic blood pressure, a fall in diastolic blood pressure, with no change in the mean arterial blood pressure (Fisher et al., 1990). The increases in ejection fraction and in heart rate in response to hypoglycaemia are mediated by $\beta$-adrenoreceptors, whereas the blood pressure responses to hypoglycaemia are mediated by $\alpha$- and $\beta$-adreno-receptors (Fisher et al., 1990).

Insulin hypoglycaemia stimulated GH secretion (i.e. from a basal level of $10\,mU\,l^{-1}$ to $48\,mU\,l^{-1}$) (Masuda et al., 1990; Popovic et al., 1990). Discordant response of GH after GH-releasing hormone (GHRH) and insulin-induced hypoglycaemia might suggest the involvement (at least partly) of somatostatin in the mechanism of GH release after hypoglycaemia and after GHRH (Popovic *et al.*, 1990). The oral clonidine test, a safer, easier and more economical test than insulin hypoglycaemia, is equally potent and can be carried out in outpatients as a GH-provocative test (Singh *et al.*, 1989).

Insulin-induced hypoglycaemia decreases luteinizing hormone (LH) secretion (Koivisto and Felig, 1978). The effect is prevented by the intravenous infusion of glucose, suggesting that neuroglycopenia and not a direct action of insulin is the cause of reduced LH secretion (Koivisto and Felig, 1978).

Insulin-induced hypoglycaemia is a strong stimulator of pituitary adrenocorticotrophin (ACTH) secretion (Caraty *et al.*, 1990). After the injection of a low ($0.2 \, \text{IU kg}^{-1}$) or high ($2 \, \text{IU kg}^{-1}$) dose of insulin, ACTH and cortisol levels in peripheral plasma increased in a dose-related manner. When the hypoglycaemia is moderate, corticotrophin-releasing factor (CRF) is the main factor triggering ACTH release, and the increased arginine-vasopressin (AVP) secretion potentiates the stimulatory effect of CRF. When hypoglycaemia is deeper, AVP secretion becomes predominant and may by itself stimulate ACTH release (Caraty *et al.*, 1990).

### 6.1.2  Frequency

The inherent risk of hypoglycaemia has increased with the modern aim of pursuing optimal glycaemic control in the hope of preventing the long-term development of diabetic complications. The frequency of hypoglycaemia is difficult to estimate accurately and probably varies according to local treatment policies which contrasts with insulin-induced hypoglycaemia, for which conservative estimates suggest that approximately 100–1000 patients per year require hospital treatment (Lawrence and Dunnigan, 1979; Potter *et al.*, 1982; Goldgewicht *et al.*, 1983).

At least one-third of all insulin-treated patients experience an episode of hypoglycaemic coma at some time, 10% have a hypoglycaemic coma in any single year, and 3% suffer frequent recurrent episodes of hypoglycaemic coma which are incapacitating.

The principal factors implicated in hypoglycaemia in the diabetic are:

(1) excessive doses of insulin (or sulphonylureas);
(2) inadequate or delayed ingestion of food;
(3) sudden or sustained exercise.

The first factor may arise as the result of decreased insulin requirement. Insulin requirement often declines during the "honeymoon" remission of IDDM after treatment is commenced in the newly diagnosed patient, and during progressive renal impairment. Failure to reduce the dose of insulin increases the risk of hypoglycaemia.

Excess insulin may also arise as the result of increased insulin bioavailability or sensitivity. Changing the insulin species or formulation administered may induce hypoglycaemia by altering the pharmacokinetic properties of insulin and enhancing its efficacy.

Dietary factors commonly predisposing to hypoglycaemia include failure to eat additional carbohydrates during strenuous domestic or sporting activities, miscalculating time intervals between insulin injections and meals, and drinking alcohol without food.

In a study involving 11 insulin-dependent diabetic subjects, leg exercise accelerated insulin absorption from a subcutaneous injection site in the leg, whereas it had no effect on insulin absorption from the arm and reduced it from the abdomen (Koivisto and Felig, 1978). Most exercise involved many muscle groups, and increased absorption was still likely. Patients who developed hypoglycaemia were advised to take extra carbohydrate before exercise rather than decrease the insulin dose (Zinman et al., 1978). Studies in five subjects suggested that absorption was increased by exercise (Koivisto, 1980a).

Studies in eight insulin-dependent diabetic men indicated that a sauna accelerated insulin absorption from the subcutaneous injection site and that, 2 h after the sauna, mean blood glucose concentration was significantly lower than on the control day (Dandona et al., 1978; Cüppers et al., 1980; Koivisto, 1980b). Hypoglycaemia and seizures were observed in one patient after the use of a sunbed (Husband and Gill, 1984).

### 6.1.3  Treatment of Insulin-induced Hypoglycaemia

In conscious and cooperative patients hypoglycaemia should be treated by the oral administration of a readily absorbable form of carbohydrate, such as sugar lumps or a glucose-based drink. Eating sugar or a sugar-sweetened product will often correct the condition and prevent more serious symptoms. If the reaction becomes more severe, breathing will be shallow and the skin will be pale. In severe hypoglycaemic reactions, intravenous dextrose may be necessary. If hypoglycaemic coma occurs, up to 50 ml of a 50% solution of glucose should be given intravenously and occasionally this may need to be repeated. If after about 1 h, blood glucose concentrations are normal and the patient has failed to regain consciousness, the possibility of cerebral oedema should be considered. In situations where the intravenous administration of glucose is impractical or not feasible, glucagon 0.5 to 1 mg by subcutaneous or intramuscular injection may be given; intravenous injection may also be employed. If the patient fails to respond to glucagon, glucose has to be given intravenously despite any impracticalities.

Following a return to consciousness, carbohydrates by mouth may need to be given until the action of insulin has ceased which, for preparations with a relatively long duration of action such as globin–zinc–insulin, isophane–insulin, some insulin–zinc suspensions, and protamine–zinc–insulin, may be several hours.

### 6.1.4 Hypoglycaemia Unawareness

The symptoms of hypoglycaemia often change with increasing duration of diabetes. Many autonomic symptoms attenuate or are even lost altogether, so that patients become unaware of the onset of hypoglycaemia and may suffer severe and prolonged neuroglycopenia as they are unable to take early corrective action (Sussman et al., 1963; Carveth-Johnson et al., 1982). In some cases, hypoglycaemia unawareness may be a consequence of autonomic neuropathy preventing the normal autonomic discharge and increased catecholamine secretion. It may also occur, however, in diabetic patients who have no evidence of autonomic dysfunction. There is a debate on this unawareness especially with respect to human insulin (Egger and Smith, 1992; Egger et al., 1992), so withdrawal of bovine and porcine insulins from the market is not justified at present.

### 6.2 MORNING HYPERGLYCAEMIA

Recent reviews of this topic include ones by Wilson (1983), Bolli and Gerich (1984), Bolli et al. (1984c), Devlin (1984), Campbell et al. (1985), Lyn (1985), Pramming et al. (1985). Morning hyperglycaemia may be the result of mere waning of subcutaneously injected insulin. It may also be rebound hyperglycaemia (post-hypoglycaemic hyperglycaemia or the Somogyi phenomenon) occurring after an episode of nocturnal hypoglycaemia. Morning hyperglycaemia has also been observed without antecedent hypoglycaemia even during constant intravenous infusion of insulin, when the waning of previously injected insulin would not be a factor and this is commonly referred to as the dawn phenomenon.

Clinically, it is important to distinguish between the dawn phenomenon, simple waning of previously injected insulin, and rebound hyperglycaemia as a cause of early-morning hyperglycaemia because their treatment differs. Management of the dawn phenomenon and insulin waning generally consists of adjusting the evening dose of insulin to provide additional coverage between 4 a.m. and 7 a.m. Management of rebound hyperglycaemia consists of reducing insulin doses or providing additional late-evening carbohydrate, or both, to avoid nocturnal hypoglycaemia. Mistaking rebound hyperglycaemia for the dawn phenomenon or mere waning of injected insulin could result in more serious nocturnal hypoglycaemia, if evening doses of insulin were increased (Cryer and Gerich, 1985).

## 6.3 LIPODYSTROPHY

Insulin, administered subcutaneously, may cause either lipoatrophy or lipohypertrophy. **Lipoatrophy** is the breakdown of adipose tissue at the insulin injection site causing a depression in the skin at the injection site and occasionally at distant sites also. It may be the result of an immune response or the use of less than pure insulin. Some findings suggest that total lipodystrophy syndrome results from the inflammatory destructive process of adipose tissue (Yanagawa et al., 1990). Injection of human or purified porcine insulin into the site over a 2–4-week period may result in subcutaneous fat accumulation.

Before purified human insulins were available, lipoatrophy occurred in about 25% of insulin-treated patients. Improvement or resolution of lesions has been noted in most patients after changing to purified porcine insulin.

Earlier insulin preparations contained a large number of protein contaminants thought to be immunogenic and hence the cause of lipodystrophy, insulin allergy and sometimes antibody-mediated insulin resistance in many patients. Monocomponent (MC)-insulin and human insulin are virtually free of these peptides and are therefore very rarely accompanied by the above-mentioned immunological side effects. In this respect, however, human insulin offers only a little advantage over MC-insulin although human insulin is the least immunogenic (Gyimesi and Ivanyi, 1989; Zenobi, 1991). One disadvantage of human insulin is that about 20% of patients treated with it experience a change in hypoglycaemia symptoms during the course of their illness. While autonomic symptoms become weaker or disappear, patients have to react to neuroglycogenic symptoms which normally remain constant. However, the incidence of hypoglycaemic events does not change during treatment with human insulin (Zenobi, 1991).

**Lipohypertrophy** is the result of repeated insulin injection into the same site. Insulin hypertrophy (lipohypertrophy) occurs as a soft dermal nodule with normal surface epidermis at the injection site, which has often been used for many years. This reaction may be due to the lipogenic action of insulin. This condition may be avoided by rotating the injection site, although it should be remembered that absorption of insulin may vary from different anatomical areas.

Lipoatrophy and lipohypertrophy were the most frequently reported local complications of conventional insulin therapy. Early reports after the introduction of highly purified insulins suggested a reduction in the frequency of lipohypertrophy and lipoatrophy. Because highly purified insulins have been in common usage for 10 years, the present frequency of these complications was assessed (McNally *et al.*, 1988). Lipohypertrophy was recorded in 27.1% of patients including three with associated lipotrophy. Lipoatrophy was found in 2.5% of cases (three porcine and four bovine insulin treated), four of which had only ever used highly purified insulins. Despite the introduction of highly purified insulins, lipohypertrophy and lipoatrophy remain prevalent in insulin-treated patients (McNally *et al.*, 1988). This common complication may be limited by routinely inspecting injection sites.

## 6.4 INSULIN ALLERGY

### 6.4.1 Introduction

Insulin, together with its polymers and other chemical derivatives, is immunogenic. Bovine insulin is more immunogenic than porcine insulin; human-sequence insulin is the least immunogenic but can nonetheless provoke antibody formation (Ganz *et al.*, 1990). Highly purified insulins have low immunogenicity. Although allergic reactions have been reported in patients receiving human insulin who were previously treated with animal insulins (Carveth-Johnson *et al.*, 1982; Frankland, 1982; Parr *et al.*, 1982; Altman *et al.*, 1983; Wiles *et al.*, 1983; Garcia-Ortega *et al.*, 1984; Grammer *et al.*, 1984; Kristensen *et al.*, 1984; von Kriegstein, 1985; Silverstone, 1986; Willms *et al.*, 1987), there does not appear to be a report of such reactions in patients treated exclusively with human insulin.

Insulin-binding antibodies are detectable in most insulin-treated patients but in most cases are clinically irrelevant. Insulin antibodies may "buffer" against sudden fluctuations in free insulin levels under experimental conditions, but generally do not seem to influence clinical insulin requirements or metabolic stability. Insulin-binding antibodies can affect the pharmacokinetics of injected insulin. Antibody-bound insulin may act as a reservoir or buffer from which free insulin can be released over a prolonged period (Stewart *et al.*, 1984; Dixon *et al.*, 1985). In the early 1960s, it was reported that, in patients taking only short-acting insulin, the daily number of injections was correlated with the disappearance rate of labelled insulin from the circulation (Bolinger *et al.*, 1964). Insulin antibody levels were generally high in insulin-treated diabetic patients at this time, and those subjects with slow insulin clearance (some of whom required only a single daily injection of soluble insulin) presumably had high levels of "buffering" antibody.

## 6.4.2   Clinical Manifestations

The clinical manifestations of insulin antibodies, now rare, include the following.

(1) **Local allergic reactions**, which are of three types. The commonest is the late-phase reaction, a biphasic **IgE** reaction characterized by immediate burning and pruritus with a wheal and flare at the injection site. It may resolve or become indurated, with pruritus continuing for hours to days. Two rarer forms are the **Arthustype reaction**, producing a pruritic painful nodule 6–8 h after injection, and the **delayed hypersensitivity reaction**, which is similar but appears 12–24 h after injection. The local reactions are characterized by swelling, erythema, pruritus and lipoatrophy at injection sites; they usually disappear with continued treatment. Generalized allergy may produce urticaria, angioedema and, very rarely, anaphylactoid reactions; if continued therapy with insulin is essential, desensitization procedures may need to be performed (Wintermantel *et al.*, 1988).

Occasionally, redness, swelling and itching at the injection site may develop. This occurs if the injection is not properly made, if the skin is sensitive to the cleansing solution or if the patient is allergic to insulin. The condition usually resolves in a few days to a few weeks. Cutaneous insulin allergy remains a clinical problem despite the use of highly purified human insulins. Regardless of the species, one manufacturer had products demonstrating aggregate levels 3- to 6-fold higher than those found in other manufacturers' preparations (Ratner *et al.*, 1990).

Local allergy was extremely common in the 1960s with the use of "impure" insulins, but the reported prevalence in patients receiving monocomponent porcine insulin was zero in one study (Arkins *et al.*, 1926) and 5% in another (Wright *et al.*, 1979). Urticarial allergic reactions to newer insulins are uncommon, with an incidence of 0.1–0.2% (Anderson and Adkinson, 1987), and anaphylaxis is very rare. Even lower frequencies should be expected with the more widespread use of human insulins, although patients sensitized to animal insulins may continue to suffer anaphylaxis even when changed to human insulin (Fineberg *et al.*, 1983).

Another manifestation of insulin allergy, which is also now rare, is a delayed local reaction to injected insulin. This presents as a tender subcutaneous lump developing at the injection site half an hour or so after injection and lasting for 12–24 h. This is a local Arthus-type reaction, mediated by IgG rather than IgE, and is due to complement activation by insulin–IgG immune complexes. It often responds to addition of hydrocortisone to the injected insulin.

(2) **Anaphylaxis**, due to IgE antibody formation; this type appears to be declining (Patterson *et al.*, 1990). Reactions to insulin and related antigens were also observed in sera of non-diabetic allergic persons without previous contact with exogenous insulin. The natural occurrence of insulin-specific

reactions makes the use of IgE as a marker of antigenicity of insulin questionable (Petersen et al., 1989). In affected subjects, insulin-specific IgE can be detected in serum and the allergen can be identified by skin-prick testing of insulin preparations; occasionally, the insulin diluent is responsible. Treatment depends on the specificity of the IgE antibody. If it does not cross-react substantially with another species of insulin, a change to that species will reduce the allergic response (Carini et al., 1982) but desensitization is required if cross-reactivity is complete.

(3) **Insulin resistance**, due to rapid clearance of injected insulin which forms large immune complexes with polyclonal antibodies. Less common, but potentially more serious, is systemic allergy to insulin, which may cause generalized urticaria, dyspnoea or wheezing and may, on continued administration of the insulin, progress to anaphylaxis. It may present as a rash, anaphylaxis or angioedema and may be life-threatening. A skin test on patients with severe systemic reactions must be performed with each new preparation before initiation of therapy with that preparation.

Erythema, swelling or pruritus may occur at injection sites. Such localized allergic manifestations usually resolve within a few days to a few weeks.

### 6.4.3 Treatment of Insulin Allergy

Treatment of these problems is by substituting another insulin species which does not cross-react with the antibodies, by desensitization, or by local or systemic administration of glucocorticoids. If a severe allergic reaction occurs, the drug has to be discontinued and the patient treated with the usual agents (e.g. adrenaline, antihistamines or corticosteroids). Patients who have experienced severe systemic allergic symptoms should be skin-tested with another insulin preparation before its initiation. Desensitization procedures may permit resumption of insulin administration.

After failure of standard desensitization measures in a patient with cutaneous allergy to insulin, desensitization was attempted by giving insulin by mouth with aspirin 1.3 g three times daily (Holdaway and Wilson, 1984; Husband and Gill, 1984). After 1 week subsequent desensitization, using insulin by injection was successful. When the patient stopped taking aspirin after 6 months the original allergic reactions recurred; aspirin was then given permanently at a dose of 1.3 g twice daily (Holdaway and Wilson, 1984).

Sometimes patients are allergic to the zinc in their insulin preparations (Feinglos and Jegasothy, 1979). Allergy may also be attributed to the protamine component of insulin injections (Asherov et al., 1979). Protamine–insulin use may immunologically sensitize patients to protamine, leading to anaphylactoid reactions upon subsequent exposure to protamine sulphate during cardiac catheterization or cardiovascular surgery (Weiss et *al.*, 1990; Vincent *et al.*, 1991). Reactions to intravenous protamine include rash, urticaria, bronchospasm, hypotension, and/or pulmonary artery pressure elevation (Sodoyez and Sodoyez-Goffaux, 1984). Intermittent insulin treatment increases the risk of immune complications (resistance and allergy) (Orlander, 1985).

6.5 ANTI-INSULIN ANTIBODY FORMATION

Patients with moderate concentrations of antibodies are also reported to show delay in recovery from induced hypoglycaemia but, conversely, lose control less quickly after insulin withdrawal and thus may be relatively protected from ketoacidosis. Yet despite these findings, neither the amounts nor the binding characteristics of insulin antibodies can usually be directly linked with the degree of diabetic control in individual patients in ordinary conditions of life.

The several other postulated adverse effects of insulin antibodies, such as causing or contributing to neonatal hypoglycaemia, have not been conclusively proved. However, recent studies do provide further evidence that the development of insulin antibodies in diabetic children is associated with a shortened "honeymoon remission period", higher dosage of insulin, and impaired endogenous secretion of insulin (Pickup, 1986).

Both pork and human insulin are definitively less immunogenic than beef insulin, producing fewer circulating insulin antibodies, but several studies have indicated no detectable change in antibody concentrations on switching from pork to human insulin or vice versa. Antibodies cause lipoatrophy and are responsible for the substantial insulin resistance seen in some patients, but both events are rare now that purified pork insulin is in common use. Interest has recently been revived in the possible contribution of antibodies in modifying metabolic control. In the short term and under hospital conditions, they are known to prolong the intravenous half-life of injected insulin and to delay the appearance in the circulation of a subcutaneously administered bolus dose.

Insulin autoantibodies also occur in 30–40% of IDDM children at presentation and in their high-risk siblings, and may be a marker for the "prediabetic" stage of IDDM. Insulin autoantibodies can develop and may cause a syndrome of postprandial glucose intolerance combined with fasting hypoglycaemia.

Insulin autoantibodies are antibodies that develop spontaneously without prior administration of exogenous insulin. These have been reported in various groups of patients, including some with Graves' disease treated with methimazole (Hirata *et al.*, 1974) and others treated with hydralazine or procainamide (Blackshear *et al.*, 1983), penicillamine (Benson *et al.*, 1985) or α-mercaptopropionylglycine (Ichihara *et al.*, 1977). In certain cases, no precipitating factor has been identified (Folling and Norman, 1972) and low-titre insulin autoantibodies may occur in a few apparently normal subjects. These antibodies may or may not have clinically apparent consequences; a syndrome of carbohydrate intolerance with fasting hypoglycaemia (see below) has been reported in association with high titres of high-affinity autoantibodies in some of the drug-induced cases described above.

### 6.5.1  Insulin Autoantibody Hypoglycaemia Syndrome

Quite different clinical manifestations are seen in certain non-diabetic patients who have high titres of insulin autoantibodies (Goldman et al., 1979). High titres of relatively high-avidity antibody lead to the formation of monovalent insulin–antibody complexes which are of relatively low molecular mass and are not cleared by the reticuloendothelial system. Instead, the antibody buffers the effect of insulin. During a meal (or glucose tolerance test), insulin release is stimulated but the free insulin concentration rises only slowly, as much of the secreted insulin is bound by antibody. Subsequently, there is prolonged release of insulin by dissociation from the antibody-bound fraction, and free insulin levels fall only slowly. The clinical result is the apparently paradoxical association of postprandial carbohydrate intolerance with hypoglycaemia during periods of fasting (Ichihara et al., 1977). In this syndrome, antibody titres usually fall spontaneously, but no specific treatment is available; steroids are ineffective.

### 6.6  INSULIN RESISTANCE

### 6.6.1  Forms of Insulin Resistance

Insulin resistance occurs rarely. Antibody-mediated resistance to insulin may be defined as an insulin requirement of more than $2\,U\,kg^{-1}\,day^{-1}$, with no apparent endocrine or other explanation and accompanied by high titres of high-avidity insulin antibody. Affected patients with insulin dosages of several thousand units per day have been reported (Field, 1979) but this syndrome is now rare. Insulin resistance is due to polyclonal antibodies (IgG) directed against separate epitopes on the insulin molecule, with the formation of stable high-molecular-mass complexes of insulin with two or more IgG molecules. Insulin dissociates extremely slowly from such complexes and is effectively destroyed as the complexes are cleared from the circulation by the reticuloendothelial system (Sodoyez and Sodoyez-Goffaux, 1984). Even large insulin dosages are unable to achieve adequate free insulin concentrations (Kurtz, 1986). Insulin resistance may also occur in obese patients, patients with acanthosis nigricans and patients with insulin receptor defects.

High titres of antibodies to exogenous insulin may be associated with severe impairment of blood glucose recovery following hypoglycaemia. These patients have increased circulating reserve of antibody-bound insulin which effectively prolongs the half-life of insulin and predisposes to more severe and protracted hypoglycaemia. Intensive insulin therapy is hazardous in these individuals.

Insulin resistance (with hyperinsulinaemia and various degrees of hyperglycaemia) is associated with several rare syndromes, either congenital or acquired, including acanthosis nigricans, "leprechaunism" and lipoatrophy. Insulin resistance with acanthosis nigricans is subdivided mainly into Type A (hereditary) and Type B (autoimmune) syndromes. The Type A syndrome, due to various genetic defects in the insulin receptor, predominantly affects young women who are grossly hyperinsulinaemic, markedly glucose-intolerant and usually virilized. **Type A** variants (including the Type C syndrome) are clinically similar but result from a post-receptor defect. The Type B syndrome, due to antibodies (usually IgG) directed against the insulin receptor, also mainly affects women who often have other features of generalized autoimmune disease. Most patients are hyperglycaemic but specific receptor-stimulating antibodies in a few may cause hypoglycaemia. **Type B** variants include other rare conditions with anti-(insulin receptor) antibodies (e.g. ataxia, telangiectasia).

"Leprechaunism" is a rare and fatal congenital syndrome of extreme insulin resistance resulting from inherited defects of the insulin receptor. Associated growth retardation and multiple somatic abnormalities may be due to coexistent resistance to other growth factors.

### 6.6.2 Management of Insulin Resistance

Hyperglycaemia may be managed by changing the source of insulin (i.e. beef or mixed beef–pork to pork or human insulin). Corticosteroids may be administered if changing the insulin is not effective. Corticosteroids may decrease IgG production or decrease insulin binding to the antibody. It has to be monitored closely for signs of hypoglycaemia and for the adverse effects of high-dose corticosteroids. Highly concentrated insulin (U-500) may also be administered to insulin-resistant patients. It should be used with caution to avoid ketoacidosis.

The dose of pork insulin for patients with insulin resistance caused by antibodies to beef insulin may be only a fraction of that of beef insulin. Insulin resistance is frequently self-limited; after several weeks or months of high dosage, responsiveness may be regained and dosage can be reduced. Insulin resistance is a common feature of insulinoma and can be shown even under near-physiological conditions such as a 24 h fast (Pontiroli *et al.*, 1990).

The effect of counter-regulatory hormones (adrenaline, noradrenaline and glucocorticoids) on insulin-induced glucose utilization in individual tissues of normal rats was investigated *in vivo*. The main effect of these hormones was to reduce the insulin-induced glucose utilization in skeletal muscles, particularly the oxidative one (Marfaing *et al.*, 1991). These results support the notion that the increase in plasma concentrations of these hormones could play a role in states of insulin resistance such as obesity and diabetes (Marfaing *et al.*, 1991).

A review of the current literature reveals that people with hypertension are also likely to suffer from insulin resistance, glucose intolerance and hyperinsulinaemia (Sowers, 1991). Likewise, hypertension is prevalent in obese and diabetic patients. Insulin deficiency at the cellular level may be a common mechanism in the development of hypertension in patients with Type-I or Type-II diabetes mellitus. Essential hypertension appears to be an insulin-resistant state (Sowers, 1991). Insulin resistance may engender hypertension by increasing peripheral vascular resistance and also by increasing salt retention at the level of the kidney. Therefore effective antihypertensive therapy should include agents that do not adversely affect carbohydrate metabolic abnormalities. Commonly used antihypertensive agents, such as thiazide, thiazide-like diuretica and β-blockers, are associated with glucose intolerance and increased insulin resistance (Sowers, 1991). In contrast, angiotensin-converting enzyme inhibitors, calcium antagonists and peripheral α-blockers (such as prazosin and terazosin) do not adversely affect glucose tolerance or insulin sensitivity. In addition, α-blockers have a positive effect on the serum lipid profile.

Dexamethasone may increase insulin resistance (Brismar *et al.*, 1991).

### 6.6.3 Biochemical Defects Causing Insulin Resistance

The reduction in receptors may be a secondary consequence of hyperglycaemia and hyperinsulinaemia and does not relate well to the impairment of insulin action. It therefore seems unlikely that a defect in the number or affinity of insulin receptors is a primary abnormality in NIDDM. However, it is possible that an abnormality of the portion of the insulin receptor projecting into the cell (β-subunit) could contribute to insulin resistance. Tyrosine kinase activity of the β-subunit appears to be intimately involved in mediating insulin action; this tyrosine kinase activity is reduced in some animal models of diabetes and there is some evidence that the same is true in human NIDDM.

Alternatively, it is possible that the primary cause of insulin resistance in NIDDM is located distally to the insulin receptor in the chain of events mediating insulin action.

6.7  EFFECTS ON THE LIVER

Transient recurrent hepatomegaly associated with hypoglycaemia in a 12-year-old diabetic girl was associated with the surreptitious administration of additional insulin injections. It was considered that the excess of insulin had led to increased storage of glycogen in the liver which was responsible for the hepatomegaly.

6.8  OEDEMA

A report of generalized oedema in one patient about 7 days after being started on insulin appeared in 1979 (Bleach et al., 1979). Further cases of fluid retention have been published (Lawrence and Dunnigan, 1979).

6.9  INTERACTION WITH OTHER DRUGS

Concomitant drug therapy may alter insulin requirements. Drugs that may **decrease insulin requirements** include alcohol, anabolic steroids, aspirin, fenfluramine and monoamine oxidase inhibitors; there have been isolated reports of decreased insulin requirements with captopril, clofibrate, cyclophosphamide, guanethidine, mebendazole, methandienone and oxytetracycline. **Increased dosage requirements** of insulin may occur with adrenaline, chlorpromazine, corticosteroids, oral contraceptives, thiazide diuretics and thyroid hormones; there have also been isolated reports of increased insulin requirements or aggravation of hyperglycaemia with chlordiazepoxide, cyclophosphamide, dobutamine and isoniazid. In most cases pharmacodynamic interactions are the reason for hyper- or hypo-glycaemias due to concomitant use of drugs and insulin; e.g. β-blockers inhibit the β-adrenergic glycogenolysis in liver and skeletal muscle and increase indirectly the insulin effect. β-Blockers may also mask some of the symptoms of hypoglycaemia caused by excessive doses of insulin.

Effective antihypertensive therapy should include agents that do not adversely affect carbohydrate metabolic abnormalities. Commonly used antihypertensive agents, such as thiazide, thiazide-like diuretics and β-blockers, are associated with glucose intolerance and increased insulin resistance (Sowers, 1991). In contrast, calcium antagonists and peripheral α-blockers (such as prazosin and terazosin) do not adversely affect glucose tolerance or insulin sensitivity.

The results of a retrospective survey indicated that patients receiving isophane insulin, which contains protamine, were subject to an increased risk of severe reactions simulating anaphylaxis when protamine was used to reverse systemic heparinization after cardiac catheterization (Gray et al., 1985).

## 7  Clinical Studies of Insulin-replacement Therapy

Clinical studies concerned with recent advances in the understanding of insulin effects predominantly applied knowledge on the physiology of insulin regulation as a prerequisite for achieving near normoglycaemic status in diabetic patients. There is now compelling evidence that a relationship exists between good metabolic control and development of late diabetic complications (DCC Trial, 1993).

Other major points of interest in clinical trials are hyperinsulinaemia and insulin resistance as a common denominator of the metabolic syndrome, hyperinsulinaemia as an independent predictor of coronary heart disease, and the efficacy of new insulin analogues.

### 7.1  STUDIES IN HEALTHY VOLUNTEERS

Physiologically, insulin, C-peptide and glucagon are released in a pulsatile fashion in metabolically healthy people (Hansen *et al.*, 1982) with a periodicity of pulses ranging from 8 to 30 min. The insulin release in the basal state ranges from 14 to 17 mU min$^{-1}$, the concentration in peripheral venous blood from 10 to 20 mU l$^{-1}$, while portal insulin concentration is three times higher. Following an oral glucose load, a total of 0.9 U insulin per 150 min and 10 g ingested glucose are secreted (1.35 U per 12 g carbohydrate).

Pulsatile insulin is more effective in suppressing hepatic glucose production while it exhibits an equipotent effect on glucose utilization (Bratusch-Marrain *et al.*, 1986). The application of pulsatile insulin may thus reduce free insulin levels (Waldhäusl *et al.*, 1985) and insulin resistance and may contribute more effectively to a reduction in hormone load in insulin-treated diabetic patients.

To shorten periods of hyperinsulinaemia in insulin-treated diabetic patients, attempts have been made to find insulin analogues with equipotent biological activities but faster absorption from subcutaneous injection sites and shorter half-lives. In addition, long-acting insulin analogues have been developed to provide a more continuous 24 h basal insulin supply than neutral protamine human insulin. The fast-acting monomeric insulin analogues Asp-B9-Glu-B27 and Asp-B10 have been tested in normal subjects by several workers (Vora *et al.*, 1988; Brange *et al.*, 1990) and exhibited a faster onset of action with a more rapid rise in plasma concentration and an earlier and more pronounced hypoglycaemic effect than human insulin. However, there was also a quicker return to preinjection levels (Jörgensen and Drejer, 1990).

Clinical trials on the effects of long-acting insulin analogues showed only a small intraindividual variation of absorption from the injection site with an appreciable advantage over Ultratard HM-insulin. The biopotency was no different from that of human insulin. Analogue Arg-B27, Gly-A21, Thr-B30 $NH_2$ was the first one chosen for clinical trials (Jörgensen and Dryer, 1990). Further studies with a diarginine-insulin (Arg-B31 and Arg-B32) exhibited almost identical insulin receptor binding and full biological activity compared with native insulin. These *in vitro* results (Zeuzem *et al.*, 1990), have not, however, been put to clinical tests.

A prolonged insulin action can also be achieved by encapsulation of insulin in liposomes before subcutaneous injection. The extended hypoglycaemic response is believed to be a result of a lower metabolic clearance rate. Currently, the encapsulation efficiency, however, is only 5% (Spangler, 1990). Further investigations are needed.

## 7.2 TYPE-I DIABETES MELLITUS

### 7.2.1 Complications

Conventional insulin treatment with its fixed insulin dosage and food intake has dominated therapy of insulin-dependent diabetes mellitus for nearly 70 years. It has sharply reduced the mortality of diabetic coma. Nevertheless diabetic coma is still the largest single cause of death in diabetic patients under the age of 20 years with an episode rate of 7%, and diabetic coma accounts for 15% of deaths in diabetics under the age of 50 years.

The occurrence of late complications is still very high. Waldhäusl (1986) reported a prevalence of 41% diabetic retinopathy, 25% neuropathy and 15% diabetic nephropathy. Normal $HBA_1$ levels were only seen in 20.7% of metropolitan and in only 4.1% of rural Type-I diabetic patients. Although definitive proof is lacking, it is now generally accepted that the microangiopathy of diabetes is related to the level of glycaemia, and near-normoglycaemia should be the outstanding aim of treatment (Tchoubroutsky, 1978). The failure of conventional insulin treatment to maintain consistently normal blood glucose was felt to be a consequence of not considering the physiological pattern of insulin release. The kinetics of plasma free insulin during a conventional regimen with one or two daily subcutaneous injections of intermediate-acting insulin is unphysiological, and appropriate meal-related plasma insulin peaks cannot be achieved. The new intensified methods of insulin delivery, multiple daily injections (MDI) and continuous subcutaneous insulin infusion (CSII), however, are more physiological. Consequently, a near-normal glycaemic control can be achieved only with these regimens (Pelkonen *et al.*, 1985).

In 1979, Phillips *et al.*, proposed the **u+n regimen**, which involved a single dose of very-long-acting ultralente insulin to act as background (u) and then several injections of variable amounts of soluble insulin (n) given when

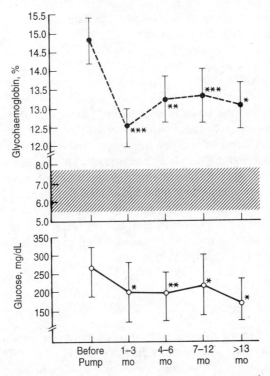

F<small>IG</small>. 13. Glycohaemoglobin and glucose values in patients undergoing continuous subcutaneous insulin infusion; mo, months. (Source: Brink and Steward, 1986.)

needed, e.g. before a meal or a snack in appropriate amounts depending upon preprandial blood glucose levels and the size of the meal to be taken (Bilous and Alberti, 1990). However, the achievement of sustained normoglycaemia using intermittent subcutaneous injections of insulin has remained elusive (Holman *et al.*, 1983).

Buysschaert *et al.* (1983) reported a better glycaemic control of totally insulin-dependent diabetic patients under continuous insulin infusion compared with conventional insulin therapy (Lager *et al.*, 1983). An improved metabolic control, an increased glucose-disposal rate and an inverse insulin resistance following a more physiological insulin regimen with continuous insulin infusion compared with conventional therapy was also reported (Jarret, 1986). Similar results were observed by Mühlhauser *et al.* (1987) where an intensified insulin injection therapy performed as routine treatment of Type-I diabetics significantly lowered $HBA_1$ levels (Fig. 13).

The importance and need for intensified insulin therapy in the treatment of insulin-dependent diabetes, however, seems to be not yet fully settled, despite the fact that nearly all clinical studies that compared CSII and/or multiple injection regimens with conventional daily insulin regimens showed a great improvement in glycaemic control.

### 7.2.2 MDI in Children

An improved metabolic control with intensified insulin therapy compared with a conventional treatment was reported by Wolf et al. (1987). A continuous insulin infusion with insulin pump therapy, monitored over 1 year, however, did not exhibit a clear advantage. The management of even preschool children with insulin pump therapy was not associated with an increased frequency or an accelerated rate of development of ketosis (Flores et al., 1984; Brambilla et al., 1987). However, Marshall et al. (1987) reported more abscesses and ketoacidosis in children on CSII, and an increased risk of developing cutaneous infections was also noted in patients treated by CSII in the Oslo Study (Dahl-Jörgensen et al., 1985).

### 7.2.3 MDI and Lipids

No additional effects of intensified insulin therapy were noted with regard to circulating lipids and lipoprotein values (Goldberg et al., 1985), but others reported an increase in HDL cholesterol and apolipoprotein A-I, without changes in serum triglycerides as a result of intensified conventional insulin therapy (ICIT) (Wilson et al., 1985).

### 7.2.4 MDI and Hypoglycaemia

Hypoglycaemic episodes were reported to be frequent following CSII and also ICIT (Arias et al., 1985). This, however, was not confirmed by others (Brunetti et al., 1984), who noted that the number of hypoglycaemic reactions, reported by home blood glucose monitoring, was similar in both therapeutic groups. No increased episodes of hypoglycaemia were also seen during physical training and CSII therapy (Mühlhauser et al., 1987).

### 7.2.5 MDI and Pregnancy

Intensified insulin therapy, started before conception in insulin-dependent women, resulted in normalized blood glucose levels in 88% cases compared with 20% in conventional treatment. The rate of congenital malformation was reduced from 7.1% to 1.1% (Fuhrmann, 1986).

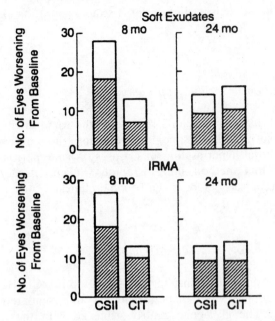

FIG. 14. Influence of continuous subcutaneous insulin infusion (CSII) and conventional treatment (CIT) on progression of soft exudates and intraretinal microvascular abnormalities (IRMA); mo, months. (Source: KROC Study Group, 1988.)

### 7.2.6 MDI and Late Diabetic Complications

Diabetic retinopathy (Oslo Study), motor nerve conduction and glomerular hyperfiltration were less progressive in patients treated with CSII or MDI compared with conventional insulin therapy (Dahl-Jörgensen, 1987). An improvement of retinopathy with CSII was reported in the KROC Study Group (1988) (Fig. 14).

### 7.2.7 Biostator

The application of an artificial endocrine pancreas (AEP=Biostator) with feedback control could be useful in the clinical management of unstable diabetics (Ohno et al., 1983). Former early closed-loop devices were large bedside machines (Pfeiffer et al., 1974) with only limited application for long-term use. More recent research has developed small glucose sensors which, however, have had only preliminarily testing for clinical application. External insulin pumps must be further miniaturized and technical failure eliminated (glucose sensor) before large-scale application in treatment of IDDM patients is feasible.

### 7.2.8  Intraperitoneal Insulin Application

Intraperitoneal insulin application represents the route of choice for insulin delivery, as absorption is physiological, being into the portal venous system, avoiding peripheral hyperinsulinaemia. Cases of acute peritonitis, however, have brought this method into disrepute (Selam et al., 1985). More experience is required before it can become clinical reality.

### 7.2.9  Insulin Analogues in Type-I Diabetics

The clinical relevance of the insulin analogues Asp-B9, Glu-B2 and Asp-B10 was also studied in Type-I diabetic patients and compared with regular human insulin. The glycaemic control achieved with the analogues was significantly improved compared with insulin administered just before the meal, indicating a potential clinical benefit of rapidly absorbed insulin analogues (Kang et al., 1990; Jörgensen and Drejer, 1990). The clinical efficacy trials of prolonged-acting insulin analogues (Arg-B27, Gly-A21, Thr-B30-NH$_2$) in Type-I diabetics showed reduced biopotency with higher overnight plasma glucose levels after subcutaneous administration (Holman and Steemson, 1989). Further work is therefore needed before any long-acting insulin analogue can be implemented for clinical use (Jörgensen and Drejer, 1990).

### 7.2.10  Nasal Absorption of Insulin

Nasal absorption of insulin has been of interest since 1983 (Moses et al., 1983). More recent clinical studies tested its long-term acceptability and efficacy in Type-I diabetic patients (Fraumann et al., 1987) and assessed the kinetics of intranasal insulin with a medium-chain phospholipid (Drejer et al., 1990). Nasal irritation was only slight and proportional to the insulin dosage. Compared with subcutaneous injection, intranasal insulin has a quicker onset of action and a much more uniform time course of absorption. Bioavailability was 8–11% and 24% in the meal-relevant period. Further studies, however, are needed before widespread clinical use can be recommended.

7.3   TYPE-II DIABETES MELLITUS

In IDDM, insulin is needed, by definition, to preserve life. It is generally agreed that near-normoglycaemia can be achieved only by MDI of short- and intermediate-acting insulin.

There is less consensus with regard to non-insulin-dependent (Type-II) diabetic patients about when to use what medication, and particularly at what point insulin therapy is appropriate. The natural history in **obese** Type-II diabetes patients usually starts with both impaired B-cell function and insulin resistance and/or basal hyperinsulinaemia resulting in elevated fasting blood glucose levels.

Reaven (1988) suggested that insulin resistance might be a common denominator for obesity, Type-II diabetes hypertension and hyperlipidaemia (metabolic syndrome) and should be treated rigorously to avoid coronary heart disease, the most common cause of morbidity and mortality in Type-II diabetes mellitus. However, it still remains to be proven that effective blood glucose control will reduce the mortality of the disease (Turner and Holman, 1990).

At this early stage, hypocaloric diet and weight loss is the primary and most important therapy for reducing basal hyperinsulinaemia and insulin resistance and improving fasting blood glucose concentration.

Exogenous insulin or insulinotropic oral agents such as sulphonylureas are not suitable for improving insulin resistance. Non-insulinotropic hypoglycaemic medication such as biguanides and/or acarbose, however, is recommended if diet alone fails to achieve sufficient metabolic control. It is still controversial, however, whether the reduction of endogenous insulin also reduces the synthesis of islet amyloid polypeptide (IAPP) sufficiently to slow down the progression of NIDDM (Clark et al., 1987).

As the exhaustion of the endocrine pancreas progresses, the initial hyperinsulinaemia decreases and oral hypoglycaemic agents in addition to diet may be insufficient to reach good metabolic control (secondary failure). At that stage insulin treatment must be started to attain better therapeutic control in NIDDM. Insulin therapy however, should only be applied to Type-II diabetes, when diet, weight normalization and oral medication (sulphonylureas and/or biguanides/acarbose) are unable to achieve satisfactory metabolic control (sulphonylurea inadequacy). In Type-II diabetes, insulin then might become a valuable therapeutic tool.

In many NIDDM patients once daily intermediate- or long-acting insulin may be adequate to render them asymptomatic, avoid the risk of nocturnal hypoglycaemic episodes (Bilous and Alberti, 1990) and produce basal normoglycaemia. A combination of intermediate-acting insulin and sulphonylureas is possible, the patients own B-cells providing the meal-time spikes. Alternatively one or two injections of a mixture of short- and intermediate-acting insulin daily is sufficient for metabolic control. In elderly diabetics with a limited life expectancy, therapeutic control should be primarily aimed at avoiding acute symptoms such as weight loss, polyuria and polydipsia, coma and foot problems. Blood glucose, however, can be tolerated up to 180 mg per 100 ml fasting and 250 mg per 100 ml postprandial and $HbA_1$ around 10%. In younger Type-II diabetics, who still have a life expectancy of more than 10 years, with long-term complications of diabetes still to come, the same degree of metabolic control should be achieved as in Type-I diabetics: near-normal blood glucose, $HbA_1$ lower than 10% and normolipidaemia. In many of these patients, after secondary failure, insulin therapy can be initially combined with oral agents which might promise some metabolic benefits for a limited time range in ca. 50% of Type-II diabetics.

Insulin alone can be applied in most Type-II diabetics with secondary failure as conventional therapy with one or two injections in the morning and evening. Only very few Type-II diabetics will finally need three and more injections daily with NPH insulin in the morning, normal insulin at supper time and basal (long-acting) insulin at night. Intensified regimens are limited to younger Type-II diabetics.

# The Secretory Machinery of Insulin Release

## 1   Introduction

Type-II diabetes is characterized by relatively deficient insulin secretion in response to glucose, peripheral insulin resistance and increased hepatic glucose production. Among oral antidiabetic drugs, sulphonylureas will be active and enhance insulin release. To understand the mechanism of the action of these drugs, we summarize here our present knowledge about the physiology of the so-called "stimulus–secretion coupling". Moreover, this chapter should also provide the physiological basis for possible future development of antidiabetic drugs which may promote discharge of insulin in a way that is different from that of sulphonylureas.

Secretion of insulin results from the action of initiators and modulators on the secretory mechanism. Whereas initiators cause the discharge of insulin by depolarization of the B-cell and subsequent influx of $Ca^{2+}$, modulation (i.e. amplification and/or attenuation) is mediated mainly by activating and/or inactivating the adenylate cyclase and/or phospholipase C systems.

Studies exploring the mechanism of insulin secretion face a number of technical and physiological problems which must be considered when scientific data on this subject are interpreted. Thus, islet tissue is only available in small amounts, its composition is not homogeneous (A-, B-, D-cells and others) and its reaction to initiating/modulating compounds may differ among species (Sundler and Böttcher, 1991; Bonner-Weir, 1991) and even between islets when localized in different areas of the pancreas. Enriched islet- derived single B-cells, on the other hand, do not react in the same way as do complete pancreatic islets (Pipeleers et al., 1982). Along with intact islets of Langerhans, clonal insulinoma cells grown in culture are used to study the physiology of the secretory mechanism. However, although a lot of basic informations about the different elements of stimulus–secretion coupling can be obtained, in physiological terms they are not completely equivalent to B cells localized in the islet tissue.


## 2   Route by which Initiators and Modulators Reach the B-Cell


From a morphological point of view the islet of Langerhans is a complicated system since it consists of different cells, with different hormones affecting secretion from different cells, the latter also being affected by nutrients, drugs and peptides/hormones which reach the islet cells via the bloodstream. Moreover, islet cells are under the control of the autonomous nervous system. As far as their distribution is concerned, B-cells are localized in the centre whereas A- and D-cells are distributed in the mantle of the islet.

A very important factor, which may give us some idea how external initiators/modulators reach their target cells and how communication between islet cells occurs, is the direction of the intraislet blood flow. Studies performed by Samols and Stagner (1988) and Samols et al. (1988) suggest that the arterial circulation first reaches the centre of the islets where B-cells are localized and from there supplies A- and D-cells in the mantle (Fig. 15). This means that B-, A- and D-cells receive information from the bloodstream and that by this route A- and D-cells also obtain messages from B-cells but not vice versa. Communication of A- and D-cells with the B-cell is assumed to occur in a paracrine manner along interstitial routes. In addition, the action of freshly released hormone on the hormone-releasing cells (i.e. direct feedback inhibition of insulin release) is possible.

# Pancreatic Islet

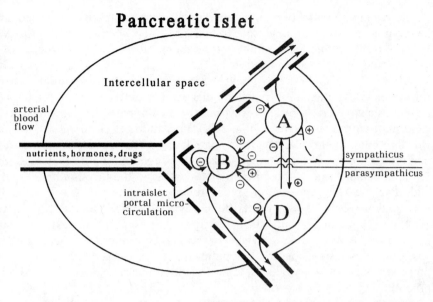

FIG. 15. Hypothetical model of how initiators and modulators that affect insulin release may reach A-, B- and D-cells. The first target of arterial blood containing nutrients, hormones, peptides and drugs is the B-cell. From there, via an intraislet portal vein system, blood which now also contains released insulin flows to the mantle where A- and D-cells are localized and from there enters the circulation. Nerves derived from the autonomous nervous system which contain neurotransmitters (acetylcholine, noradrenaline) and neuropeptides (including vasoactive intestinal peptide (VIP), gastrin-releasing peptide (GRP), galanin) are connected to islet cells. Glucagon (A-cells) and somatostatin (D-cells) reach other endocrine cells in the islet in a paracrine manner. The B-cell may also be the target of previously released insulin via a short loop.

## 3  Initiation of Insulin Secretion

Initiators of insulin secretion switch on the secretory machinery. Thereafter modulators derived from nutrient metabolism, hormones/peptides and neurotransmitters determine how fast or slow the machine will run.

### 3.1  MEMBRANE POTENTIAL AND PERMEABILITY TO K$^+$

It is now well accepted that initiation of insulin release in response to glucose and other nutrients is caused by depolarization of the B-cell as a first step followed by subsequent $Ca^{2+}$ influx.

The resting potential of mouse pancreatic B-cells perifused with a medium containing non-stimulatory glucose (0 or 3 mM) is between $-60$ and $-70$ mV. It is the result of high permeability of the membrane to $K^+$ (Meissner et al., 1978). Raising the concentration of glucose above 3 mM progressively depolarizes the membrane by about 7–8 mV to a threshold potential. When this threshold potential is reached, electrical activity appears. Electrical activity is characterized by slow waves of the membrane potential with spikes superimposed on the plateau (Fig. 16). The pattern of electrical activity of B-cells is thus quite different from that observed during depolarization of nerve or muscle cells for instance. It is well established that the decrease in $K^+$ conductance causes the initial depolarization to the threshold potential, and that the slow waves and spikes reflect the influx of $Ca^{2+}$ through voltage-dependent $Ca^{2+}$ channels (for a review see Henquin and Meissner, 1984). In agreement with this, the fact that removal of extracellular $Ca^{2+}$ abolishes most spike and slow-wave activity underlines the fact that $Ca^{2+}$ influx is responsible for this pattern of electrical activity. During the presence of stimulatory glucose there is no repolarization to the resting potential between the slow waves.

As far as other ions are concerned available evidence suggests that specific permeability to $Na^+$, $Cl^-$, $Ca^{2+}$ or $Mg^{2+}$ is not involved in the initial depolarization (for a review see Henquin et al., 1992).

By employing patch-clamp techniques, several types of $K^+$ channels have been identified (for a review see Henquin et al., 1992): (1) ATP-sensitive $K^+$ channels which are closed when ATP increases at the inner surface of the membrane – these channels are also closed by sulphonylureas and opened

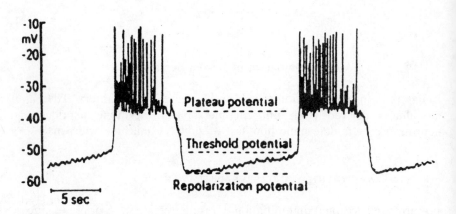

FIG. 16. Slow waves of membrane potential induced by 10 mM glucose in a single mouse B-cell (Henquin and Meissner, 1984.)

by diazoxide; (2) voltage-dependent $K^+$ channels ("delayed rectifiers") – these are not sensitive to ATP or sulphonylureas and are closed by tetraethylammonium; (3) voltage- and $Ca^{2+}$-dependent $K^+$ channels which are activated by depolarization and by the increase in cytosolic $Ca^{2+}$.

Perforated patch records suggest that about 10–25% of total $K^+$–ATP conductance is activated at rest in mouse B-cells (Ashcroft and Rorsman, 1989) and rather less (about 4%) in rat B-cells (Cohen et al., 1990). Cell-attached patch recordings have established that 50% of the channels are inhibited at 2 mM glucose and more than 90% at 5 mM (Misler et al., 1986; Ashcroft et al., 1988; Rorsman and Trube, 1990). For depolarization only the ATP-sensitive $K^+$ channels are responsible. This means that closure occurs when the intracellular ATP and/or the intracellular ATP/ADP ratio (Section 3.3.4) increases in response to increased nutrient (mainly glucose) metabolism (Fig. 17).

The major changes in channel activity and ATP content both occur between zero and 8 mM glucose. The effect of glucose on channel activity in cell-attached patches of intact B-cells resembles that found for ATP in inside-out patches (Rorsman and Trube, 1985).

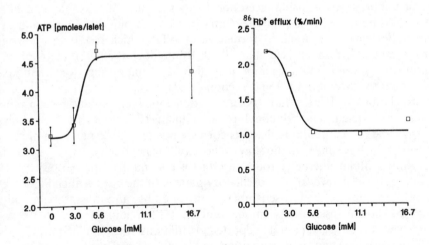

FIG. 17. Effect of glucose on ATP levels and $^{86}Rb^+$ efflux of rat pancreatic islets. The increase in ATP and the inhibition of $K^+$ (here $^{86}Rb^+$) efflux caused by glucose occur in a concentration range up to approximately 5.6 mM. Interestingly, in contrast to insulin secretion and other islet parameters (see Fig. 18), no further change is observable at glucose concentrations above 5.6 mM (Ammon and Wahl, 1994.)

3.2 $Ca^{2+}$ FLUXES AND CALCIUM–CALMODULIN-ACTIVATED PROTEIN KINASE(CaCaMK)

It is commonly agreed that cytosolic $Ca^{2+}$ serves as a second messenger in stimulus–secretion coupling of insulin release (for a review see Hellman *et al.*, 1992).

The pancreatic B-cells in general are rich in $Ca^{2+}$. When calculated in terms of intracellular water, the concentration of $Ca^{2+}$ in mouse B-cells ranges from 16 to 25 mM (Hellman, 1986 ). Conversely, $Ca^{2+}$ in the cytosolic compartment which serves as a second messenger is only in the nanomolar range.

Glucose is a potent stimulator of $Ca^{2+}$ uptake, but it has been found that most of this accumulation is due to increased $Ca^{2+}$ turnover, and that the effect is relatively small when isotopic equilibrium is maintained (Bergsten and Hellman, 1984). In mouse islets, $Ca^{2+}$ turnover rate has been calculated to exceed 5% per min after glucose stimulation (Hellman, 1986). Direct measurements have failed to demonstrate any glucose-induced increase in the total amount of intracellular $Ca^{2+}$ (Anderssen *et al.*, 1982; Wolters *et al.*, 1982).

After depolarization, influx of $Ca^{2+}$ occurs from the extracellular into the intracellular space where its concentration increases about 5–10 times during maximal stimulation. From the presently identified $Ca^{2+}$ channels in insulin-producing cells, N-, T- and L-type channels have been described (Velasco, 1987; Aicardi *et al.*, 1991) but only the L-type channels appear to be of importance for insulin secretion (Yaney et al., 1991; Rönfeldt *et al.*, 1992). Although glucose promotes entry of $Ca^{2+}$ through depolarization of the cytoplasmic membrane by formation of ATP, which results in opening of L-type $Ca^{2+}$ channels (Hellman, 1988; Rönfeldt *et al.*, 1992), metabolism of glucose beyond ATP formation may also be of importance for the influx of $Ca^{2+}$ (Smith *et al.*, 1989 and section 3.3.4).

Oscillations of $[Ca^{2+}]_i$ have been reported following initiation of insulin release by nutrients and sulphonylureas (Hellman *et al.*, 1992). The frequency of these large-amplitude oscillations corresponds to 0.2–0.5 $min^{-1}$ in mouse B-cells, which is similar to the slow cyclic variations in burst activity recorded with intracellular microelectrodes in intact islets and also the periodicity of insulin release. However, this oscillatory pattern of the electrical and $[Ca^{2+}]_i$ responses induced by glucose is not accompanied by, and thus probably not due to, similar oscillations in metabolism (Gilon and Henquin, 1992). However, Longo *et al.* (1991) reported oscillations with similar periods in insulin secretion, oxygen consumption and $[Ca^{2+}]_i$. Since oscillations appear *in vivo* as well as *in vitro* there must be a pacemaker in the islet tissue itself (Goodner *et al.*, 1991).

In addition to $Ca^{2+}$ influx, $Ca^{2+}$ release from intracellular stores (endoplasmic reticulum) also participates in its physiological functions (Prentki *et al.*, 1984a). It appears, however, that this intracellular release modulates rather than initiates insulin secretion, since compounds that cause insulin release only by releasing intracellular $Ca^{2+}$ have little insulin-secretory effect but amplify the action of initiators causing discharge of insulin via depolarization. Except for intracellular stores, mitochondria and insulin granules are not involved in the regulation of cytosolic $Ca^{2+}$ (Prentki et al., 1984b; Carafoli, 1987). Perhaps they take part in sequestration of intracellular $Ca^{2+}$ (Henquin, 1985).

Immediately following the elevation of cytosolic $[Ca^{2+}]$, efflux of this cation is enhanced. There are several possible mechanisms. Most of the $Ca^{2+}$ is excreted by a $Ca^{2+}$/calmodulin-activated $Ca^{2+}$-ATPase with high affinity for $Ca^{2+}$ and could represent a $Ca^{2+}$-extrusion pump, able to maintain low levels of free $Ca^{2+}$ in resting B-cells (Colca et al., 1983a). Endoplasmic reticulum and mitochondria do not appear to be involved in buffering of $Ca^{2+}$ at submicromolar levels (Colca et al., 1983a,b; Prentki et al., 1983). Insulin granules are also $Ca^{2+}$ pools. Their role has been underlined (Anderssen et al., 1982; Wolters et al., 1982; Hutton et al., 1983).

It has been shown by several authors, as summarized by Henquin (1985), that pancreatic islets as well as insulinoma cells contain $Ca^{2+}$/calmodulin-activated protein kinase which phosphorylates endogenous proteins. In fact, stimulation of islets with glucose causes phosphorylation. Among the candidates to be phosphorylated is myosin light-chain kinase which couples the ionic events to the process of granule movement (MacDonald and Kowluru, 1982; Penn et al., 1982). The $\alpha$- and $\beta$-subunits of tubulin (Colca et al., 1983c) are other possible sites of phosphorylation by calmodulin-dependent protein kinase. It has also been proposed that calmodulin modulates the interaction between insulin granules and the inner face of the cytoplasmic membrane (Watkins and Cooperstein, 1983). Such an effect would be compatible with the phosphorylation of a protein on the granule membrane (Brocklehurst and Hutton, 1983).

## 3.3   ISLET METABOLISM, IONIC EVENTS AND INSULIN SECRETION

### 3.3.1   Initiating Events

The most potent initiator of insulin secretion is glucose. Under physiological conditions its action is modulated by hormones, peptides and neurotransmitters as discussed later.

The mode of initiation of insulin release is unique. As in other excitable tissues, B-cell function is triggered through depolarization and subsequent opening of $Ca^{2+}$ channels, but unlike other tissues, depolarization is caused by a nutrient – glucose – which at the same time is a metabolizable substrate providing the cell with energy. The mechanism by which glucose initiates the cascade of events that finally lead to exocytosis remained obscure for a long time. However, the matter has recently become clear. Penetration of glucose into the intracellular space of the B-cell is not limited under physiological conditions and does not depend on insulin. Glucose is carried across the cytoplasmic membrane with the help of a glucose transporter, GLUT-2, with a $K_m$ of 15–20 mM (Bell et al., 1990; Mueckler, 1990). Once inside the cell it is not the glucose molecule itself that causes depolarization and subsequent insulin release, but its actual metabolism. This is demonstrated by the fact that inhibitors of glucose phosphorylation block both depolarization and insulin secretion, indicating that a step or critical metabolite located before glucose-6-phosphate might be responsible for initiating the secretion.

Unlike other tissues, but like the liver, B-cells contain two glucose-phosphorylating enzymes, i.e. hexokinase and glucokinase. Whereas hexokinase with a $K_m$ of 50 $\mu$M is maximally active at glucose concentrations below physiological values, phosphorylation of glucose at physiological concentrations in the islet can be mediated by glucokinase, an enzyme with a $K_m$ of approx. 10 mM. Therefore glucokinase can be regarded not as the glucose receptor, but as a glucose acceptor or the first key allowing the concentration-dependent metabolism of this substrate (German, 1993).

If not glucose itself, what is responsible for providing the signal to produce glucose-concentration-dependent (parallel) insulin secretion? A candidate could be a metabolite of the glycolytic pathway, as suggested by Malaisse (1992), a change in pH (Best, 1992), increased production of reduced nicotinamide nucleotides (Ammon and Wahl, 1994), reduced glutathione and/or other thiols (Ammon and Wahl, 1994), or just the final product of oxidative glucose metabolism which is ATP (Ashcroft and Rorsman, 1989). For a long time the idea was accepted that only the production of the signal metabolite and therefore its concentration would decide how much insulin would be released. However, opinion on this matter has changed in so far as the possibility is no longer excluded that, along with the production of a signal metabolite (ATP and/or ATP/ADP) leading to depolarization, modulating factors – their concentration also depending on glucose concentration – are also formed during metabolism which, in addition to the signal, regulate the secretory response at a step beyond depolarization. And it may be speculated that the signal acts by causing depolarization to a threshold value sufficient to open voltage-dependent $Ca^{2+}$ channels, whereas changes in the concentration of other metabolites may act more like an "electric light dimmer".

### 3.3.2 Glucose Metabolism

Following phosphorylation of glucose by hexokinase and glucokinase, approximately 90–95% of the glucose passes through the aerobic glycolytic pathway whereas 5–10% undergoes metabolism via the pentose phosphate

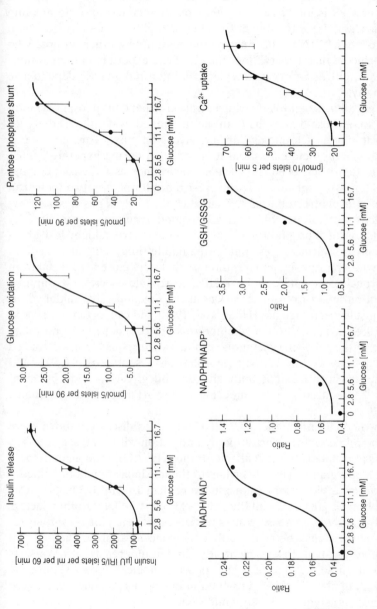

FIG. 18. Effect of glucose on insulin release, glucose oxidation, pentose phosphate shunt, NADH/NAD[+], NADPH/NADP[+], GSH/GSSG ratios and Ca[2+] uptake of rat pancreatic islets. In a concentration range up to 16.7 mM, glucose-mediated stimulation of insulin secretion is closely parallelled by increases in glucose oxidation, pentose phosphate shunt activity, the NADH/NAD[+], NADPH/NADP[+], GSH/GSSG ratios and Ca[2+] uptake (Ammon and Wahl, 1994).

shunt (PPS). Both pathways depend on glucose concentration (Fig. 18). In this connection it is interesting to note that in static incubations of islets the activity of the PPS is inhibited by insulin freshly secreted into the medium (Verspohl *et al.*, 1979), probably at the glucose-6-phosphate dehydrogenase step (Akhtar *et al.*, 1977). This may be the reason why other groups, who did not consider this observation under their experimental conditions (Ashcroft *et al.*, 1972; Giroix *et al.*, 1985), did not find glucose dependence of this pathway.

Whereas glucokinase allows the concentration-dependent phosphorylation of glucose to glucose-6-phosphate in an unlimited way, the activity of phosphofructokinase determines further glycolytic flux. This enzyme is regulated by several metabolites and it is activated during hyperglycaemia. In this connection it has been shown that glucose increases the islet content of fructose-2,6-bisphosphate and glucose-1,6-bisphosphate, two powerful activators of phosphofructokinase (Malaisse *et al.*, 1982). Thus it is conceivable that activation of fructokinase is a second regulatory event in islet glucose metabolism. Phosphofructokinase generates glyceraldehyde-1-phosphate and dihydroxyacetone phosphate, the equilibrium being at the site of glyceraldehyde-1-phosphate, and it is thought that steps close to or distal from glyceraldehyde-1-phosphate may be related to stimulus–secretion coupling. This assumption arises from observations that exogenous glyceraldehyde is a powerful insulin secretagogue (Hedeskov, 1980) and causes depolarization (Ashcroft, 1988). The question of whether or not glyceraldehyde-1-phosphate itself or one of the following metabolic products is responsible has attracted many investigators. Glyceraldehyde-phosphate is a source of NADH, and it has been demonstrated that both glucose and glyceraldehyde augment fluorescence of reduced nicotinamide nucleotides (Panten and Christians, 1973).

Elevation of ATP and/or the ATP/ADP ratio – as discussed above – are thought to be related to depolarization by interaction with ATP-sensitive $K^+$ channels. As also stated above, ATP and/or the ATP/ADP ratio increase only up to about 8 mM glucose (Fig. 17) whereas the maximal stimulatory glucose concentration in rat islets for instance is more than 16.7 mM. This suggests that metabolism of glucose in addition to ATP must generate other factors which finally guarantee glucose concentration-dependency of insulin secretion. If this is so, it may be claimed that the concentration of such critical factors correlates with glucose concentration and insulin release. Conversely, a decrease in these factors, e.g. by pharmacological tools, should be associated with inhibition of insulin secretion in response to glucose. Among relevant factors are reduced nicotinamide nucleotides.

Here, special attention should be paid to the $NADPH/NADP^+$ ratio with regard to the fact that this ratio, in contrast to the $NADH/NAD^+$ ratio, is not directly linked to ATP production. It has been demonstrated that not only the $NADH/NAD^+$, but also the $NADPH/NADP^+$, ratio depends on glucose concentration (Fig. 18) (Ammon *et al.*, 1980, 1983a). A major source of NADPH formation is the PPS, the activity of which is also increased during hyperglycaemia (Verspohl *et al.*, 1979). It is interesting to note that methylene blue, under conditions where it decreased islet NADPH/NADP$^+$ ratio but left the NADH/NAD$^+$ ratio unaffected, inhibited glucose- and tolbutamide-induced secretion of insulin (Ammon and Verspohl, 1979; Ammon *et al.*, 1979a).

Thus, when trying to put the pieces together with regard to glucose as an initiator and modulator of insulin secretion, it appears that formation of ATP switches on the system, but changes in metabolism including the redox state of nicotinamide nucleotides modulate the system in its response to depolarization.

### 3.3.3   Possible Role of Thiols

If we accept that the redox state of nicotinamide nucleotides is a modulating system, we need to know how this works. An attractive idea involves the fact that the NADPH/NADP$^+$ ratio is in equilibrium with the GSH/GSSG ratio which itself is of importance for the redox state and therefore the activity of functional proteins (Barron, 1951).

In pancreatic islets the thiol status seems to behave quite differently from other tissues. Thus the GSH/GSSG ratio is comparatively low and varies only between 1.0 (Ammon *et al.*, 1980) and 6.7 (Anjaneyulu *et al.*, 1982). Furthermore, and this is also in contrast to other tissues, this ratio depends on the glucose concentration and is raised by hyperglycaemic glucose (Ammon *et al.*, 1980; Anjaneyulu *et al.*, 1982) (Fig. 18), an effect that occurs quickly (in less than 1 min) (Ammon *et al.*, 1979a, 1980; Pralong *et al.*, 1990), thus preceding the onset of hormone secretion. This raises the possibility that this ratio may be involved in regulatory processes associated with the secretion of insulin. Besides glucose, leucine, which is an initiator of insulin release, also produces an increase in islet NADPH/NADP$^+$ (Ammon *et al.*, 1979b) and GSH/GSSG ratios (Ammon *et al.*, 1981). In addition other nutrients/factors have been reported to increase islet GSH, e.g. D-glyceraldehyde, $\alpha$-ketoisocaproate, anoxia and KCN (Anjaneyulu *et al.*, 1982).

Whereas elevation of the GSH/GSSG ratio is accompanied by stimulation of insulin secretion, thiol reagents that decrease this ratio inhibit release of insulin when triggered by a variety of initiators. In this connection diazenedicarboxylic acid bis-($N'$-methylpiperazide) (DIP), an oxidant of GSH (Kosower *et al.*, 1976), has been shown to lower islet GSH/GSSG ratio and to depress glucose-induced insulin secretion (Ammon *et al.*, 1983b) (Fig. 19). Similar results were achieved by using diamide, an oxidant of GSH (Kosower *et al.*, 1969), and other oxidants including *tert*-butyl hydroperoxide

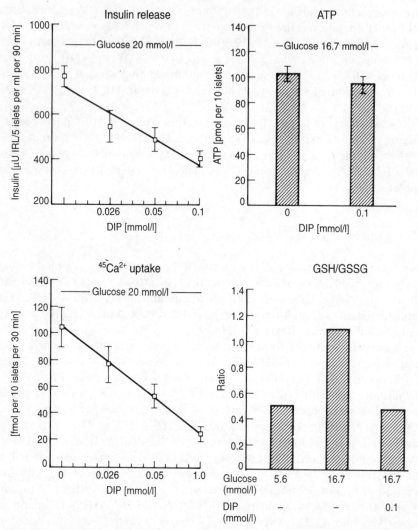

FIG. 19. Effect of diazenedicarboxylic acid bis-($N'$-methylpiperazide) (DIP) on insulin release, ATP concentration, GSH/GSSG ratio and $Ca^{2+}$ uptake of rat pancreatic islets. DIP, an oxidant of GSH at the concentration used here, did not affect islet ATP concentration but inhibited glucose-induced increases in GSH/GSSG ratio, $^{45}Ca^{2+}$ uptake and insulin release (Ammon and Wahl, 1994).

(t-BHP) (Ammon *et al.*, 1977, 1979a) and 2-cyclohexen-1-one (Sener *et al.*, 1986). Methylene Blue, an oxidant of NADPH, has also been shown to decrease the GSH/GSSG ratio of pancreatic islets (Ammon *et al.*, 1979a). The action of methylene blue was associated with inhibition of glucose-/leucine-mediated insulin secretion, again suggesting a role for the

NADPH/NADP$^+$ and/or GSH/GSSG systems in insulin release (Ammon et al., 1979b; Ammon and Verspohl, 1979).

Previous evidence suggests that it is the change in the GSH/GSSG ratio rather than that in GSH levels as such that modulates insulin secretion: buthionine-sulphoximine (BSO), an inhibitor of glutathione synthesis (Griffith and Meister, 1979), dramatically decreased islet GSH in rats when administered in vivo, but did not affect its GSH/GSSG ratio. Under these conditions, glucose-induced release of insulin was not affected (Klumpp and Ammon, 1988).

With other compounds that promote insulin secretion, whether or not their action was inhibited by thiol reagents, it transpired that the insulin-releasing capacity of only some of them was blocked, whereas the action of others was not. This led to the concept of thiol-dependent and non-thiol-dependent stimulation of insulin secretion (Ammon et al., 1984). From the published data it appears that only the effect of those compounds that initiate insulin release via depolarization of the B-cell (glucose, sulphonylureas, leucine, glyceraldehyde, arginine and KCl) was depressed by thiol reagents, whereas the insulin secretory action of others that do not follow this cascade (isoprenaline, dibutyryl cyclic adenosine monophosphate (db-cAMP), theophylline, Ca$^{2+}$ ionophore A23187) was not (Ammon et al., 1984). This suggests that variation of the redox state of intracellular thiols may be related to the cascade of events starting with depolarization and finally leading to Ca$^{2+}$ uptake whereas it is of less importance at the level of the adenylate cyclase system and distal to the increase in [Ca$^{2+}$]$_i$.

### 3.3.4 Coupling of Metabolic Events to Ion Fluxes

The links between metabolism and ion fluxes have been summarized by Henquin (1980a). At that time it was considered that a fall in pH and/or increased production of reduced nicotinamide nucleotides and GSH could be important coupling factors between glucose metabolism and the change in ion permeabilities in B-cells. As far as pH is concerned, it was found that glucose does not decrease but even increases the overall pH in islet cells (Deleers et al., 1983; Lindström and Sehlin, 1984).

#### 3.3.4.1 K$^+$ Efflux.
After introduction of patch-clamp techniques, new insights into the coupling of metabolic events to ion fluxes were gained especially with regard to the impact of islet ATP on inhibition of K$^+$ efflux and subsequent depolarization. Thus, using the patch-clamp technique, Cook and Hales (1984) found that ATP (0.5 mM) caused an almost complete inhibition of K$^+$ channel activity. Since an increase in glucose concentration from 0 to 5.6 mM produced the most pronounced increase in islet ATP levels, it was claimed that ATP might be the initiating signal in glucose-induced

insulin secretion (Petersen and Findlay, 1987; Fig. 17; see also section 3.1). Another idea is that it is not the changes in ATP levels as such, but the change in ATP/ADP ratio that is the critical factor. In this case, the local concentration of both is of no consequence. In fact, Malaisse and Sener (1987) have demonstrated that an increase in glucose concentration increased islet ATP/ADP ratio.

However, it is unlikely that the extent of inhibition of $K^+$ efflux alone determines the amount of insulin released, suggesting that additional factors are involved. This view is impressively supported by data shown in Figs. 18 and 19 presenting relationships between glucose concentration on the one hand and insulin release, glucose oxidation, activity, $NADPH/NADP^+$, $NADH/NAD^+$ and GSH/GSSG ratios, and ATP and $^{86}Rb^+$ efflux on the other. It is clear from Fig. 17 that ATP levels reach their maximum at about 5.6 mM glucose, which is a concentration close to that causing maximal inhibition of $K^+$ efflux, whereas the other parameters have a maximum close to 16.7 mM glucose and above and their increase runs parallel to the rate of insulin release.

*3.3.4.2   $Ca^{2+}$ Uptake.* At present, the stimulation of $Ca^{2+}$ entry into pancreatic islet cells is thought to be due to gating of voltage-dependent $Ca^{2+}$ channels (Prentki and Wollheim, 1984) in response to a shift in the membrane potential from the resting to a threshold potential. These $Ca^{2+}$ channels have been identified as being of the L-type in mice (Plant, 1988; Ashcroft *et al.*, 1989) and in rat (Findlay *et al.*, 1989; Yaney *et al.*, 1991; Rönfeldt *et al.*, 1992). However, not only changes in the electrical potential, but also other metabolically derived factors may be involved in $Ca^{2+}$ entry.

Hellman and co-workers (1975) were the first to propose that by employing thiol reagents, a change in the thiol/disulphide balance of membrane-associated proteins may alter their participation in ionic movements. Since then, this matter has been further investigated with membrane-penetrating thiol oxidants. From these studies, it is evident that DIP, diamide and t-BHP, reagents that decrease intracellular GSH/GSSG ratio (Ammon *et al.*, 1979b), inhibit the glucose-induced net uptake of $Ca^{2+}$ and insulin secretion (Ammon *et al.*, 1983b, 1986). Similar observations have been reported using 1,3-bis-(2-chloroethyl)-1-nitrosourea (BCNU) which lowers the islet GSH/GSSG ratio not through direct oxidation but by inhibition of glutathione reductase (Malaisse *et al.*, 1985a).

Methylene blue, an oxidant of NADPH, also decreased $Ca^{2+}$ uptake in response to glucose (Ammon *et al.*, unpublished data). As could be expected from the data discussed so far, the thiol oxidant DIP diminished net $^{45}Ca^{2+}$ uptake and insulin secretion, not only in response to glucose but also in response to other depolarizing agents including glyceraldehyde, leucine, BCH, α-ketoisocaproate, arginine, KCl, glibenclamide and tolbutamide (Ammon *et al.*, 1986).

The fact that it is the depolarization-mediated uptake of $Ca^{2+}$ that is related to the intracellular thiol system is supported by data showing that $Ca^{2+}$ uptake mediated by the ionophore A23187 was not affected by DIP (Ammon et al., 1983b). This suggests that stimulation of $Ca^{2+}$ entry in response to depolarization may be related to the redox system of the intracellular thiols, regardless of whether the uptake of $Ca^{2+}$ was induced by metabolizable or non-metabolizable agents.

The intracellular thiol redox status may be related to $Ca^{2+}$ uptake in two different ways. First, a particular basal redox ratio present in the B-cell during normoglycaemia is necessary if $Ca^{2+}$ uptake is to function at all after depolarization. Secondly, an additional increase in this ratio, caused by the metabolism of nutrients, may enhance $Ca^{2+}$ uptake in response to depolarization.

Further indirect evidence supporting a possible role for the above-mentioned redox ratios comes from studies with a cholecystokinin analogue ($CCK_8$) and from studies with islets cultured at low glucose.

The cholecystokinin analogue amplifies glucose-mediated insulin release (Verspohl et al., 1986b), but it is ineffective at non-stimulatory glucose concentrations. Further studies have shown that $CCK_8$ did not affect [86]$Rb^+$ efflux but markedly increased glucose-mediated [45]$Ca^{2+}$ uptake (Verspohl et al., 1987). This action was associated with stimulation of islet PPS activity and an increase in NADPH/NADP$^+$ ratio (Verspohl et al., 1989).

In a previous study (Verspohl et al., 1988), it was found that, if islets were cultured for 5 days in the presence of 5.6 mM glucose, their secretory response to high glucose decreased. Since the inhibitory action of glucose on [86]$Rb^+$ efflux was still intact, the diminished secretory response could not be explained by the fact that the "glucose signal" as such was not recognized by the B-cell. However, although the depolarization of the B-cell was possible, glucose-mediated net uptake of [45]$Ca^{2+}$ was significantly depressed. As far as the metabolic response of islets cultured at low glucose is concerned, it was found that an increase in glucose concentrations here did not enhance PPS activity and the NADPH/NADP$^+$ ratio.

Further indirect support for this idea comes from experiments conducted by Pralong et al. (1990). These authors studied the time sequence of events and found that in single B-cells, a rise in glucose concentration produced an increase in redox state of nicotinamide nucleotides which preceded the increase in cytosolic $Ca^{2+}$.

From the present data, it is not possible to conclude whether or not critical thiols and/or the redox state of nicotinamide nucleotides are directly linked to voltage-dependent $Ca^{2+}$ channels or related to close proteins. Nevertheless, if the concept is true, it is unique since pancreatic islets are the only tissue where $Ca^{2+}$ uptake is predominantly regulated by glucose and its metabolism. However, it must be stated that the available evidence needs to be confirmed by further investigation.

# 4    Modulation of Insulin Secretion via Adenylate Cyclase and Phospholipase C (PLC)

As discussed in section 3, insulin secretion is initiated through depolarization and subsequent opening of L-type $Ca^{2+}$ channels. It has also been suggested that here insulin secretion and $Ca^{2+}$ uptake may be modulated by nutrient metabolism, especially glucose, probably by changing islet nicotinamide nucleotide/thiol redox status. Other possibilities for modulation of insulin release come from factors affecting the adenylate cyclase and PLC systems through activation of protein kinases and release of $Ca^{2+}$ from intracellular stores. The modulating agents include hormones from the entero–insular axis, neurotransmitters and neuropeptides from pancreatic nerves and last but not least intraislet hormones (see also section 2).

## 4.1    ADENYLATE CYCLASE–cAMP SYSTEM

Similar to other tissues, insulin-producing cells possess an adenylate cyclase–cAMP system including stimulatory and inhibitory G-proteins and phosphodiesterases.

It is generally agreed that the role of cAMP in insulin secretion is not an initiating one, but, by activation of PKA, it potentiates the insulin-releasing capacity of initiators (for a review see Hughes and Ashcroft, 1992). Thus cAMP in the B-cell is important for potentiating its response to glucose and other initiators of insulin release (Malaisse and Malaisse-Lagae, 1984; Hellman, 1986; Hellman and Gylfe, 1986; Prentki and Matschinsky, 1987). In addition to the action of some hormones and neuropeptides, the cAMP content also increases when isolated islets are exposed to glucose and other fuel secretagogues (Charles et al., 1975; Grill and Cerasi, 1976). However, the effect of glucose is small and is only found in islets of rats but hardly at all in islets of mice (Thams et al., 1982). Thus the physiological role of glucose here is questionable. In requiring extracellular $Ca^{2+}$, the nutrient-induced accumulation of cAMP has been attributed to the elevation of $[Ca^{2+}]_i$ (Valverde et al., 1979; Sharp et al., 1980).

Adenosine, an agonist of $A_1$ and $A_2$ receptors, interacts with the adenylate cyclase system such that low concentrations cause inhibition whereas high concentrations stimulate this enzyme by interfering with respective G-proteins. The stable adenosine analogues D- and L-phenylisopropyladenosine (PIA) inhibited glucose-induced insulin release from rat islet cells (Hillaire-Buys et al., 1987). This effect was abolished by 8-phenyltheophylline, a potent $A_1$-receptor antagonist. In another study Bertrand et al. (1989) reported that high concentrations of L-PIA augmented, whereas low concentrations decreased, glucose-induced electrical activity and insulin secretion. Also, forskolin action on insulin secretion was blocked by low L-PIA whereas the action of db-cAMP was not. It is therefore possible that these effects of adenosine analogues on insulin release are brought about via cAMP.

Inhibition of the adenylate cyclase system is also derived from somatostatin and $\alpha$-adrenergics which interact with the inhibitory receptor of this enzyme system.

As to the mode of action of cAMP in insulin release, it has long since been considered that cAMP contributes to the rise in cytosolic $Ca^{2+}$ in B-cells by an effect on $Ca^{2+}$ stores. However, in agreement with earlier reports, cAMP did not exert an effect on $Ca^{2+}$ sequestration by insulinoma mitochondria (Prentki et al., 1983) or by endoplasmic reticulum from islet cells (Colca et al., 1983a). Conversely, electrophysiological and other experiments suggest that cAMP augments glucose-induced $Ca^{2+}$ influx into B-cells (Henquin and Meissner, 1983; Henquin et al., 1983; Wang et al., 1993). Another possibility is that cAMP sensitizes the exocytotic machinery to the action of increased $[Ca^{2+}]_i$ (for a review see Hughes and Ashcroft, 1992). Since it seems unlikely that cAMP itself will have a major impact on ionic events, it is reasonable to assume that activation of PKA is the major target of cAMP. In fact, the presence of PKA has been established (Montague and Howell, 1972; Sugden et al., 1979). There is agreement that cAMP or cAMP-raising agents induce phosphorylation of a large number of islet proteins. However, none of these phosphorylations could be directly related to insulin release (Harrison and Ashcroft, 1982; Schubart, 1982; Suzuki et al., 1983; Christie and Ashcroft, 1984). Recently, Ämmälä et al. (1993) showed that cAMP, by activating PKA, increases $Ca^{2+}$ influx through voltage-dependent L-type $Ca^{2+}$ channels thereby elevating $[Ca^{2+}]_i$ and accelerating exocytosis. And also Wang et al. (1993) suggested that cAMP may regulate $Ca^{2+}$ entry along voltage-dependent $Ca^{2+}$ channels, and this may be a possibility for potentiating glucose-induced insulin release.

## 4.2 PHOSPHOLIPID METABOLISM

The role of metabolism and/or metabolic products of membrane phospholipids under the influence of PLC and $PLA_2$ has been reviewed by Henquin (1985) and Morgan and Montague (1992).

There is general agreement that glucose and cholinergic agents accelerate phospholipid turnover in islet cells. Meanwhile other secretagogues, including $CCK_8$, that amplify insulin secretion have also been found to increase metabolism of phospholipids (Zawalich et al., 1987).

### 4.2.1 Phospholipase C

Activation of PLC generates diacylglycerol (DAG) and inositol trisphosphate $(Ins(1,4,5)P_3)$. In contrast with many cells, islet PLC may also be directly activated by $Ca^{2+}$. Thus, in an isolated membrane preparation, raising the $Ca^{2+}$ concentration from 1 to 10 $\mu M$ resulted in a significant increase in enzyme activity (Dunlop and Malaisse, 1986). This suggests the possibility that the enzyme cannot only be activated by signal–receptor interaction but also by changes in the cytosolic $Ca^{2+}$ concentration, i.e. in response to depolarization and subsequent $Ca^{2+}$ influx. However, the experimental evidence for this is still controversial (for review see Morgan and Montague, 1992). It appears that as far as the effect of glucose is concerned, metabolic events are involved. For receptor-mediated activation, participation of G-proteins is discussed. A PLC activity able to hydrolyse inositol-containing phospholipids has been described in the guinea pig (Schrey and Montague, 1983) and rat (Dunlop and Larkins, 1988) islets.

DAG and $Ins(1,4,5)P_3$ are thought to possess regulatory functions in the process of insulin release. Further products of inositol phosphate metabolism will not be discussed here. Phosphoinositol turnover is, however, neither necessary nor sufficient to initiate insulin release (Axen et al., 1983; Layschock, 1983), but it has been found to augment glucose-induced secretion of insulin.

### 4.2.2 Ins(1,4,5)P₃

$Ins(1,4,5)P_3$ induces release of $Ca^{2+}$ from membrane-bound stores and thereby promotes a rise in the cytosolic free $Ca^{2+}$ concentration (Wollheim and Biden, 1986). It is supposed to release $Ca^{2+}$ from the endoplasmic reticulum into cytoplasm from which it is taken up by an $Ins(1,4,5)P_3$-insensitive compartment (pool 2). The stored $Ca^{2+}$ is then recycled to pool 1, a process that occurs within 20 min at a basal $[Ca^{2+}]_i$ value (for review see Hellman et al., 1992).

### 4.2.3 Diacylglycerol

DAG, which is the second product of PLC activation, may be an important signal molecule in the pancreatic B-cell for several reasons. First, it could be involved in stimulating PKC by lowering the $Ca^{2+}$ sensitivity of the enzyme and translocating it from the cytosol to the cytoplasmic membrane. Second, DAG can increase the fusogenic potential of biological membranes which may be important for exocytosis. Addition of exogenous DAG to isolated islets induces insulin secretion (Malaisse et al., 1985b). DAG can be formed in two ways: first by metabolism of glucose (for a review see Persaud et al., 1992), and second via PLC. In the first case glucose has been shown to increase islet DAG (Peter-Reisch *et al.*, 1988). However, although DAG is formed as an early response to glucose and PLC activation, we do not yet know how far DAG is involved in signal transduction.

### 4.2.4 PKC

A possible role for DAG in insulin secretion has been discussed above. The target of DAG is the $Ca^{2+}$/phospholipid-dependent PKC which is activated by this intracellular second messenger. PKC is present in insulin-producing cells, including pancreatic islets (Tanigawa *et al.*, 1982) in individual B-cells (Onoda *et al.*, 1990) and the clonal tumour cell line RINm5F (Mosbacher, 1992). At physiological $Ca^{2+}$ concentrations PKC is not only activated by DAG but also by tumour-promoting phorbol esters which have been used as tools to study PKC effects.

Activation of PKC is accompanied by its translocation from the cytosol to the cytoplasmic membrane. In fact, as in other tissues, phorbol esters and DAG analogues stimulate translocation of PKC in rat islets (Easom *et al.*, 1989; Persaud *et al.*, 1989a) and insulin-secreting tumour cells (Yamatani *et al.*, 1988; Thomas *et al.*, 1989; Mosbacher, 1992). There is some evidence that receptor-mediated insulin secretagogues that activate PLC induce PKC translocation (for a review see Persaud *et al.*, 1992). Interestingly, carbachol stimulates translocation of PKC activity in rat islets at both 2 and 20 mM glucose concentrations. Since insulin secretion was not affected at 2 mM glucose, it is suggested that activation and translocation of PKC *per se* may not be sufficient to stimulate insulin release (Persaud *et al.*, 1989b). The effects of nutrient secretagogues on PKC translocation are much less clear. Thus glucose is without any effect on PKC translocation (Easom *et al.*, 1989; Persaud *et al.*, 1989a).

There are numerous reports that agents that directly activate PKC stimulate insulin secretion from both islets and insulin-secreting tumour cells (for a review see Persaud *et al.*, 1992). The mechanism of this action is, however, unclear. Different modes are under discussion but are still unconfirmed; these include effects on ATP-sensitive $K^+$ channels (Wollheim *et al.*, 1988) and influx and efflux of $Ca^{2+}$ (Malaisse *et al.*, 1985b; Berggren *et al.*, 1989; Yada *et al.*, 1989). It has also been claimed that activation of PKC may sensitize the secretory mechanism to $Ca^{2+}$ (Jones *et al.*, 1985; Tamagawa *et al.*, 1985; Vallar *et al.*, 1987), but other possibilities may exist. Since PKC-depleted islets did not show diminished response to glucose, Jones *et al.* (1992) suggested that PKC-mediated phosphorylation is not essential for nutrient-induced insulin secretion. Conversely, Wang *et al.* (1993) suggested that PKC may regulate $Ca^{2+}$ entry along voltage-dependent $Ca^{2+}$ channels and thus potentiate glucose-induced insulin secretion.

## 4.2.5 $PLA_2$/Arachidonic Acid Metabolism

The release of arachidonic acid has been attributed to $PLA_2$ and depends on glucose metabolism (Konrad et al., 1993). The activity of $PLA_2$ is increased during glucose stimulation (Layschock, 1982; Konrad et al., 1993) and by carbachol (Konrad et al., 1992a). Glucose-induced insulin secretion is diminished by the use of a $PLA_2$ inhibitor (Konrad et al., 1992b). Arachidonic acid amplifies both voltage-dependent $Ca^{2+}$ entry and depolarization-induced insulin release (Ramanadham et al., 1992). However, other hand, arachidonic acid also causes insulin release in the absence of extracellular $Ca^{2+}$ (Band et al., 1992). Phosphorylation induced by arachidonic acid which is independent from PKC activation has been reported by Basudev et al. (1992).

The metabolism of arachidonic acid via cyclo-oxygenase and lipoxygenase has been demonstrated in pancreatic islets (Evans et al., 1983; Metz et al., 1983; Yamamoto et al., 1983). Exogenous arachidonic acid increases insulin release (Falck et al., 1983; Metz et al., 1983) and this effect is blocked by inhibitors of the lipoxygenase, but not of the cyclo-oxygenase pathway. However, there were doubts about whether arachidonic acid metabolism is of physiological relevance in stimulating insulin secretion, since, in arachidonic acid-depleted RINm5F cells, depolarization (KCl) produced the same insulin release as in controls (Safayhi et al., 1993). In fact, this means only that depolarization per se does not need the metabolism of arachidonic acid, and does not exclude the possibility that additional stimulation of $PLA_2$ may produce a modulating effect.

Of the products of arachidonic acid metabolism, leukotrienes have been reported to inhibit glucose-induced insulin secretion (Nathan and Pek, 1990). The same holds for $PGE_2$ (Layschock and Bilgin, 1989).

## 4.3 ROLE OF PHOSPHATASES

As discussed above, protein phosphorylation caused by CaCaMk, PKA and PKC may induce a variety of functions in the machinery of stimulus–secretion coupling. This, however, implies that to keep the system functional for regulation, dephosphorylations must also take place. Dephosphorylations in general are the result of phosphatase activity. To date, little is known about the function of such phosphatases in insulin-producing cells, or whether they are regulated.

Okadaic acid, a toxin of marine origin, is a specific inhibitor of type 1 and 2A phosphatases. In a previous study, type-1 and/or -2A phosphatases have been shown to be present in RINm5F cells (Heurich et al., 1992). When okadaic acid was added to these cells, activity of type-1 and/or -2A phosphatases was decreased. This was associated with inhibition of KCl-stimulated increases in $[Ca^{2+}]_i$ and insulin secretion. Since insulin secretion in response to the calcium-ionophore A23187 was not affected, it was concluded that inhibition of dephosphorylation must be somehow related to $Ca^{2+}$ entry (Heurich et al., 1992).

## 4.4 MODULATION OF INSULIN SECRETION BY HORMONES, NEUROPEPTIDES AND NEUROTRANSMITTERS

### 4.4.1 Introduction

Although glucose is the most important initiator of insulin secretion, its effect is modified by a variety of factors, e.g. hormones/peptides derived from the entero–insular axis and released into the blood during food intake, neurotransmitters released from nerves related to islet tissues (cholinergic, adrenergic, peptidergic), catecholamines reaching the islet via blood, and intrainsular hormones (glucagon, somatostatin). Cholinergic mechanisms are responsible for the early insulin response to a meal in the so-called "cephalic phase" which is independent of nutrient absorption (Ahrén et al., 1986). The pancreas is also innervated by peptidergic neurons, many of which contain gut peptides that function as neurotransmitters. Cholecystokinin (CCK)-, vasoactive intestinal peptide (VIP)- and gastrin-releasing peptide (GRP)- containing neurones have all been implicated in the peptidergic stimulation of insulin release, and galanin in its suppression (Dockray, 1987). In quantitative terms neuronal-mediated secretion accounts for approximately 20% and hormone-mediated secretion 30% of the insulin response to a fast liquid meal (Berthoud, 1984).

Modulators that augment insulin secretion in response to glucose also seem to have a priming effect on insulin release when given in advance of glucose. This has been demonstrated for $GLP-1_{(7-36)}$, GIP, $CCK_8$ and cholinergic agonists (Zawalich et al., 1989b; Fehmann et al., 1991).

### 4.4.2 The Entero–insular Axis

It is generally accepted that oral glucose is much more effective in raising circulating insulin levels than intravenous glucose, when given in amounts sufficient to produce similar degrees of arterial hyperglycaemia (Elrick et al., 1964; McIntyre et al., 1964; ). McIntyre and co-workers have postulated that nutrients taken orally stimulate the secretion of one or more gastrointestinal hormones, which in term modulate insulin secretion. Gastrointestinal hormones are also called "incretins". The incretin effect is mediated by both increased secretion and decreased hepatic extractions of insulin (Hampton et al., 1986; Shuster et al., 1988).

Many peptides that can stimulate insulin release have been isolated from intestinal and nervous tissues. However, not all of them may be of physiological relevance as, in addition to possessing an insulin-releasing capacity, they must be secreted into the circulation during food intake and the concentration reached thereby in the blood must be high enough to affect insulin-producing cells. Moreover, it is reasonable to assume that not all insulin-releasing peptides are secreted after ingestion of the same carbo-hydrates. In this connection it is interesting to note that the release of CCK, for instance, is stimulated not so much by protein but rather by glucose (for a review see Morgan, 1992). It is also notable that the effects on insulin secretion in most cases depend on the presence of more or less stimulatory concentrations of glucose. Nevertheless, it is conceivable that deficient release of these hormones may be a factor involved in the pathogenesis of Type-II diabetes. Indeed, a reduced incretin effect has been reported in NIDDM which could contribute to the delayed and impaired insulin secretion found in this condition (Tronier et al., 1985; Nauck et al., 1986). This interesting area is obviously not fully understood, but it may offer possibilities for drug development.

Hormones related by the entero–insular axis which may be of significance for insulin release are CCK, gastric inhibitory peptide (GIP) and glucagon-like peptide (GLP).

**CCK** is a peptide with 33 amino acids originally isolated from pork intestine. Its action on insulin secretion is very weak in humans. Several smaller molecular forms, however, have been isolated from gut mucosa and from brain. Both the C-terminal octapeptide ($CCK_8$) and the tetrapeptide ($CCK_4$) stimulate insulin release in vitro (Okabayashi et al., 1983; Herman-sen, 1984; Verspohl et al., 1986b; Zawalich et al., 1987).

Infusions of $CCK_8$ at physiological concentrations have been shown to augment insulin secretion in response to arginine and various amino acids but not to glucose, suggesting a physiological role after protein ingestion (Rushakoff et al., 1987). Studies carried out by Reimers et al. (1988) in which mixtures of amino acids were infused in human subjects could not confirm an augmenting role for CCK.

In in vitro studies with rat pancreatic islets, the effect of $CCK_8$ on insulin secretion depends on the presence of stimulatory concentrations of glucose (Verspohl et al., 1986b). As far as its mechanism of action is concerned, $CCK_8$ did not affect $K^+$ efflux (Verspohl et al., 1987) but enhanced glucose-induced uptake of $Ca^{2+}$, an effect that is reduced by nifedipine (Wang et al., 1992). In the absence of a stimulatory glucose concentration, no such effect could be observed (Verspohl et al., 1987). $CCK_8$ also affected glucose metabolism of islet tissue. Here, it increased activity of the PPS and the $NADPH/NADP^+$ ratio, suggesting that by its action on the islet redox system it might sensitize $Ca^{2+}$ entry in response to glucose (Verspohl et al., 1989).

In the presence of stimulatory concentrations of glucose, $CCK_8$ promoted a biphasic release of insulin (Zawalich *et al.*, 1987). When $Ca^{2+}$ influx was inhibited, $CCK_8$ produced only a small first phase of insulin secretion, suggesting a dual effect of $CCK_8$. The first effect is probably on glucose metabolism, while the second concerns stimulation of receptor-linked polyphosphoinositide hydrolysis. An increase in $IP_3$ has been described by Zawalich (1987) and Florholmen *et al.* (1989) and this is supported by recent data (Fridolf *et al.*, 1992) showing that $CCK_8$ also increased $[Ca^{2+}]_i$ in the absence of extracellular $Ca^{2+}$. In $^{45}Ca^{2+}$-prelabelled islets in the presence of a non-stimulatory concentration of glucose, $CCK_8$ increased $^{45}Ca^{2+}$ efflux which could be due to liberation of $Ca^{2+}$ from intracellular stores by $IP_3$ (Zawalich *et al.*, 1987).

**GIP** (also called glucose-dependent insulinotropic peptide) is generally recognized as being a major component of the entero–insular axis. GIP, isolated from porcine intestine (predominantly the jejunum), stimulates insulin secretion under physiological conditions in both dogs and men (Brown *et al.*, 1975; Jones *et al.*, 1987). GIP potentiates glucose-mediated secretion of insulin. In rodents it appears to account for about 50% of the augmentation of insulin release after intraduodenal glucose when compared with intravenous glucose (Ebert and Creutzfeld, 1982). Of the different forms of GIP, the 5 kDa form seems to be the most important one (Krarup, 1988).

GIP is released by carbohydrates (Sykes *et al.*, 1980), amino acids (Penman *et al.*, 1981) and long-chain fatty acids (Kwasowski *et al.*, 1985). In humans, fats are a more potent stimulant than carbohydrates (Penman *et al.*, 1981).

GIP stimulates insulin secretion only in the presence of mild to moderate hyperglycaemia (Andersen *et al.*, 1978; Wahl *et al.*, 1992), but not in the presence of normal glucose concentrations. In addition to secretion of insulin, GIP augments insulin-dependent inhibition of hepatic glycogenolysis (Elahi *et al.*, 1986; Hartman *et al.*, 1986). It also activates adipose tissue lipoprotein lipase (Eckel *et al.*, 1978) and has been shown to stimulate fatty acid synthesis *de novo* in rat adipose tissue (Oben *et al.*, 1991).

GIP stimulates the adenylate cyclase system in pancreatic B-cells (Szecowka *et al.*, 1982). This suggests that GIP potentiates insulin release by promoting formation of cAMP. Recent data (Wahl *et al.*, 1992) suggest that amplification of insulin release by GIP is based on enhancement of $Ca^{2+}$ uptake.

**GLP** is secreted from the lower gut in response to oral glucose, and GLP-$1_{(7-36)}$ amide also increases in the blood after feeding (Kreymann *et al.*, 1988). GLP-$1_{(7-36)}$ amide has been found to be a potent stimulator of insulin secretion *in vitro* (Holst *et al.*, 1987; Mojsov *et al.*, 1987), equivalent to or even greater than GIP (Shima *et al.*, 1988). Studies with the isolated perfused pancreas show a synergistic stimulatory effect of GLP-$1_{(7-36)}$ amide and GIP, suggesting, that several "incretin factors" may act simultaneously on the secretory mechanism, probably via different mechanisms of action (Fehman et al., 1989).

In addition to its effect on insulin secretion, GLP-1$_{(7-36)}$ amide stimulates de novo fatty acid synthesis in adipose tissue (Oben et al., 1991). GLP-1$_{(7-36)}$ activates adenylate cyclase (Drucker et al., 1987; Conlon, 1988); this peptide probably stimulates insulin release in a similar manner to glucagon.

### 4.4.3 Classical and Peptidergic Neurotransmitters of Insulin Secretion

*4.4.3.1 Introduction.* It is well-known that the hypothalamus participates in the regulation of carbohydrate metabolism via the autonomic nervous system. As far as the secretion of insulin is concerned, vagal stimulation causes release of insulin whereas adrenergic stimulation is inhibitory. Moreover, in addition to the classical neurotransmitters, neuropeptides present in the efferent autonomic nerves (GRP, VIP, peptide histidine-isoleucinamide (PHI), neuropeptide Y (NPY), CCK, galanin) are also of importance. The subject has previously been reviewed by Holst (1992). The existence of a cephalic phase of insulin secretion, i.e. reflex-stimulated secretion, has been well established in rats (Strubbe and Steffens, 1975), and there is also evidence for a cephalic-phase insulin response in humans (Bruce et al., 1987; Loud et al., 1988).

In addition to vagal stimulation, adrenergic stimulation is of physiological importance through inhibition of insulin secretion (for a review see Holst, 1992) and avoiding hypoglycaemia especially under conditions of psychological and physical stress. Here, it should be underlined that anxiety or surgical stress are important situations in which impaired carbohydrate metabolism in diabetics may dramatically worsen. The inhibition of insulin secretion, together with the increase in glucagon release, appears to be essential for proper adjustment of hepatic glucose production to augmented needs (Issekutz, 1980; Wolfe et al., 1986). Furthermore, adrenergic stimulation increases availability of glucose via hepatic glycogenolysis.

The naturally mediated inhibition of insulin secretion in response to hypoglycaemia is probably elicited after activation of cerebral "glucoseceptors" (Rohner-Jeanrenaud et al., 1983) and through central noradrenergic pathways (McCaleb and Myers, 1982). The nerve fibres that enter the pancreas are mixed nerves (i.e. sympathetic and parasympathetic) derived from the splanchnic area and the N. vagus. These nerves generally accompany the superior pancreatic–duodenal vessels. Autonomic nerves have their terminals in close proximity to A- and B-cells (Ahrén et al., 1986).

Islet tissue contains a variety of peptides which are stored in pancreatic neurons, nerve fibres and secretory cells and which may, when released, also modulate insulin secretion. Among these are VIP, PHI, GRP, NPY, galanin, CCK, calcitonine-gene-related peptide (CGRP), substance P and opioid peptides (for a review see Holst, 1992). Practically all these peptides are known to have some effect on pancreatic endocrine secretion.

*4.4.3.2 Vagal Nerve Stimulation.* There is general agreement that **acetyl-choline** released from parasympathic nerves modulates insulin secretion in a variety of species and pancreatic islet preparations (for a review see Holst, 1992), an effect that can be blocked by atropine. The effect appears to be mediated via muscarinic receptors of the $M_3$ subtype (Verspohl *et al.*, 1990b). Nevertheless, substantial insulin secretion after vagal stimulation remains despite excessive atropinization, suggesting that non-cholinergic mechanisms are also operative (Miller and Ullrey, 1987; Nishi *et al.*, 1987). As recently discussed (for a review see Berggren *et al.*, 1992), the mechanism of action consists of activation of the PLC system with subsequent formation of $Ins(1,4,5)P_3$ and DAG which in turn activate release of endoplasmic $Ca^{2+}$ and may stimulate PKC respectively.

**VIP** is released from pancreatic neurons by vagus stimulation (Holst *et al.*, 1984). It increases insulin secretion in a glucose-dependent manner (Jensen *et al.*, 1978; Ahrén *et al.*, 1986; Holst *et al.*, 1987; Wahl *et al.*, 1993). Although released by vagus stimulation, its action is not related to a cholinergic effect. Previously, Wahl *et al.* (1993) reported that VIP increased glucose-mediated $Ca^{2+}$ uptake into pancreatic islets which paralleled insulin secretion. This effect was not caused by interference with $K^+$ efflux.

Another pancreatic neuropeptide released during vagus stimulation is **GRP**. It is structurally related to bombesin, a tetradecapeptide isolated from frog skin. GRP increases glucose-induced insulin release in a glucose-dependent manner (Ipp and Unger, 1979; Martindale *et al.*, 1982; Knuhtsen *et al.*, 1986; Hermansen and Ahrén, 1990; Wahl *et al.*, 1991). It specifically binds to mouse pancreatic islets and enhances glucose-induced $Ca^{2+}$ uptake without affecting $^{86}Rb^+$ efflux. It appears that increased formation of $IP_3$ is involved in the mechanism of the synergistic action of insulin and GRP (Wahl *et al.*, 1991, 1992).

*4.4.3.3 Adrenergic Nerve Effects.* **Catecholamines: $\beta$-adrenergic effects.** It is well known that insulin secretion is modified by $\beta$-receptor agonists which cause release via stimulation of adenylate cyclase, as well as by $\alpha_2$-receptor agonists which cause inhibition of insulin secretion (for a review see Holst, 1992). Since noradrenaline is the predominating hormone of sympathetic nerve fibres it must be assumed that, since catecholamines act via nerve stimulation but not via the circulation, stimulation of sympathetic nerves will inhibit insulin secretion. This has in fact been shown by several authors in *in vivo* studies stimulating splanchnic nerves (for a review see Holst, 1992). Whether or not this holds also for catecholamines that come from the circulation is not clear, but such an effect should be markedly concentration-dependent. A-cells but not B-cells are equipped with $\beta$-

receptors (Schuit and Pipeleers, 1986). This implies that $\beta$-receptor agonists stimulate insulin secretion through a mechanism involving glucagon. Upon $\beta$-adrenoceptor activation of A-cells, the increase in cAMP will lead to stimulation of glucagon release (Zielmann et al., 1985).

$\alpha_2$-Adrenergic agonists. The endocrine pancreas has a rich supply of catecholaminergic nerves originating from the splanchnic trunc (Miller, 1981). Inhibition of insulin release by catecholamines (adrenaline and noradrenaline) is mediated through activation of $\alpha$-adrenergic receptors (Schuit and Pipeleers, 1986). Although a lowering of both cAMP and $[Ca^{2+}]_i$ has been suggested to account for this inhibitory action (for a review see Berggren et al., 1992), the exact mechanism remains unclear. Inhibition of insulin secretion by catecholamines is mediated via the $\alpha_2$-receptors. Thus the typical $\alpha_2$-agonist, clonidine, inhibits glucose-induced insulin release, an effect that is parallelled by membrane repolarization and decrease in $[Ca^{2+}]_i$. This is similar to the action of somatostatin. $\alpha_2$-Agonists, via $R_i$, stimulate the action of the inhibitory GTP-binding protein ($G_i$). Whether $\alpha_2$-agonists interact in this way with ion fluxes remains to be established. The possibility has been suggested that $\alpha_2$-adrenoceptor activation promotes the opening of a $K^+$ channel that is distinct from the ATP-sensitive $K^+$ channel, and which results in repolarization (Rorsmann et al., 1991; Wåhlander et al., 1991).

*4.4.3.4  Galanin.* Galanin is a 29-amino acid peptide initially isolated from porcine small intestine (Tatemoto et al., 1983) and localized in nerve fibres innervating the endocrine as well as the exocrine pancreas (Dunning et al., 1986). It is also present in pancreatic neurones and nerve fibres (for a review see Holst, 1992), but non-adrenergic nerves may also contain it (Lindskog et al., 1991). Galanin suppresses insulin secretion under certain conditions *in vitro* and *in vivo* (Ahrén et al., 1991). The action of galanin is mediated via its interaction with galanin receptors (Amiranoff et al., 1987; Sharp et al., 1989). The possible mechanism of action of galanin has been extensively reviewed (Berggren et al., 1992). It appears that it does not directly interfere with the initiation site (depolarization and subsequent $Ca^{2+}$ uptake) of the secretory machinery, but there may be the possibility of an interaction with G-proteins related to adenylate cyclase- and G-protein-regulated $K^+$ efflux.

*4.4.3.5  γ-Aminobutyric acid (GABA).* By causing hyperpolarization by opening $Cl^-$ channels GABA is known to have inhibitory functions in the nervous system. In rat pancreatic islets, a suppressive effect of GABA on the glucose-induced rise of $[Ca^{2+}]_i$ and insulin secretion has been reported (Gu et al., 1993).

*4.4.3.6  Other Pancreatic Peptides.* Other peptides that have been found in endocrine cells and/or nerve fibres are CGRP, Substance P, CCK-like immunoreactivity and endorphins/enkephalins (for a review see Holst, 1992). However, their physiological involvement in controlling insulin release is unclear.

CGRP has been reported to inhibit insulin secretion in rat B-cells and in pigs. Substance P was found to stimulate the secretion of insulin from perfused canine pancreas, but inhibits glucose-induced insulin secretion in mice *in vivo*. The action of CCK has already been discussed.

Pancreastatin, a peptide isolated from porcine pancreas, inhibits insulin secretion and pancreatic secretion *in vivo*. It also inhibits insulin release from rat pancreatic islets and $Ca^{2+}$ uptake in response to glucose without affecting $K^+$ efflux (Lindskog *et al.*, 1992), suggesting modulation of insulin release at the level of $Ca^{2+}$ entry.

Enkephalins and endorphins have been found to stimulate insulin release (Ipp *et al.*, 1978; Hermansen, 1983, Verspohl *et al.*, 1986a). In this connection it was also demonstrated that opioid $\mu$-receptors do not play a role in pancreatic islets but that the insulinotropic effect of low concentrations of Met-enkephalin is mediated via $\delta$-receptors (Verspohl *et al.*, 1986a).

### 4.4.4  Interactions Between Islet Hormones

*4.4.4.1  Introduction.* The main hormones localized in islet tissue are insulin (B-cells), glucagon (A-cells) and somatostatin (D-cells). The subject has been reviewed by Marks *et al.* (1992). *In vitro*, addition of all these hormones to pancreatic islets affects insulin secretion. Whereas glucagon is stimulatory, somatostatin and insulin act as inhibitors. However, from a morphological point of view there is unequal distribution of A-, B-, D- and PP-cells in the islet mass (Fig. 15). Whereas A-cells, D-cells and pancreatic polypeptide (PP) containing cells are mainly localized in the periphery of the islet, B-cells are localized in the centre. This raises the question whether, or by what mechanisms, secreted hormones reach their target cells in the islet in order to stimulate or inhibit their secretory function. Moreover, from a quantitative point of view, there is quite a difference in the percentage of various cell types. Thus, B-cells account for about 60–80%, A-cells for 15–20%, and D-cells for 5–10%. In 1983 Reichlin proposed that A-, B- and D-cells regulate each other's secretion through the intraislet interstitial fluid they all share. The inhibition of both insulin and glucagon by somatostatin would then be the main feature. However, more recent observations, especially on the structure and function of islet vasculature, have made it less likely that the paracrine hypothesis is able to provide a complete and fully satisfactory explanation of all the major intraislet cell relationships (Samols, 1983; Samols *et al.*, 1988; Samols and Stagner, 1988; Marks *et al.*, 1990). On the basis of new information on the microvasculature of the islets of Langerhans, Samols *et al.* (1988) proposed the existence of an intraislet portal vein system where blood perfusing the central core of B-cells picks up insulin. This is then delivered downstream to the A- and D-cells constituting the mantle, where it serves to regulate the secretion of glucagon and somatostatin respectively. Thus, these observations, which were later strengthened (Samols *et al.*, 1988; Stagner *et al.*, 1988, 1989), provide little evidence for the paracrine hypothesis, at least as far as the effect of insulin on A- and D-cells is concerned.

The above hypothesis does not cover the route by which A- and D-cells communicate with each other and affect insulin secretion. Here, the possibility of paracrine interaction via the interstitial fluid cannot be ruled out, especially when we consider the important role of glucagon in amplifying the insulinotropic action of glucose (Pipeleers *et al.*, 1982).

*4.4.4.2  Glucagon.* Glucagon secreted by the pancreatic A-cells stimulates insulin release, at least in part, by activating adenylate cyclase and promoting the formation of cAMP (Schuit and Pipeleers, 1986). This mechanism is regulated by a stimulatory GTP-binding protein ($G_s$) (Ui, 1984). The action of glucagon is most prominent at stimulatory concentrations of glucose. Thus glucagon is a modulator of insulin secretion rather than an initiator. It is released during hypoglycaemia and $\beta$-adrenergic stimulation, its secretion being inhibited by hyperglycaemia, insulin and somatostatin (Samols and Harrison, 1976). The importance of glucagon in insulin secretion is underlined by studies of Pipeleers *et al.* (1982) employing single B- and A-cells. Here, glucose-stimulated insulin secretion by B-cells was markedly higher in the presence of A-cells.

*4.4.4.3  Somatostatin.* Somatostatin is present in numerous tissues including pancreatic D-cells and pituitary cells. Its secretion appears to be mediated via increases in cAMP (Patel *et al.*, 1991). The peptide inhibits insulin and glucagon release in a paracrine or intercellular fashion involving inhibition of cAMP formation (Pipeleers, 1987). Somatostatin, like $\alpha_2$-agonists such as clonidine, stimulates inhibitory $G_i$-protein in B-cells. Moreover, somatostatin induces repolarization and decreases $[Ca^{2+}]_i$ in the B-cell (for a review see Berggren *et al.*, 1992). Previously, Hsu *et al.* (1991) reported that somatostatin inhibits insulin secretion by a G-protein-mediated decrease in $Ca^{2+}$ entry via a voltage-dependent $Ca^{2+}$ channel in the B-cell.

*4.4.4.4  Feedback Inhibition of Insulin Secretion.* Whether or not feedback inhibition of insulin secretion occurs is still under debate since the data from many studies are contradictory. In particular, *in vivo* administration of insulin has given controversial results. However, *in vitro* where exogenous insulin was added to pancreatic islets or to the perfused pancreas, it showed inhibition of glucose-induced insulin release (Ammon and Verspohl, 1976;

Verspohl *et al.*, 1982; Ammon *et al.*, 1991). Conversely, glucose-mediated insulin secretion was augmented when freshly released insulin was rapidly removed from a perfusion system by increasing the flow rate and/or addition of insulin antibody (Ammon *et al.*, 1991). This led to the concept of a short-loop feedback, where freshly released insulin acts on B-cells (Ammon *et al.*, 1991).

Specific binding of insulin to B-cells has been reported (Verspohl and Ammon, 1980). Moreover, exogenous insulin has been found to affect islet cell metabolism, i.e. insulin prevented the increase in PPS activity and the NADPH/NADP$^+$ ratio in the presence of high levels of glucose (Akhtar *et al.*, 1977). Inhibition of inositol phosphate turnover has been proposed as a possible mechanism of action (Verspohl *et al.*, 1990a). Feedback inhibition of insulin gene expression and insulin biosynthesis have also been suggested (Koranyi *et al.*, 1992).

The controversy about negative feedback may be explained by the fact that, *in vivo* at least, insulin levels in the circulation following its administration are not as high as its local concentration around the B-cell during stimulation of its release.

### 4.4.5  Cytotoxicity of Interleukin-1 (IL-1)

IL-1, an important macrophage-derived cytokine, has been shown to decrease insulin secretion. Thus, Zawalich and Diaz (1986) reported inhibition of glucose-mediated discharge of insulin from rat islets by 100 U ml$^{-1}$ IL-1. But potentiation of glucose-induced insulin release together with increased phosphoinositide hydrolysis was also reported when islets had been pre-exposed to IL-1 (Zawalich *et al.*, 1989a).

Inhibition of insulin release by 25 U ml$^{-1}$ IL-1 was associated with a decrease in its biosynthesis and oxidative metabolism. Using light micros-copy, marked signs of degeneration indicating cytotoxic action on the B-cells were seen (Sandler *et al.*, 1987). The early steps of impairment of B-cell function by IL-1 seem to be due to protease activation (Eizirik *et al.*, 1991a). The effects of IL-1 on insulin-producing cells can be prevented by IL-1 receptor antagonists (Eizirik *et al.*, 1991b). A 6–9 kDa IL-1 inhibitor was also shown to prevent IL-1 islet toxicity (Kawahara *et al.*, 1991). The data therefore seem to indicate that the effects of IL-1 are mediated via IL-1–receptor interaction. Bergmann *et al.* (1992) and Corbett *et al.* (1991) claim formation of NO to be responsible for IL-1 cytotoxicity against islet cells. This is supported by the findings of Welsh and Sandler (1992) of NO formation associated with inhibition of the Krebs cycle enzyme aconitase.

Thus, taken together, these data indicate that IL-1 is not a physiological modulator of insulin secretion but may have pathophysiological implication during destruction of B-cells leading to Type-I diabetes.

## 5 Concept of Initiation and Modulation of Insulin Secretion

A hypothetical scheme for the machinery of insulin release assuming coupling of initiation and modulation to the process of granule movement–exocytosis is given in Fig. 20.

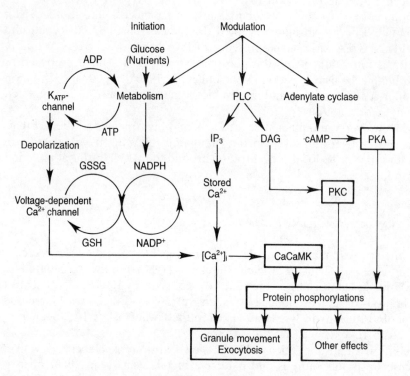

FIG. 20. Hypothetical model of how insulin secretion is regulated. The most important event is the depolarization of the B-cell which causes $Ca^{2+}$ influx along L-type $Ca^{2+}$ channels and subsequent increase in cytosolic $Ca^{2+}$. Depolarization is produced by nutrient (glucose) metabolism via an increase in B-cell ATP and/or ATP/ADP ratio which closes $K_{ATP}$ channels. Also, sulphonylureas, at a distinct location, close $K_{ATP}$ channels. The increase in $[Ca^{2+}]_i$ activates CaCaMK. $Ca^{2+}$ uptake appears to be modulated by nutrient metabolism (redox state of NAD(P)H and GSH). Insulin release in response to depolarization is also modulated by factors affecting PLC and adenylate cyclase. Here, production of $IP_3$ leads to release of stored $Ca^{2+}$ from the endoplasmic reticulum. DAG activates PKC whereas cAMP activates PKA. CaMK, PKC and PKA cause protein phosphorylations which finally cause granule movement and exocytosis. But there will also be other effects of phosphorylations related to stimulus–secretion coupling, e.g. a possible interaction with voltage-dependent $Ca^{2+}$ channels.

# Compounds Acting on Insulin Secretion: Sulphonylureas

The hypoglycaemic activity of sulphonylureas was detected by chance as a side effect of certain sulphonamides used for the treatment of typhoid fever (Janbon *et al.*, 1942a,b). These observations led to clinical trials that promoted the development of sulphonylureas as oral hypoglycaemic agents. Very soon it was clear that the site of action was the B-cell because the blood-sugar-lowering action was not observed in animals whose pancreas had been removed (Loubatieres, 1944, 1957). Since in Type-I diabetics these compounds were not active, it was concluded that the presence of a pancreas is necessary for the hypoglycaemic action of these drugs.

Sulphonylureas have been used for the treatment of Type-II diabetes for more than 30 years. Two actions are thought to be responsible for their ability to lower glucose concentration in blood: (1) their action on B-cells which causes insulin secretion; (2) the so-called extrapancreatic effects which have been mainly demonstrated in *in vitro* experiments.

Orally administered hypoglycaemic sulphonylureas provide effective treatment for Type-II diabetes (for a review see Gerich, 1989; Boyd and Huynh, 1990; Melander *et al.*, 1990).

# 1  Chemical Structure

Two generations of sulphonylureas (Fig. 21) have been developed which differ in chemical structure and potency. The first-generation compounds have an aliphatic side chain. By replacement of the aliphatic side chain with a cyclohexyl group and by addition of a benzene ring linked to glycine, second-generation agents were derived of which glibenclamide (glyburide) and glibizide are the most frequently used. The most prominent difference between first- and second-generation sulphonylureas is the higher affinity of specific binding of the latter which in turn causes much higher stimulation of insulin secretion and therefore significantly decreases the doses needed.

# 2  Actions

## 2.1  PANCREATIC EFFECTS

### 2.1.1  Action on Insulin Release
Numerous studies have demonstrated that addition of sulphonylureas to rat pancreas (Bouman and Goorenstroom, 1961), isolated pancreatic islets

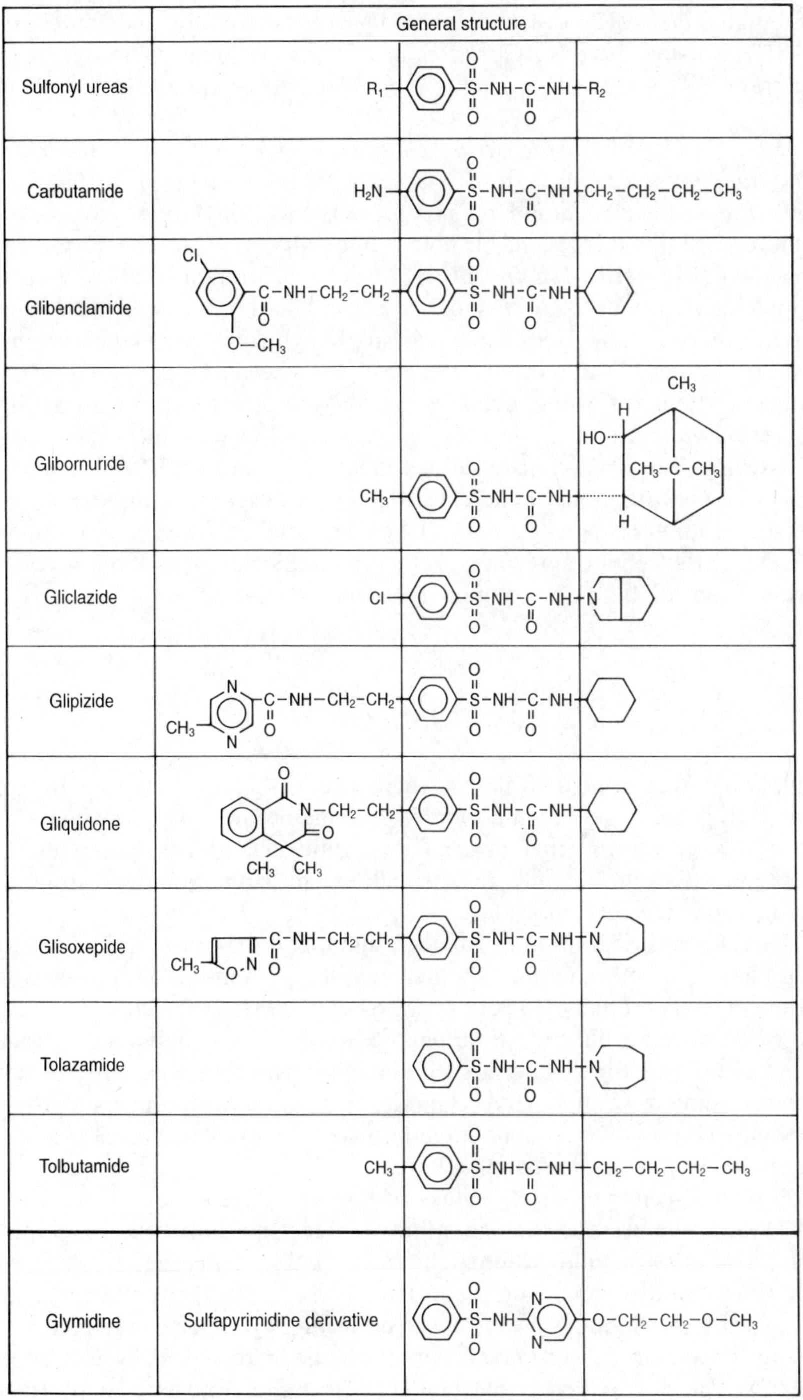

| | General structure |
|---|---|
| Sulfonyl ureas | $R_1$—⟨phenyl⟩—$S(=O)_2$—NH—C(=O)—NH—$R_2$ |
| Carbutamide | $H_2N$—⟨phenyl⟩—$S(=O)_2$—NH—C(=O)—NH—$CH_2$–$CH_2$–$CH_2$–$CH_3$ |
| Glibenclamide | Cl, $O$–$CH_3$ substituted phenyl—C(=O)—NH—$CH_2$–$CH_2$—⟨phenyl⟩—$S(=O)_2$—NH—C(=O)—NH—⟨cyclohexyl⟩ |
| Glibornuride | $CH_3$—⟨phenyl⟩—$S(=O)_2$—NH—C(=O)—NH—⟨bornane-OH, CH₃, CH₃–C–CH₃⟩ |
| Gliclazide | Cl—⟨phenyl⟩—$S(=O)_2$—NH—C(=O)—NH—N⟨bicyclic⟩ |
| Glipizide | $CH_3$, N, N pyrazine—C(=O)—NH—$CH_2$–$CH_2$—⟨phenyl⟩—$S(=O)_2$—NH—C(=O)—NH—⟨cyclohexyl⟩ |
| Gliquidone | isoquinolinedione ($CH_3$ $CH_3$, =O)—N—$CH_2$–$CH_2$—⟨phenyl⟩—$S(=O)_2$—NH—C(=O)—NH—⟨cyclohexyl⟩ |
| Glisoxepide | $CH_3$, O, N isoxazole—C(=O)—NH—$CH_2$–$CH_2$—⟨phenyl⟩—$S(=O)_2$—NH—C(=O)—NH—N⟨ring⟩ |
| Tolazamide | ⟨phenyl⟩—$S(=O)_2$—NH—C(=O)—NH—N⟨ring⟩ |
| Tolbutamide | $CH_3$—⟨phenyl⟩—$S(=O)_2$—NH—C(=O)—NH—$CH_2$–$CH_2$–$CH_2$–$CH_3$ |
| Glymidine | Sulfapyrimidine derivative | ⟨phenyl⟩—$S(=O)_2$—NH—⟨pyrimidine⟩—$O$–$CH_2$–$CH_2$–$O$–$CH_3$ |

FIG. 21. Chemical structure of sulphonylureas.

(Steinke *et al.*, 1972), isolated perfused pancreas (Ammon and Abdel-Hamid 1981), isolated B-cells (Gorus *et al.*, 1988) or hamster insulin-secreting tumour (HIT) cells (Nelson *et al.*, 1987) results in rapid insulin release.

### 2.1.1.1 Use of Bovine Serum Albumin (BSA) in Incubation Media and Sulphonylurea Actions.

For all studies with sulphonylureas *in vitro* and *in vivo* the following should be considered. Sulphonylureas possess a high binding affinity for plasma proteins, but only the unbound form is pharmacologically active. In *in vitro* studies incubation media are frequently supplemented with BSA to stabilize cells. This holds also for experiments on insulin secretion. Bound and free sulphonylureas are in equilibrium. The use of BSA is therefore responsible for the fact that relatively high concentrations of sulphonylureas have been employed to study insulin secretion *in vitro*. Panten *et al.* (1989) developed a filtration assay for measuring free drug concentrations in the presence of BSA. In perfusion experiments with mouse pancreatic islets, they observed half-maximal insulin secretion for free glibenclamide (0.4 nM), glibizide (4 nM) and tolbutamide (5 $\mu$M), in excellent agreement with the equilibrium dissociation constants established for high-affinity binding.

### 2.1.2 Binding to and Uptake in Islet Cells

Sulphonylureas appear to induce their insulin secretory effect mainly from the extracellular site of the cytoplasmic membrane. Thus Hellman *et al.* (1984) have shown that, except for glibenclamide, sulphonylureas do not enter B-cells or only to a small extent (tolbutamide, carbutamide, chlorpropamide and glibizide).

This raises the question of whether sulphonylureas specifically bind to the cytoplasmic membrane and whether or not such binding induces a cascade of events which finally leads to exocytosis. In 1982 Kaubisch and colleagues reported specific binding of sulphonylureas to crude membrane fractions from brain and B-cell tumours. Studies performed by Geisen *et al.* (1985) showed similar results. Here, binding correlated with the hypoglycaemic action. Verspohl *et al.* (1990c) demonstrated the existence of more than one binding site for various sulphonylureas.

For rat B-cell tumour $K_d$ values of 0.03 nM were reported by Geisen *et al.* (1985). The presence of high-affinity binding sites in B-cells was confirmed for RIN cells (Schmid-Antomarchi *et al.*, 1987), HIT cells (Gaines *et al.*, 1988) and mouse pancreatic islets (Panten *et al.*, 1989). In all three studies, a high-affinity binding site was observed using [³H]glibenclamide ($K_d$) in the range 0.3–0.8 nM. Receptor isolation has been reviewed by Nelson *et al.* (1992). There is evidence that binding of sulphonylureas to their receptors occurs from the lipid phase of the B-cell membrane rather than from the cytoplasm (Zuenkler et al., 1989).

An important location of the sulphonylurea receptor is the ATP-sensitive $K^+$ channel. Here, in contrast to ATP action, the binding site for sulphonylureas is not on the intracellular side but on the extracellular side of this channel (Niki et al., 1990). Niki et al. (1989, 1990) have provided evidence that ADP also binds to and competitively displaces glibenclamide from high-affinity HIT-cell sulphonylurea-binding sites. They also showed that ADP inhibited $^{86}Rb^+$ efflux, elicited a rapid and sustained increase in $[Ca^{2+}]_i$ and caused insulin secretion. Since ADP is unable to cross the cytoplasmic membrane, they concluded that ADP and sulphonylureas have common binding sites on the outer cell surface.

Recently, $\alpha$- and $\beta$-endosulfines, peptides isolated from brain, have been shown to bind to sulphonylurea receptors of brain membranes (Virsolvy-Vergine et al., 1992). The question arises whether they and/or ADP are physiological ligands of sulphonylurea receptors.

### 2.1.3  Binding to Other Tissues

2.1.3.1   Brain.  In rat cortical membranes [$^3$H]gliquidone binding was specific, and could be displaced by other sulphonylureas. Dissociation constants were estimated for glibenclamide (0.06 nM), unlabelled gliquidone (0.9 nM), tolbutamide (1.4 $\mu$M) and chlorpropamide (2.8 $\mu$M). The binding affinities were correlated with the rank order of the therapeutic doses (for a review see Nelson et al., 1992). A binding site for glipizide was also reported in rat cerebral cortex (Lupo and Bataille, 1987) with a $K_d$ of 1.5 nM. Other areas of sulphonylurea (glibenclamide) binding in the brain (including substantia nigra, globus pallidus, hippocampus, etc.) have been identified (Treherne and Ashford, 1991).

In brain cells sulphonylurea-sensitive ATP-regulated $K^+$ channels are present which play a role in neurosecretion at nerve terminals. ATP-regulated $K^+$ channels in substantia nigra, a brain region that shows high sulphonylurea binding, are inactivated by high glucose concentrations and by antidiabetic sulphonylureas and are activated by ATP depletion and anoxia. ATP-regulated $K^+$ channel inhibition leads to activation of GABA. These channels may be involved in the response of the brain to hyper- and hypo-glycaemia (in diabetes) and ischaemia or anoxia (Amoroso et al., 1990).

2.1.3.2   Other Tissues.  Sulphonylurea receptors have also been described for cardiac muscle, skeletal muscle and smooth muscle but do not appear to be of therapeutic benefit for lowering blood sugar (Panten et al., 1992). Specific binding to membranes isolated from other rat tissues (liver, lung, kidney, heart, spleen, diaphragm, duodenum, colon and stomach) was negligible. A sulphonylurea-binding protein in the plasma membrane of adipocytes has been proposed (Martz *et al.*, 1989).

### 2.1.4 Membrane Potential and Ion Fluxes

*2.1.4.1 Membrane Potential.* As early as 1970 Matthews and Dean reported depolarization of the B-cell by tolbutamide and glibenclamide. This observation was confirmed by others. Thus, in the presence of a non-stimulating glucose concentration (3 mM), tolbutamide and glibenclamide produced depolarization and spike activity (Meissner and Atwater, 1976; Meissner *et al.*, 1979; Henquin and Meissner, 1982). These effects were not due to $Na^+$ influx (Kawazu *et al.*, 1980).

*2.1.4.2 $K^+$ Efflux.* As discussed above, inhibition of $K^+$ efflux along the ATP-sensitive $K^+$ channel causes depolarization. In fact, it has been shown that tolbutamide, in the presence of a glucose concentration (3 mM) that does not stimulate insulin secretion, inhibits $^{86}Rb^+$ efflux, used as a measure of $K^+$ efflux (Boschero and Malaisse, 1979; Henquin, 1980b; Henquin and Meissner, 1982). A similar effect was observed in the presence of glibenclamide (Gylfe *et al.*, 1984). It was also reported that the addition of glibenclamide (20 $\mu$M) or tolbutamide (1 mM) to the bathing medium of excised B-cell plasma membrane patches reduced the number of single ATP-sensitive $K^+$-channel openings (Sturgess *et al.*, 1985). Similar results were obtained in excised RIN-cell patches using 20 nM glibenclamide (Schmid-Antomarchi *et al.*, 1987).

Mb 699, a benzoic acid derivative similar to the non-sulphonylurea moiety of glibenclamide, also inhibits $^{86}Rb^+$ efflux, depolarizes the B-cell membrane and accelerates $^{45}Ca^{2+}$ efflux from islet cells (Garrino *et al.*, 1985). The authors suggest that a sulphonylurea group is not required to trigger the sequence of events finally leading to insulin release.

That inhibition of $K^+$ efflux by sulphonylureas along ATP-sensitive $K^+$ channels does not depend on ATP is evident from studies in which RIN cells were depleted of ATP by the use of 2-deoxy-D-glucose and oligomycin which block glycolysis and oxidative phosphorylation. Here, sulphonylureas such as glibenclamide inhibited $^{86}Rb^+$ efflux (Schmid-Antomarchi *et al.*, 1987). Similar results were obtained by Niki *et al.* (1989) using glibenclamide in HIT cells. Thus the evidence discussed so far indicates that sulphonylurea-induced depolarization is the result of inhibition of $K^+$ permeability (Henquin, 1980b).

Chronic treatment of rats with glyburide (3 mg per kg per day; intra-peritoneal injection every hour for 9 days) increased its binding to heart and brain membranes. The authors concluded that $K_{ATP}$ channels can be regulated after chronic treatment (Gopalakrishnan and Triggle, 1992). Whether this holds also for B-cells remains to be established.

*2.1.4.3   $Ca^{2+}$ Fluxes.* As can be expected, sulphonylureas increase net $Ca^{2+}$ uptake along voltage-dependent $Ca^{2+}$ channels (Henquin, 1980b; Ammon et al., 1986) and, as far as the chemical structure is concerned, only those sulphonylureas that produce insulin release enhance uptake of $Ca^{2+}$ (Hellman, 1981). Uptake of $Ca^{2+}$ is associated with increased $[Ca^{2+}]_i$ (Abrahamson et al., 1985). In HIT cells, membrane depolarization effected by the addition of glibenclamide or tolbutamide increased intracellular $Ca^{2+}$ by activating voltage-dependent $Ca^{2+}$ channels (Nelson et al., 1987).

It thus seems clear that the initiating mechanism by which sulphonylureas promote insulin secretion is depolarization and subsequent uptake of $Ca^{2+}$ which is similar to the mode of action of glucose. However, and here is the difference, sulphonylureas cannot replace the metabolism of glucose in B-cells. In contrast, their action on $Ca^{2+}$ uptake, but not $K^+$ efflux, depends on the concentration of glucose; in other words, it depends on the metabolism of glucose which seems to modulate the action of sulphonylureas on the B-cell.

## 2.1.5   Modulating Systems

The interrelationships between sulphonylureas and modulating systems of the B-cell can be seen from two aspects. First, do modulating systems interfere with the initiating action of sulphonylureas? Second, do sulphonylureas affect the modulating systems? As discussed in chapter 6, section 4, there are at least three modulating systems, i.e. glucose metabolism, the adenylate cyclase system and the PLC system.

*2.1.5.1   Glucose Metabolism.* It has been extensively discussed in chapter 6, section 3.3.2, that glucose metabolism not only produces a signal (ATP) which, by interfering with the ATP-sensitive $K^+$ channel, inhibits $K^+$ efflux and thus causes depolarization, but also delivers one or more metabolic products which distally to the $K_{ATP}$ channel, and perhaps close to $Ca^{2+}$ uptake, are involved in modulating $Ca^{2+}$ influx and thus insulin secretion. Such metabolic products/factors were suggested to be the redox ratios of nicotinamide nucleotides and/or thiols (glutathione) (for a review see also Ammon and Wahl, 1994). In the case of sulphonylureas it was shown that Methylene Blue and thiol reagents that decrease these redox ratios diminished $Ca^{2+}$ uptake and insulin secretion in response to tolbutamide and glibenclamide (Ammon et al., 1984, 1986). Since these compounds did not change ATP levels of pancreatic islets and failed to affect tolbutamide-induced inhibition of $^{86}Rb^+$ efflux (Ammon and Wahl, 1994), it seems possible that the redox ratios of $NAD(P)H/NAD(P)^+$ and GSH/GSSG are involved in sulphonylurea-mediated $Ca^{2+}$ uptake and insulin secretion distal to depolarization.

The question of whether or not sulphonylureas interact with the metabolism of pancreatic islets has also been studied. It was found that tolbutamide changed neither glucose metabolism nor the above redox ratios (Ammon, 1975), indicating that, in contrast with glucose, which initiates *and* modulates insulin release, sulphonylureas, as far as metabolism is concerned, possess only initiating activity. Moreover, they have even been found to decrease ATP levels (Hellmann *et al.*, 1969; Kawazu *et al.*, 1980).

*2.1.5.2 Adenylate Cyclase System.* In the presence of sulphonylureas some increase in cAMP has been observed to occur in islet tissue. This effect seems, however, not to be of relevance for insulin secretion (Gylfe *et al.*, 1984) because it is small (Täljedal, 1982). The effect on cAMP is probably due to $Ca^{2+}$ influx (Malaisse and Malaisse-Lagae, 1984). Another possibility comes from the observation that sulphonylureas inhibit low-$K_m$ phosphodiesterase (Malaisse and Malaisse-Lagae, 1984).

As discussed above (see chapter 6, section 4.1), initiation of insulin secretion via depolarization can be modulated by compounds that affect the adenylate cyclase system. It is therefore not surprising that glucagon and db-cAMP potentiate tolbutamide-induced insulin secretion (Ammon, 1975). This also holds for methylxanthines which, at the concentrations used *in vitro*, inhibit phosphodiesterase and thus cAMP (Lambert *et al.*, 1971; Ammon, 1975).

## 2.2 EXTRAPANCREATIC EFFECTS

### 2.2.1 Introduction

While the pancreatic effects of sulphonylureas on their hypoglycaemic action are beyond doubt, the relevance of extrapancreatic effects is controversial. In this connection, the increased sensitivity of Type-II diabetics to insulin in response to sulphonylureas has been addressed repeatedly. One argument among others for the possibility of extrapancreatic effects is the observation that, on one hand, normalization of blood glucose levels after a long period of therapy with sulphonylureas does not necessarily correlate with increased plasma levels of insulin (Reaven and Dray, 1967; Barnes *et al.*, 1974), but, on the other hand, hyperglycaemia returns after withdrawal of sulphonylureas. Moreover, sulphonylureas were observed to save some insulin in insulin-treated pancreactomized dogs (Beyer *et al.*, 1972). In the same experimental animal sulphonylureas increased the effect of an intravenous insulin-tolerance test (Beck-Nielsen, 1988).

From a theoretical point of view there are three possible reasons for the extrapancreatic effects of sulphonylureas that lead to a lowering of blood glucose: (1) they increase insulin action; (2) they have insulin-like effects; (3) they have indirect effects.

## 2.2.2 Increase in Insulin Actions and Insulin-like Effects

Target tissues for the enhancement of insulin effects and/or direct effects of sulphonylureas are adipose tissue, skeletal muscle and liver.

### 2.2.2.1 Insulin Receptors.
Insulin mediates its effects after binding to insulin receptors. Olefsky and Reaven (1976) reported that, in Type-II diabetes, treatment of patients with chlorpropamide increased the number of insulin receptors of monocytes. Similar results were achieved with human fibroblasts after treatment with glibenclamide (Prince and Olefsky, 1980). However, further studies carried out by others (for a review see Beck-Nielsen, 1988) have produced contradictory results. The major criticism was that some of the tissues studied are not involved in blood glucose lowering and that the questionable effect of sulphonylureas on insulin receptors may be of an indirect nature. Furthermore it was claimed that the doses of the sulphonylureas used were very high, leading to maximal secretion of insulin (Joost, 1985) or were even higher than necessary for blood glucose lowering (Maloff and Lockwood, 1981). It seems therefore unlikely that an increased number of insulin receptors is responsible for the potentiation of insulin action by sulphonylureas.

### 2.2.2.2 Post-receptor Effects.
Biological effects of insulin after binding to its receptor have been discussed elsewhere. Some of the post-receptor effects of insulin have been studied in the presence of sulphonylureas. The problem of dosage and binding of sulphonylureas to proteins added to incubation media has already been discussed. In connection with insulin release, first-generation sulphonylureas have been found to be effective in the micromolar range whereas second-generation sulphonylureas are effective in the nanomolar range. The studies discussed now must be seen in this light.

### 2.2.2.3 Insulin Receptor Metabolism.
Frank et al. (1985) determined the turnover rate of insulin receptors in liver of rats. They found a doubling after 6 days of treatment with $5 \, mg \, kg^{-1}$ glibenclamide daily. If this is true, a longer-lasting insulin receptor binding would be conceivable. In this connection it should be mentioned that glibenclamide ($10–1000 \, ng \, ml^{-1}$) inhibited degradation of insulin in endothelial cells (Kaiser et al., 1983).

### 2.2.2.4 Glucose Transporter.
Glucose is carried from the extracellular site to the interior of cells by so-called glucose transporters. One of them (GLUT-4) operates only after binding of insulin to its receptor. One measure for transporter-mediated hexose uptake is the determination of the cellular uptake of 3-O-methylglucose and 2-deoxyglucose. Unlike glucose which undergoes metabolism immediately after its uptake (and therefore measurement of tissue concentrations of glucose are not valid as a parameter of glucose uptake), 3-O-methylglucose and 2-deoxyglucose are transported by

GLUT-4 but are then not metabolized. In fact, in adipocytes glibenclamide ($2 \, \mu g \, ml^{-1}$) increases insulin-induced translocation of glucose transporters from the microsomes to the cytoplasmic membrane (Jacobs and Jung, 1985). This might be an explanation for the increase in insulin-mediated uptake of 3-$O$-methylglucose and 2-deoxyglucose into adipocytes caused by tolazamide ($3$–$300 \, \mu g \, ml^{-1}$) and glibenclamide ($1 \, \mu g \, ml^{-1}$) (Lockwood, 1983). Results similar to those in adipose tissue were obtained in skeletal muscle (Jacobs and Jung, 1985).

*2.2.2.5 Glucose Metabolism.* As far as the metabolism of glucose is concerned it is interesting to note that sulphonylureas in liver and skeletal muscle *per se* (absence of insulin) increase fructose 2,6-bisphosphate, a metabolite of glycolysis. In perfused liver experiments, Hatao *et al.* (1985) reported stimulation of fructose 2,6-bisphosphate formation by first- and second-generation sulphonylureas, the maximum effect being produced by tolbutamide at 1 mM and glibenclamide at $1 \, \mu M$. This action is synergistic with that of insulin ($50 \, \mu M$ glipizide, $300 \, \mu g \, ml^{-1}$ tolbutamide) (Matsutani *et al.*, 1984; Monge *et al.*, 1985; Lopez-Alarcon *et al.*, 1986). An increase in fructose 2,6-bisphosphate stimulates the activity of phosphofructokinase, increases glycogen synthesis and inhibits gluconeogenesis. Consequently, in hepatocytes an increase in insulin-mediated synthesis of glycogen, and inhibition of gluconeogenesis and glucose output from liver were seen in response to gliquidon ($5 \, mg \, ml^{-1}$) and glibenclamide ($1.6 \, \mu g \, ml^{-1}$) (Fleig *et al.*, 1984; Rinninger *et al.*, 1984; McGuinness *et al.*, 1987).

Insulin-stimulated 3-$O$-methylglucose uptake and glucose oxidation in adipocytes were potentiated when the tissue had been taken from rats given a daily dose of gliclazide ($8 \, mg \, kg^{-1}$) for 6 days (Hoich and Ng, 1986). Activation of glucose transport associated with activation of PKC in rat adipocytes by tolbutamide ($1$–$2 \, mM$) and glyburide ($20$–$40 \, \mu M$) was also reported (Farese *et al.*, 1991). Similar effects of both have also been demonstrated in myocytes (Cooper *et al.*, 1990b). In cultured hepatocytes, glyburide ($2 \, mg \, l^{-1}$) directly inhibited glycogenolysis, stimulated glycogen synthesis and glycogen synthase and potentiated the action of insulin on glycogen synthesis at a post-binding site (Davidson and Sladen, 1987).

Since most of these extrapancreatic effects of sulphonylureas are coupled to the presence of insulin, it would be attractive to conclude that sulphonylureas possess an extrapancreatic action in Type-II diabetes where insulin secretion is still possible.

*2.2.3 Critical Evaluation*

In 1985 Joost pointed out that the extrapancreatic effects of sulphonylureas can be observed with tolbutamide at concentrations of 0.5–5 mM and with glibenclamide at 1–10 $\mu$M, whereas for maximal insulin secretion only 0.1 mM and 0.1 $\mu$M respectively are necessary. Panten (1987), in a review, also raised this discrepancy considering that only a few per cent of a given drug are unbound and therefore biologically active. These facts make it difficult to conclude that *in vitro* data are transferable to the situation *in vivo*. This sceptical view is supported by the study of Mooradian (1987), who observed no improvement in insulin-mediated glucose uptake into liver, adipose tissue and skeletal muscle in rats given daily doses of 5 mg kg$^{-1}$ glipizide.

If increasing insulin sensitivity is a common feature of sulphonylureas, then these compounds should act synergistically with insulin treatment in Type-I diabetes. However, this is not the case.


### 2.2.4  Indirect Effects

Taking into account that hyperglycaemia as such can cause insulin resistance, it is conceivable that, primarily through an increase in insulin secretion caused by sulphonylureas, hyperglycaemia and then normoglycaemia are decreased. Since sulphonylureas are more effective during hyperglycaemia and since after long-term treatment with sulphonylureas normoglycaemia can be achieved, it is also possible to understand why at a later phase of treatment no increase in plasma insulin is detectable.


### 3  Pharmacokinetics

Variations in the pharmacokinetics of the sulphonylureas are clinically relevant because of the differences in their rate of onset and their duration of action. Differences in the rate of onset are important because they relate to the capacity to reduce the delay in acute insulin release after nutritional challenge and therefore their capacity to reduce the evaluation and prolongation of the postprandial hyperglycaemia. Differences in the duration of action are important because they relate to the risk of causing chronic hyperinsulinaemia, long-lasting hypoglycaemia, and possibly desensitization to sulphonylureas (Melander *et al.*, 1990).


### 3.1  DOSAGE AND APPLICATION

Treatment with a sulphonylurea is begun with a small dose of medication and a progressive build-up over a 1–2-week period (Asmal and Marble, 1984). This is important in order not to induce hypoglycaemia. Furthermore, the progress of the patient must be followed closely in the first weeks of treatment. The dose must be increased progressively in order to avoid side effects. After treatment for 6 months or 1 year, reduction of the dose or complete withdrawal of the treatment must be considered (Beck-Nielsen, 1991).

The most appropriate dosage schedules for the application of sulphonylureas are not yet established. Available data suggest that once-daily (morning) administration 30 min before breakfast may improve the efficacy of sulphonylurea treatment, but only if the exposure to the drug is continuous (Samanta et al., 1984). If postprandial hypoglycaemia ensues in the early part of the day, or if inadequate glycaemic control occurs in the later part of the day, a divided dosage schedule could be tried (Melander et al., 1990).

The optimal daily dosage is difficult to define, as it is dependent on the degree of impairment of $\beta$-cell function before treatment and also the degree of compliance with diet regulation. Furthermore, the dose–response curve may be bell-shaped, and the steady-state concentrations of several, if not all, sulphonylureas show a large interindividual variation following standard doses (Melander et al., 1989).

### 3.2   PHARMACOKINETIC PARAMETERS (TABLE 5)

#### 3.2.1   Absorption

Absorption of both first- and second-generation sulphonylureas is rapid and complete except for gliclazide and tolazamide, which are absorbed more slowly. The maximal plasma concentrations are usually reached within 2–4 h. The kinetics of absorption depend on the formulation and crystalline structure of the drug. Absorption of chlorpropamide may also depend on pH and therefore on food intake, which appears not to be true for the other sulphonylureas (Sartor et al., 1980). The absorption of glibenclamide, although rapid and almost complete, can be improved by an appropriate formulation (Haupt et al., 1984) which leads to a reduction in the daily dosage required.

At least for some sulphonylureas (gliclazide and glipizide), intra- and inter-individual variations in absorption are pronounced, perhaps explaining the large variations observed in their responses (Hartling et al., 1987).

#### 3.2.2   Distribution

The volume of distribution of the sulphonylureas is between 0.1 and $0.3 \, l \, kg^{-1}$. Their plasma protein binding is about 95–99%, but decreases for tolbutamide with age in healthy volunteers showing concentration-dependence (Adir et al., 1982). Displacement from plasma-binding sites is uncharac-

TABLE 5[a]

Pharmacokinetic characteristics of oral hypoglycaemic agents

| Drug | Time of absorption (h) | Volume of distribution ($l\,kg^{-1}$) | Protein binding (%) | Renal excretion (% of dose) | Dosage (number daily) |
|---|---|---|---|---|---|
| Acetohexamide | 0.8–2.4[b] 4–6[c] | – | 75 | – | 0.25–1.5 g (2) |
| Chlorpropamide | 24–48 | 0.1–0.27 | 88–96 | 6–60 | 100–500 mg (1) |
| Glibenclamide | 1.4–2.9 | 0.3 | 99 | 50 | 2.5–20 mg (1–2) |
| Glibornuride | 5–12 | 0.25 | 95 | 65 | 12.5–25 mg (1–2) |
| Gliclazide | 6–15 | 0.2 | 94 | 60–70 | 40–320 mg (1–2) |
| Glipizide | 1–5 | 0.16 | 92–99 | 70 | 2.5–40 mg (1–3) |
| Gliquidone | 24 | 0.15 | 99 | 8 | 15–180 mg (2–3) |
| Glisoxepide | 1.7 | 0.1 | 93 | 50 | 2–16 mg (2–3) |
| Glymidine | 4 | – | 90 | 1 | 0.5–2 g (2) |
| Tolazamide | 4–7 | – | 87–94 | 33–66 | 25–100 mg (1–2) |
| Tolbutamide | 3–28 | 0.1–0.15 | 95–97 | 100 | 1–3 g (2–3) |

[a]Adapted from Asmal and Marble (1984), Jackson and Bressler (1981) and Ferner and Chaplin (1987). [b]Parent drug. [c]Active metabolite (hydroxyhexamide).

teristic for glipizide, which is less readily displaced by anionic drugs than tolbutamide (Crooks and Brown, 1975).

Fitting of plasma-concentration data for glibenclamide is done by single-, two- or three-compartment methods, although the existence of a "deep" third compartment is questionable, at least in the single-dose application experiments (Ferner and Chaplin, 1987).

### 3.2.3   Metabolism

Metabolism of the sulphonylureas is mainly via hepatic oxidation (Table 6) leading to metabolites that are inactive or have very low activity or are present only in low concentrations.

TABLE 6

Metabolism of sulphonylureas

| Drug | Metabolites |
|---|---|
| Chlorpropamide | p-Chlorobenzenesulphonylurea (?) |
| | 2-Hydroxychlorpropamide (?) |
| | 3-Hydroxychlorpropamide (?) |
| Glibenclamide | 4-trans-Hydroxyglibenclamide (a) |
| | 3-cis-Hydroxyglibenclamide (i) |
| | One unidentified metabolite (i) |
| Glibornuride | Five monohydroxy derivatives (i) |
| | One carboxy derivative (i) |
| Gliclazide | Eight hydroxylated or N-oxygenated compounds (i) |
| Glipizide | Two hydroxycyclohexyl derivatives |
| | N-(2)-acetylaminoethylphenylsulphonyl-N'-cyclohexylurea (i) |
| | Two unidentified metabolites |
| Gliquidone | Five hydroxylated and demethylated derivatives (i) |
| Glisoxepid | Four derivatives (i) |
| | Desmethylglymidine (a) |
| Glymidine | Carboxylic acid (i) |
| Tolazamide | p-Carboxytolazamide (a) |
| | Two hydroxy derivatives (a,i) |
| | p-Toluenesulphonamide (a) |
| | One unknown metabolite |
| Tolbutamide | Hydroxytolbutamide (a) |
| | Carboxytolbutamide (i) |

Metabolites: (a) active; (i) inactive; (?) uncharacterized.

### 3.2.4  Elimination

The inactivation and disappearance of sulphonylureas is dominated by their metabolism. An enterohepatic recirculation is postulated for gliclazide from animal experiments but seems to be absent in humans (Benakis and Glasson, 1980).

### 3.3  PATHOLOGICAL CHANGES IN THE PHARMACOKINETICS OF SULPHONYLUREAS

In the elderly patient, the elimination half-life is significantly increased for most sulphonylureas, although this effect is compensated by reduced absorption and volume of distribution. Owing to the mainly hepatic elimination of the sulphonylureas, their accumulation and therefore hypoglycaemia may be expected. Nevertheless, the clinical significance of this accumulation is questionable, since the metabolic function of the liver is maintained even in severe liver diseases, and elimination of the metabolites

COMPOUNDS ACTING ON INSULIN SECRETION: SULPHONYLUREAS   121

can be compensated for by renal excretion. This has been shown for gliquidone, for example. In diabetics with damaged liver function without cholestasis, gliquidone was eliminated from plasma after 24 h, and in patients with cholestasis it was eliminated after 48 h; the urinary elimination of gliquidone in the first group was about 5%, and that in the second about 20%; the rest was eliminated in the faeces (Nelson, 1964; Koss et al., 1976; Williams et al., 1977).

Sulphonylureas should ideally be avoided when the glomerular filtration rate is below 30 ml min$^{-1}$, since hypoglycaemia may be expected in patients with renal failure associated with impaired liver function. Although tolbutamide can be given in normal doses to patients with renal failure (Hasselblatt, 1989), it is generally recommended not to be used in patients with severe impairment of renal function (Martindale, 1989).

## 4   Toxic Effects

Overdosage can produce hypoglycaemia. In order of general appearance, the signs and symptoms associated with hypoglycaemia include: hunger; nausea; diminished cerebral function (lethargy, yawning, confusion, agitation, nervousness); tingling of lips and tongue; increased sympathetic activity (tachycardia, sweating, tremor); and ultimately, convulsions, stupor and coma. Hypoglycaemic coma may lead to permanent brain damage if consciousness is not regained after some months (Lazner, 1970).

### 4.1   TREATMENT

Mild hypoglycaemia without loss of consciousness or neurological findings should be treated with oral glucose and closely monitored adjustments in drug dosage or meal patterns. Severe hypoglycaemic reactions require immediate hospitalization. If hypoglycaemic coma is suspected, concentrated (50%) dextrose has to be rapidly injected intravenously. A continuous infusion of more dilute (10%) dextrose at a rate that will maintain the blood glucose at a level above 100 mg dl$^{-1}$ is necessary. Hypoglycaemia may recur after apparent clinical recovery.

Because of the prolonged hypoglycaemic action of chlorpropamide, patients who become hypoglycaemic from this drug require close supervision for a minimum of 3–5 days, others for a minimum of 24–48 h.

In acute poisoning the stomach should be emptied by aspiration and lavage. Activated charcoal probably adsorbs sulphonylureas and so may be of benefit in acute poisoning (Neuvonen et al., 1983; Neuvonen and Kärkkäinen, 1983; Kannisto and Neuvonen, 1984). Glibenclamide is cytotoxic in vitro (Popiela and Moore, 1991).

## 5  Side Effects

All sulphonylureas may produce severe hypoglycaemia (Seltzer, 1979, 1989; Melander et al., 1989; Binder and Bendtson, 1992). In particular, chlorpropamide and glibenclamide, either alone or with a second hypoglycaemic or potentiating agent, account for 63% of all earlier cases (Seltzer, 1989) which were severe, prolonged and sometimes fatal (see section 4). Because of the long half-life of chlorpropamide and glibenclamide, patients who become hypoglycaemic during therapy require careful supervision of the dose and frequent feeding for at least 3–5 days. Hospitalization and intravenous glucose may be necessary.

Of 204 episodes of severe hypoglycaemia in adults, recorded during a 1-year prospective survey of admissions to a hospital accident and emergency department, 200 occurred in insulin-treated diabetics, three in elderly patients receiving sulphonylureas, and one in a patient with insulinoma (Potter et al., 1982). In a similar study, two of 77 episodes of hypoglycaemia occurred in patients taking oral hypoglycaemic drugs and the remainder in patients receiving insulin therapy (Moses et al., 1985). A report of severe hypoglycaemia, at first thought to be due to insulinoma but later found to be due to adult nesidioblastosis (proliferation of the islet cells), was observed in a woman covertly taking chlorpropamide (Rayman et al., 1984).

It is not necessarily only the sulphonylurea that is responsible for the side effects, the circumstances of drug intake and disposition also have to be recognized: restricted carbohydrate intake is by far the most frequent predisposing factor, followed by age. Hypoglycaemia is more likely to occur when caloric intake is deficient, after severe or prolonged exercise, when alcohol is ingested or when more than one glucose-lowering drug is used. Patients over 60 years of age are particularly at risk. Abnormal liver or kidney functions are important contributing factors, depending on the drug administered (Seltzer, 1979). Renal or hepatic insufficiency may elevate blood drug levels and the latter may also diminish gluconeogenic capacity, both of which increase the risk of serious hypoglycaemic reactions. Elderly, debilitated or malnourished patients, and those with adrenal or pituitary insufficiency, are particularly susceptible to the hypoglycaemic action of glucose-lowering drugs. Hypoglycaemia may be difficult to recognize in the elderly, and in patients taking β-adrenergic-blocking drugs. Proper patient selection, dosage and instructions are important to avoid hypoglycaemic episodes.

Moreover, the threshold for hormonal counter-regulatory responses of adrenaline, growth hormone and cortisol is lowered after a period of strict metabolic control in insulin-dependent diabetic patients. The glucose level at which patients become subjectively aware of hypoglycaemia is correspondingly reduced (Binder and Bendtson, 1992).

When a patient stabilized on any diabetic regimen is exposed to stress such as fever, trauma, infection or surgery, a loss of **blood glucose control** may occur. At such times, it may be necessary to discontinue the drug and administer insulin. The effectiveness of any oral hypoglycaemic in lowering blood glucose to a desired level decreases in many patients over time (**secondary failure**); this may be due to progression of the severity of the diabetes or to diminished drug responsiveness. Primary failure occurs when the drug is ineffective in a patient when first given. Certain patients who demonstrate an inadequate response or true primary or secondary failure to one sulphonylurea may benefit from a transfer to another. Sulphonylureas have been reported to have a high failure rate with time (Harrower and Wong, 1990). The age at onset of diabetes and the duration of effective treatment were found to be inversely proportional. The treatment of patients who develop diabetes before the 50th year of age has been found to be effective for longer (mean $10.1 \pm 5.3$ years) (Stryjek-Kaminska et al., 1989). Secondary failure to treatment with oral hypoglycaemic agents is determined by the disease itself rather than by patient-related factors. Treatment of secondary drug failure should therefore aim at ameliorating both hepatic and peripheral insulin resistance (Groop et al., 1989).

**Combined insulin–sulphonylurea** therapy appears to be an interesting alternative for treating diabetic patients with secondary failure to sulphonylureas (Berger, 1971; Mezitis et al., 1992). In addition to better glucose profiles and/or decreased insulin needs, which have been shown to persist after 1 year or more, the risk of hypoglycaemic episodes is rather small when insulin doses are adapted at the beginning of the combined therapy (Berger, 1971).

Although sulphonylureas are selective blockers of ATP-sensitive $K^+$ channels, their ability to prevent cellular $K^+$ loss and shortening of action potential duration during ischaemia or hypoxia in the intact heart is modest compared with their efficacy at blocking $K^+$ channels in excised membrane patches (Venkatesh et al., 1991). The first-generation sulphonylureas were found to exert a positive inotropic effect in dogs, in contrast to second-generation compounds (Ballagi-Pordany et al., 1991; Groop et al., 1989). Work on tolbutamide has suggested that the sulphonylureas might be associated with an increase in cardiovascular mortality; this has been the subject of considerable debate (Paice et al., 1985).

Other severe effects may be **allergic** in nature. They include cholestatic jaundice, leucopenia, thrombocytopenia, aplastic anaemia, agranulocytosis, haemolytic anaemia, erythema multiforme or the Stevens–Johnson syndrome, exfoliative dermatitis and erythem anodosum. Rashes are usually allergic reactions and may progress to more serious disorders.

Among the mild adverse effects (mostly dose-dependent) observed with sulphonylureas we find gastrointestinal disturbances such as nausea, vomiting, heartburn, anorexia, constipation, diarrhoea and a metallic taste, and there may be headache, dizziness, weakness, paraesthesia and tinnitus. Skin rashes and pruritus may occur and photosensitivity has been reported.

The **second-generation** oral hypoglycaemic agents such as glibenclamide and glipizide are more potent osmotic agents than their predecessors and may give rise to crystalline lens changes and refractive error shifts (Lightman *et al.*, 1989).

Acute porphyriasis may be exacerbated; chlorpropamide was considered to be unsafe in patients with acute porphyria as it has been associated with acute attacks (Moore *et al.*, 1987). Tolazamide was considered to be unsafe in patients with acute porphyria because it has been shown to be porphyrinogenic in animals and *in vitro* systems (Moore *et al.*, 1987).

The sulphonylureas, particularly chlorpropamide, may infrequently induce a syndrome of inappropriate secretion of antidiuretic hormone (augmenting hypothalamic–pituitary release of this hormone) characterized by water retention, hyponatraemia, low serum osmolality and high urine osmolality, and central nervous system signs. Water retention and dilutional hyponatraemia have occurred after administration of chlorpropamide and tolbutamide to NIDDM patients, especially those with congestive heart failure or hepatic cirrhosis. Glipizide, acetohexamide (Moses *et al.*, 1973), tolazamide, glibenclamide are mildly diuretic.

## 5.1 WHILE DRIVING

Hypoglycaemic events are the most common cause of drug-induced acute illness while driving. Drivers needing insulin should not drive vocationally. Vocational drivers needing oral hypoglycaemic drugs have a difficult problem especially if they are on rotating shifts, if the amount of physical exercise varies greatly, or if they change jobs frequently. If they are to be allowed to drive, they should be taking a biguanide or a short-acting sulphonylurea (Raffle, 1981).

## 5.2 DURING PREGNANCY

Reproduction studies with glibenclamide in animals at higher than recommended human doses have revealed no evidence of impaired fertility or fetal harm. Other sulphonylureas are teratogenic in animals. There are no adequate studies in pregnant women. They should only be used during pregnancy if clearly needed, and it is better to switch to insulin. In general, they will not provide good control in patients who cannot be controlled by diet alone. Because abnormal blood glucose levels during pregnancy may be associated with a higher incidence of congenital abnormalities, insulin is recommended to maintain blood glucose levels as close to normal as possible. However, fetal mortality and major congenital anomalies generally occur 3 to 4 times more often in offspring of diabetic mothers.

## 5.3 DURING LABOUR

Prolonged severe hypoglycaemia (4–10 days) has been reported in neonates born to mothers who were receiving a sulphonylurea at the time of delivery. This has been reported more frequently with agents with prolonged half-lives. If sulphonylureas are used during pregnancy (even though they should not), they must be discontinued at least 2 weeks (chlorpropamide and glipizide, 1 month) before the expected delivery date.

## 5.4 DURING LACTATION

Chlorpropamide and tolbutamide are excreted in breast milk. Data on other sulphonylureas are not available. Because of the potential for hypoglycaemia in nursing infants, it has to be decided whether to discontinue nursing or to discontinue the drug.

## 5.5 IN CHILDREN

Safety and efficacy in children have not been established.

## 5.6 SPECIAL REMARKS WITH RESPECT TO INDIVIDUAL SULPHONYLUREAS

### 5.6.1 Chlorpropamide

More than 50% of reactions to chlorpropamide have been related to skin reactions including the Stevens–Johnson syndrome, exfoliative dermatitis, eczema, photodermatitis, erythema nodosum and purpuric and papular rashes. Blood disorders include aplastic anaemic (5%), agranulocytosis (3%), pancytopenia (5%), leucopenia (6%), thrombocytopenia (8%) and haemolytia anaemic (3%). Liver damage occurs in 12% of patients and is mainly of the cholestatic type accompanied by jaundice (Harris, 1971). A 5-day challenge with chlorpropamide results in a mild decrease in acuity followed by return to baseline values when treatment is again stopped. Drug-induced optic neuropathy sometimes may occur (Wymore and Carter, 1982). Nephrotic syndrome, glomerular lesions (of an immunocomplex nature) and Stevens–Johnson syndrome have all been described (Kanefsky and Medoff, 1980).

### 5.6.2 Glibenclamide

A review of 57 instances of hypoglycaemia associated with glibenclamide exists. Coma or disturbed consciousness was observed in 46 patients and in

10 there was a fatal outcome. Death occurred up to 20 days after presentation. In discussing their review, the authors reported that, including the present series of 57 cases, there have been published reports on 101 severe hypoglycaemias, 14 with a fatal outcome (Asplund *et al.*, 1983). There was a significant increase in nocturia in diabetic patients given glibenclamide compared with those treated with chlorpropamide or insulin or by dietary control (Shaw *et al.*, 1977).

### 5.6.3   Glymidine

Gastrointestinal disturbances, skin eruptions and urticaria, leucopenia, and thrombocytopenic purpura have been reported. Patients allergic to the other sulphonylureas may not be sensitive to glymidine.

### 5.6.4   Tolbutamide

Mortality from cardiovascular causes has been reported by the University Group Diabetes Program (UGDP) to be higher (ca. 2.5 times) in patients receiving tolbutamide (1.5 g per day) than in patients receiving insulin. The administration of other oral hypoglycaemic drugs is expected to be associated with increased cardiovascular mortality over treatment with diet alone or diet plus insulin. This long-term prospective clinical trial involving 823 patients evaluated the effectiveness of glucose-lowering drugs in preventing or delaying vascular complications in patients with non-insulin-dependent diabetes. While this has been accepted by the Food and Drug Administration (FDA), the outcome of the association of sulphonylurea treatment with cardiovascular complications has been the subject of intense and continued debate. The reports from the UGDP have aroused prolonged controversy not entirely settled by detailed reassessment of relevant studies. The FDA is about to make it a requirement that sulphonylureas be labelled with a specific warning about the possibility of increased cardiovascular mortality associated with the use of these drugs. Thrombophlebitis has occurred following the intravenous injection of tolbutamide sodium; too rapid injection may cause a transient sensation of heat in the vein.

### 5.7   PRECAUTIONS

Diet and exercise remain the primary considerations of diabetic patient management. Caloric restriction and weight loss are essential in the obese diabetic. These drugs are an adjunct to, not a substitute for, dietary regulation. In patients with Type-II diabetes who have few or no symptoms but do not respond satisfactorily to diet, a sulphonylurea should be introduced at a low dose with gradual increases until a satisfactory response occurs, thus avoiding hypoglycaemia. Abuse of sulphonylureas occurs when patients who could benefit from diet alone are treated with the drug unnecessarily or, more often, when patients with poorly controlled disease continue to take maximum doses of the drugs (Davidson, 1992).

5.8 MONITORING THERAPY

Patients should be kept under continuous medical supervision. During the initial test period the patient should communicate with the physician daily, and report at least weekly for the first month for physical examination and evaluation of diabetic control. After the first month, examination should be at monthly intervals or as indicated. Uncooperative individuals may be unsuitable for treatment with oral agents.

5.9 HEPATIC AND RENAL IMPAIRMENT

Oral hypoglycaemic agents are metabolized in the liver. The drugs and most of their metabolites are excreted by the kidneys. Hepatic impairment may cause inadequate release of glucose to balance hypoglycaemia. Renal impairment may cause decreased elimination of sulphonylureas leading to accumulation producing hypoglycaemia; therefore these agents should be used with caution in NIDDM patients with renal or hepatic impairment. Renal and liver function should be monitored frequently.

## 6 Interaction with Other Drugs

Many compounds have been reported to interact with sulphonylureas. Most of the interactions result from changes in absorption, displacement from plasma proteins, alterations in their metabolism, or from the interacting drug having its own effect on blood sugar. Oral sulphonylureas with high plasma protein binding (e.g. glibenclamide, glibornuride, glipizide, gliquidone and tolbutamide) may be displaced from binding proteins by chloramphenicol, clofibrate, coumarins, phenylbutazone, salicylates and sulphonamides with the risk of hypoglycaemia. It has been suggested that interactions due to displacement from binding sites may be less likely with glibenclamide than with other sulphonylureas. Sometimes these effects are not clinically significant with respect to inhibition of plasma protein binding.

Compounds that may **increase the hypoglycaemic effect** of sulphonylureas and cause a reduction in their dosage requirement include: antibiotics and anti-infective agents such as chloramphenicol (Christensen and Skovsted, 1969) and sulphonamides including co-trimoxazole (Berger, 1971; Wing and Miners, 1985); coumarin anticoagulants (Berger, 1971; Judis, 1973); anti-inflammatory agents and analgesics including azapropazone, phenylbutazone and salicylates (Schulz, 1968; Harris, 1971; Andreasen *et al.*, 1981; Karsh, 1990); lipid-regulating agents such as clofibrate and halofenate (Jain *et al.*, 1975; Ferrari *et al.*, 1976). Other compounds implicated in increasing the hypoglycaemic effect of sulphonylureas are cimetidine and ranitidine (Dey *et al.*, 1983; Feely and Peden, 1983; MacWalter *et al.*, 1985), fenfluramine (Verdy *et al.*, 1983), indobufen (Elvander-Stahl *et al.*, 1984), methyldopa (Gachàlyi *et al.*, 1980), miconazole (Meurice *et al.*, 1983) and sulphin-pyrazone (Birkitt *et al.*, 1982). β-Blockers may mask some of the symptoms of hypoglycaemia. While there has been a report of β-blockers reducing the hypoglycaemic action of glibenclamide (Zaman *et al.*, 1982), other studies have failed to observe an interaction with β-blockers and glibenclamide or tolbutamide (Davies, 1984; Miners *et al.*, 1984).

Compounds that may **diminish the hypoglycaemic effect** and thus cause an increase in the dosage requirement of sulphonylurea include rifampicin (Syvälahti *et al.*, 1974). There is a theoretical risk of a diminished hypoglycaemic effect with corticosteroids and with oral contraceptives. It has been stated that the absorption of glibenclamide from the gastrointestinal tract may be reduced if it is taken together with guar gum.

The elimination of renally excreted sulphonylureas (e.g. carbutamide, chlorpropamide, glisoxepide) may be diminished by probenecide and salicylates.

It is considered that any interaction between sulphonylureas and $Ca^{2+}$-channel blockers such as nifedipine and verapamil is not significant.

Instead of first-generation sulphonylureas, second-generation drugs must be preferred in cardiac glycoside-treated diabetics (Ballagi-Pordany *et al.*, 1989). In rabbits and rats, glibenclamide decreased, while tolbutamide and carbutamide increased, strophantidin toxicity and myocardial ischaemia-induced transitory ventricular fibrillation in a dose-dependent manner (Pogatsa *et al.*, 1988).

## 6.1   DISULFIRAM-LIKE SYNDROME

A sulphonylurea-induced facial flushing reaction may occur when some sulphonylureas are administered with alcohol. This syndrome is characterized by facial flushing and occasional breathlessness but without the nausea, vomiting and hypotension seen with a true alcohol–disulfiram reaction. The facial flushing reaction occurs in approximately 33% of NIDDM patients taking chlorpropamide and alcohol. It is uncertain whether glibenclamide and glipizide can cause the facial flushing reaction.

It has been proposed that the symptom of facial flushing could be used as a diagnostic test for NIDDM (Leslie and Pyke, 1978; Raffle, 1981; Wiles *et al.*, 1984). However, there have been reports of the test not being specific (de Silva and Tumbridge, 1981; Fui *et al.*, 1983) and despite a great deal having been published on the chloropropamide–alcohol flushing test (CPAF), its value is not clearly defined. Alcohol, as well as provoking a flushing reaction with chlorpropamide, has been reported both to increase and decrease the half-life of tolbutamide, depending on whether the alcohol administration was acute or chronic (Sellers and Holloway, 1978).

## 7  Clinical Studies

### 7.1  HEALTHY VOLUNTEERS

Oral hypoglycaemic agents have been in clinical use since 1956 in the United States. Despite more than 35 years of clinical practice and thousands of scientific papers, controversy still exists with regard to the exact mode of their hypoglycaemic action and the best clinical use of sulphonylurea agents. Recent advances mainly have been made in the understanding of clinical efficacy, long-term actions and effects on hypoglycaemia and lipoproteins as well as on late complications. More information has also been gained on secondary failure and the combined therapy with insulin.

### 7.1.1  Comparison of Various Sulphonylureas

Despite a seemingly fundamental differentiation between first- and second-generation sulphonylureas, very few basic differences are demonstrable between these groups from a clinical perspective, with the exception of potency on a molar basis (Melander *et al.*, 1989). The therapeutic usefulness of the second-generation drugs must also be questioned in view of the fact that most of them are ineffective in the treatment of secondary failure to first-generation sulphonylureas (Lev *et al.*, 1987). Glibenclamide at 5 mg increases serum insulin for as long as 250 mg chlorpropamide, and in long-term therapy (8 weeks) the two drugs show similar efficacy (Ylitalo *et al.*, 1985).

These findings were confirmed by Pendergast (1984), who noted that second-generation glyburide and glipizide do not seem to be more effective in controlling blood glucose than first-generation chlorpropamide and tolazomide, and that these agents do not appear to offer a major therapeutic advantage over first-generation sulphonylureas. Conversely, Harrower (1985) examined the effects of five different sulphonylureas over a period of 1 year and noted differences that could well be of clinical advantage in certain diabetic patients. Gliclazide was found to produce normal $HbA_1$ levels in a significantly greater number of patients than chlorpropamide and gliquidone, while gliquidone and gliclazide were more effective in lowering $HbA_1$ than glipizide.

Glipizide, 15 mg, potentiated insulin action and amplified plasma insulin response to meals more than glyburide, 15 mg, which improved insulin sensitivity, as assessed by an insulin-tolerance test, more than glyburide. The two agents both improved glucose control by 25% compared with placebo (Groop et al., 1985).

Glyburide, unlike other sulphonylureas, is inactivated by the liver and kidneys and excreted in the faeces and urine. It should therefore not be prescribed in patients with liver and renal disease. Glyburide appears to decrease resistance to insulin and sensitize the receptor while utilizing the patients available endogenous insulin (Krall, 1984).

Because diabetes is a heterogeneous disease, each patient must be treated individually. More studies, however, are necessary to determine which of several available sulphonylureas is most appropriate in clinical treatment. The evidence of the relative efficacy of sulphonylureas, however, is still inconclusive. The blood glucose-lowering effect has always been primarily attributed to their insulinotropic action. In subjects not previously exposed to sulphonylureas, close association between the appearance of the drug in the plasma after a single dose and the release of insulin has been amply demonstrated. Sulphonylureas, however, also seem to exert potent extra-pancreatic effects. This may explain why, in two recent reports, these agents were found to also be beneficial in the management of insulin-dependent diabetes.

## 7.2   TYPE-I DIABETES MELLITUS

IDDM patients are not suitable candidates for sulphonylurea therapy. In insulin deficiency, these drugs (e.g. glyburide) produced no changes in $24^-$ h glucose level, glucosuria, $HbA_1$ or basal hepatic glucose production (Simonson et al., 1987). However, in patients who were C-peptide secretors, glibenclamide was found to induce a fall in daily blood glucose and improve $HbA_1$ markedly. There was no change in any of the measurements, however, in C-peptide non-secretors and no evidence was seen for any extrapancreatic effects of glibenclamide (Burke et al., 1984).

In 1988, Kabachi and Birkenholz, noted that sulphonylureas enhanced the effect of endogenous insulin. In a double-blind clinical trial with tolazamide and insulin for 3 months, fasting plasma glucose and $HbA_1$ markedly improved compared with placebo administration. In general, however, the enhancement of insulin sensitivity by sulphonylureas in IDDM patients is only minor and clinically without importance (Stocks et al., 1988); a combination of insulin and sulphonylureas therefore does not seem to be warranted in the treatment of Type-I diabetic patients!

## 7.3   TYPE-II DIABETES MELLITUS

### 7.3.1   Monotherapy

The majority of Type-II diabetics are obese (II b) and suffer predominantly from an impairment of insulin action due to heterogeneous mechanisms. Decreased insulin responsiveness of peripheral tissues may be due to (1) a post-receptor defect with secondary hyperinsulinaemia, (2) down-regulation of the number of insulin receptors, or (3) the glucotoxic effect of hyper-glycaemia caused by accelerated hepatic glucose production. An additional impairment of insulin secretion is present, however, only in non-obese Type-II-a diabetics.

The cornerstone of management of Type-II (NIDDM) diabetics is diet and exercise. The majority of these patients, however, will remain hyperglycaemic and are candidates for oral hypoglycaemic agents.

Sulphonylurea compounds have been shown to lower blood glucose effectively in Type-II diabetics on acute administration and chronic applica-tion as well. The mechanisms responsible for this effect are controversial and determined by the type of NIDDM, and the nature and the duration of treatment.

Sulphonylureas increase endogenous insulin secretion and are therefore the drug of choice in non-obese NIDDM patients with prevailing impaired islet cell function. B-cell sensitivity to glucose is improved by sulphonylureas during acute administration, and hyperinsulinaemia is maintained for 3–6 months. Following a 3-month treatment, glycaemic control is markedly improved and accompanied by an increase in insulin secretion (Kolterman and Olefsky, 1984). Similar results were reported by Peacock and Tattersall (1984), who noted that, after 6 months treatment with sulphonylureas, glucagon-stimulated pancreatic insulin secretion was much higher than in patients on insulin with identical glycaemic control. After 18 months, however, when plasma glucose had improved significantly, the glucotoxic effect disappeared and insulin effectiveness improved, and sulphonylurea-induced hyperinsulinaemia was no longer demonstrable. At that time, Faber et al. (1990) did not find any additional effects of glyburide on insulin- and C-peptide response to a meal or during continued fasting in patients treated with sulphonylureas. Good metabolic control, however, was still main-tained.

As plasma glucose fell, the stimulating sulphonylurea effect on insulin secretion was still present although masked and could only be detected if the challenge (sulphonylurea) was given at the previous glucose levels (Fig. 22).

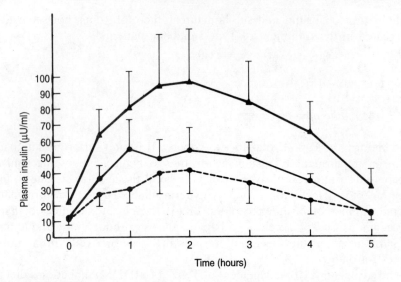

FɪG. 22. Plasma insulin concentrations achieved during oral glucose tolerance test before and during therapy with glyburide. The concentrations were increased at 2 months but returned to control values by 6 months. Controls (---●---), 2 months (—▲—), 6 months (—●—). (Source: Feldman, 1985.)

With loss of the sulphonylurea-induced hyperinsulinaemia, down-regulation of insulin receptors improved and an additional aspect of peripheral insulin resistance in NIDDM improved with sulphonylurea treatment.

In obese Type-II diabetics, however, where peripheral insulin resistance is the most prevailing and clinically dominating defect, weight reduction and exercise are the most effective means of achieving hypoglycaemia and lasting reduction of insulin resistance. Sulphonylureas should not be applied as the first-choice drug. Non-insulinotropic hypoglycaemic drugs such as acarbose or biguanide should be preferred if patients stay hyperglycaemic. Nevertheless, sulphonylureas also seem to ameliorate metabolic control acutely in obese diabetics by suppression of hepatic glucose output and insulin-stimulated glucose transport (DeFronzo and Simonson, 1984). Sulphonylureas do not increase the number of insulin receptors because of a further increase in insulin secretion in these patients (Pfeifer et al., 1984). In a later phase, however, insulin binding may also be increased. Decreased insulin receptor degradation has only been noted in vitro by Prince and Olefsky (1980).

Post-receptor effects are still controversial. Kolterman and Olefsky (1984) felt that an increase in post-receptor function appears to be a crucial determinant of the clinical response to sulphonylureas (Fig. 23). Extra-pancreatic mechanisms in obese NIDDM patients may vary with the

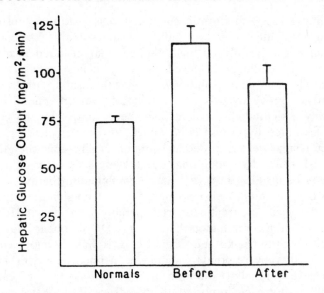

FIG. 23. Basal hepatic glucose production rates in normal subjects and in Type-II diabetic patients before and after 3 months of glyburide therapy. (Source: Kolterman and Olevsky, 1984.)

sulphonylurea and the duration of treatment. Glipizide potentiates the effects on glucose disposal but does not alter insulin effects on hepatic glucose production (Putnam *et al.*, 1981) while glibenclamide may also reduce hyperglycaemia by inhibiting the absorption of glucose from the gastrointestinal tract (Teale and Love, 1972).

Glycaemic control of Type-II diabetics, however, is by no means perfect after sulphonylurea therapy. Many patients continue to have hyperglycaemia on maximal sulphonylurea therapy. This may be called "secondary failure", which develops at a rate of ca. 5% per year in Type-II diabetics (Thoelke and Ratzmann, 1989). To achieve the prime aim of normal fasting glucose concentration in these diabetics, different options are available.

## 7.3.2   Combination Therapy

According to modern pathophysiological understanding of Type-II diabetes and the mechanism of sulphonylurea action, combined insulin–sulphonylurea therapy appears to be an interesting alternative for treating NIDDM patients with secondary failure to sulphonylureas. Several recent clinical trials confirmed favourable results (Stenman *et al.*, 1988). Holman *et al.* (1987) studied the metabolic profiles of 24 Type-II diabetics who were treated with sulphonylureas + metformin, sulphonylureas + ultralente insulin, insulin alone and ultralente + soluble insulin. The mean $HbA_1$ concentration was reduced significantly only by the treatment that included insulin. Fasting normoglycaemia could be achieved easily by means of basal insulin supplementation. Combining sulphonylureas with insulin, however, did not significantly improve overall glucose control over treatment with insulin alone. Only a slight improvement in diabetic control by the combination therapy was noted by Groop et al. (1984, 1985) and Schade et al. (1987). Long-term results were recorded as being uncertain, since the effect tended to vanish with time. No additional effects were seen on insulin binding to erythrocytes or insulin sensitivity due to combination therapy.

Quatraro et al. (1986) also pointed out that combination therapy may increase the cost of treatment considerably and concluded that sulphonylurea–insulin combination therapy in NIDDM appears warranted only in selected patients (Falko and Osei, 1985). It was therefore claimed that combination therapy responders should be defined as having high fasting C-peptide levels and short duration of diabetes (less than 8 years). Lewitt et al. (1989), however, reported that 31 Type-II diabetics treated with insulin + glyburide compared with insulin alone had a significant improvement in glycaemic control and reduction of $HbA_1$. Casner (1988) noted that an improvement in fasting glucose and $HbA_1$ levels as well as an increase in C-peptide after insulin–glyburide combination therapy in NIDDM patients was maintained over a period of at least 3–6 months. Similar results were obtained by Quatraro et al. (1986) in Type-II diabetics treated with gliclazide combined with insulin for 12 months. The diurnal glucose profile and $HbA_1$ improved significantly.

Lotz et al. (1988) treated their patients with secondary failure for 2 years with either insulin alone or glibenclamide 3.5 mg every 2 days, plus small amounts of intermediate-acting insulin. Nearly identical metabolic control was achieved with 14 units in the combined-therapy group. A reduction of daily insulin doses by 25% in the combination therapy with a significant lowering of fasting glucose and an increase in C-peptide was also observed (Stenman et al., 1988). Most authors now agree that combination therapy may be an appropriate treatment regimen in Type-II diabetics with secondary failure, who still secrete some endogenous insulin.

### 7.3.3 Sulphonylureas and Hypoglycaemic Reaction

Hypoglycaemic reactions may appear after acute and chronic sulphonylurea application. The incidence of hypoglycaemia was examined for two different periods (1960–1969 and 1975–1984) by Berger et al. (1986) and was shown to be constant and quite comparable with 0.22 versus 0.25 per 1000 patients per year. However, the risk was significantly higher with glibenclamide and chlorpropamide treatment than with glibornuride and tolbutamide. Some 6.5% of the hypoglycaemic episodes were fatal in the years 1960–1969, compared with 4.3% for the later period.

Data on relative safety suggest that chlorpropamide is the most toxic sulphonylurea (Ferner, 1988), but glyburide causes more dangerous hypoglycaemias than chlorpropamide. Glibenclamide has been shown to have a delayed effect on stimulating insulin secretion and this may be responsible for many unexpected severe hypoglycaemic episodes (Turner et al., 1987).

No significant difference was seen in the calculated mortality risk for metformin-associated lactacidosis and glibenclamide-associated hypoglycaemia. Sulphonylureas were no less dangerous than metformin and both should be used with care in non-insulin-dependent diabetics, especially in elderly subjects and those with impaired renal or hepatic function (Campbell, 1985).

## 7.3.4  Sulphonylureas and Lipoproteins

Patients with diabetes frequently have elevated plasma concentrations of triglycerides and low-density lipoprotein (LDL) cholesterol concentration, together with reduced high-density lipoprotein (HDL) cholesterol concentration. Studies of the effect of sulphonylureas on lipid metabolism in Type-II diabetes, however, are quite controversial and the results have been discussed widely during the last few years. Glibenclamide and metformin were found to have no primary effect on serum triglycerides (Rains et al., 1988). Neither drug altered HDL cholesterol or subfraction cholesterol. Metformin alone, however, reduced LDL cholesterol.

Glyburide caused a significant reduction in VLDL cholesterol in patients with NIDDM and Type-IV hyperlipoproteinaemia along with a variable change in HDL cholesterol, independent of its effect on plasma glucose. The best study on the effect of glipizide exhibited a correlation in plasma glucose with a reduction in plasma triglycerides and LDL cholesterol. There was also a significant increase in the plasma HDL cholesterol/total cholesterol ratio (Greenfield et al., 1982). Tolazamide had no effect on serum cholesterol, although serum triglyceride concentration tended to increase (Gunderson et al., 1975).

## 7.3.5  Sulphonylureas and Late Complications of Diabetes

Apart from the amelioration of acute symptoms, a major aim of the treatment of NIDDM should be the prevention of cardiovascular complications. Since the studies of the university groups diabetes programme (UGDP) in 1970, the initial advice of the American Diabetes Association (ADA) concerning caution in the use of sulphonylureas was later withdrawn because it was felt that there was insufficient evidence to prove that sulphonylurea therapy might induce an associated increased risk from cardiac death. In the meantime a new prospective randomized study has been set up (UK-P.D.S.). Until these results become available it is reasonable to continue to use diet and sulphonylureas to reduce hyperglycaemia if diet alone has failed to produce a normal fasting plasma glucose.

However, the two biochemical abnormalities that predispose to increased macrovascular disease in diabetes are hyperlipidaemia and hyperglycaemia. Both parameters improve with the application of sulphonylureas in metabolically uncontrolled Type-II diabetes. In addition a reduction in increased platelet aggregation in NIDDM was noted by glyburide and glicazide (Klaff et al., 1979). It is not clear, however, if this is solely due to the reduction in hyperglycaemia or if sulphonylureas have a direct effect on platelet function (Feldman, 1985).

Akanuma et al. (1988) compared the effect of gliclazide and other sulphonylureas on diabetic microangiopathy. In long-term comparative clinical trials, it was claimed that gliclazide has additional properties in preventing deterioration of diabetic retinopathy and particular progression to proliferative retinopathy. Jerums et al. (1987), however, did not observe a reversal of early diabetic microangiopathy in a prospective double-blind controlled study over 2 years in insulin- and non-insulin-treated diabetics comparing gliclazide and placebo. There was also no effect when comparing gliclazide and placebo with regard to any parameter of platelet function (Larkins et al., 1988), while Holmes et al., (1984) reported a reduction of platelet adhesiveness and aggregation.

A decrease in basement membrane thickening in diabetics to levels close to these found in subjects without diabetes was reported by Camerini-Davalos et al. (1988), who treated 35 patients with Type-II diabetes and compared the results with those obtained with placebo. However, since plasma glucose and HbA$_1$ also decreased significantly, basement-membrane changes were felt to be a consequence of effective oral medication and not due to a specific sulphonylurea agent.

### 7.3.6 Conclusion

When appropriately used, sulphonylureas can provide a safe and effective adjunct to diet in the management of patients with NIDDM.

# Compounds Acting on Glucose Uptake: Biguanides

## 1 Chemistry

Metformin and phenformin are biguanides. It has been known for six decades that guanidine and derived structures possess hypoglycaemic effects. Most of them, such as decamethylenbiguanid, have been withdrawn because of toxic effects. Unlike other glucose-lowering biguanides, there is no lipophilic side chain, no intramolecular N–H–N binding and no ring formation with metformin (Fig. 24); under physiological conditions the predominant form of the molecule is singly protonated on the central amino group; taken together, these properties may lead to fewer side effects of metformin, since it enters the cell to a lesser extent than other biguanides.

138 ANTIDIABETIC AGENTS

## 2 Pharmacology

Phenformin is a hypoglycaemic (better to say antihyperglycaemic) agent that was formerly used in the treatment of NIDDM. It is associated with an unacceptably high incidence of lactacidosis that has often proved fatal. Metformin is still on the market in Canada and Europe, but the sulphonylureas comprise the only class of oral agents that are commercially available for the treatment of Type-II diabetes in the United States.

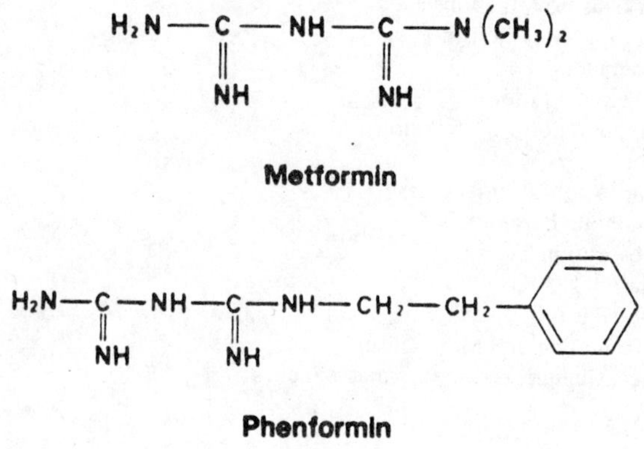

$$H_2N - C - NH - C - N(CH_3)_2$$
$$\quad\quad \| \quad\quad\quad \|$$
$$\quad\quad NH \quad\quad\quad NH$$

**Metformin**

$$H_2N - C - NH - C - NH - CH_2 - CH_2 - \langle \rangle$$
$$\quad\quad \| \quad\quad\quad \|$$
$$\quad\quad NH \quad\quad\quad NH$$

**Phenformin**

Fig. 24. Chemical structure of two biguanides.

2.1 MECHANISMS OF ACTION

The mode of action of metformin is complex and not fully understood (Hermann, 1979). It decreases blood glucose levels of diabetics and adipose non-diabetics, but not of normal subjects. It does not stimulate insulin release but does require that some insulin be present for it to exert a hypoglycaemic effect. It appears to act directly on insulin target cells to enhance insulin action. Some data indicate that metformin increases the number of low-affinity insulin-receptor-binding sites on the erythrocytes of obese patients with Type-II diabetes (Lord et al., 1983). Similar results were obtained using monocytes (Trischitta et al., 1983). Accordingly, the drug potentiates insulin suppression of hepatic gluconeogenesis (Wollen and Bailey, 1988a) and increases insulin-mediated peripheral glucose uptake and metabolism, anaerobic glycolysis, glucose efflux and increase in lipolysis.

Interpretation of the changes in insulin binding after metformin dosing is still controversial. Although metformin may increase insulin receptor binding, its main effect appears to be directed at the post-receptor level of insulin action (Bailey and Natrass, 1988; Gregorio et al., 1990; Bailey, 1992). The change in binding may be secondary to pH changes (see section 5.1 on lactacidosis). The increase in insulin binding in various cell types by metformin is not universal and does not correlate with stimulation of glucose utilization. Furthermore, changes in insulin binding and insulin internalization by isolated monocytes do not correlate with the improvement in glycaemic control. In addition, direct effects of the drug on the glucose-transport system have been demonstrated. Metformin elevates the uptake of non-metabolizable analogues of glucose in both non-diabetic rat adipocytes and diabetic mouse muscle. In the latter, the stimulatory effect of the drug is additive to that of insulin. In human and rat muscle cells in culture, metformin increases glucose-analogue transport independently of and additively to insulin. Most of these results suggest that the basis for the hypoglycaemic effect of this biguanide is probably at the level of skeletal muscle by increasing glucose transport across the cell membrane (Klip and Leiter, 1990). It was proposed that the molecular basis of metformin action in skeletal muscle involves the subcellular redistribution of GLUT-1 proteins from an intracellular compartment to the plasma membrane; such a recruitment process may form an integral part of the mechanism by which the drug stimulates glucose uptake and utilization in skeletal muscle and facilitates lowering of blood glucose in the management of Type-II diabetes (Hundal et al., 1992). The presence of insulin is required, and enhancement of insulin action at the post-receptor level occurs in peripheral tissues such as muscle.

In peripheral tissues metformin increases insulin-mediated glucose uptake and oxidative metabolism. Metformin also increases glucose utilization by the intestine, primarily via non-oxidative metabolism. The extra lactate produced is largely extracted by the liver and serves as a substrate to sustain gluconeogenesis. This limits the extent to which metformin reduces hepatic glucose production but provides a safeguard against excessive glucose lowering (Bailey, 1992).

Biguanides inhibit the enteric absorption of glucose. Owing to appetite loss the patient is forced to take smaller meals. They do not work when given parenterally.

The effect of metformin on insulin binding and insulin action in the presence of anti-insulin receptor antibodies was investigated in a case of type B extreme insulin resistance (DiPaolo, 1992). Addition of metformin to antibody in preincubation buffer strongly enhanced basal glucose incorporation into lipids, but did not prevent insulin unresponsiveness (DiPaolo, 1992). Controversial recent data show that metformin and phenformin potentiate, at least in rats, the late phase of the insulin-secretory response to high glucose (16.7 mM) mainly by facilitating the transmembrane $Ca^{2+}$ ion influx responsible for the second phase of insulin release (Gregorio et al., 1989).

Metformin profoundly alters the sensitivity of adenylate cyclase to inhibition by insulin, with inhibition being increased to some 32% using liver membranes from either lean or obese animals (Gawler et al., 1988, 1989). Metformin also changes the kinetics of inhibition of adenylate cyclase by insulin (Gawler et al., 1988).

Metformin achieves a 23% lower mean $HbA_1$ than placebo (Dornan *et al.*, 1991). Unlike sulphonylureas, it is not bound to plasma proteins (no drug interactions), is not metabolized and is eliminated rapidly by the kidney (Bailey, 1992).

## 2.2 EFFECTS ON GLUCOSE METABOLISM

Metformin treatment has no significant effect on basal glucose uptake but increases insulin-stimulated glucose transport of isolated adipocytes (Matthaei *et al.*, 1991). Its effects on intestinal glucose absorption, insulin secretion and hepatic glucose production are insufficient to explain its hypoglycaemic action, with most evidence suggesting that the major effect of the drug is on glucose utilization. *In vivo* and *in vitro* studies have demonstrated that metformin stimulates the insulin-induced component of glucose uptake into skeletal muscle and adipocytes in both diabetic individuals and animal models. This increase is more significant in diabetic than in non-diabetic animals, suggesting an enhanced action of the drug in the hyperglycaemic state. The increase in glucose uptake is also reflected in an increase in the insulin-dependent portion of glucose oxidation.

Insulin-stimulated glucose uptake measured during hyperinsulinaemic clamp studies was similar before and after metformin treatment. Thus, the ability of metformin to lower plasma glucose concentration in NIDDM does not appear to be secondary to an improvement in insulin action (Wu *et al.*, 1990).

A clamp study revealed that metformin treatment was associated with an enhanced insulin-mediated glucose utilization, whereas insulin-mediated suppression of hepatic glucose production was unchanged (Hother-Nielsen, 1989). Also basal glucose clearance was improved whereas basal hepatic glucose production was unchanged. Metformin treatment in obese Type-II diabetic patients therefore reduces hyperglycaemia without changing the insulin secretion (Hother-Nielsen, 1989).

## 2.3 EFFECTS ON LIPID METABOLISM

Metformin treatment of patients with NIDDM led to an improvement in both glycaemic control and lipoprotein metabolism (Wu *et al.*, 1990). Triglycerides are reduced by 40% in patients with hyperlipoproteinaemia. Metformin helps combat hypertriglyceridaemia (Bailey, 1992) and has been ascribed some vasoprotective properties (Bailey, 1992). Metformin prevents experimental atherosclerosis and induces structural changes in lipoproteins in experimental animals. The reduction in total and LDL cholesterol levels was shown for diabetic patients with hypercholesterolaemia (Rains *et al.*, 1989; Pentikäinen *et al.*, 1990; Landin *et al.*, 1991). While a reduction in VLDL is observed together with improved glucose control irrespective of the applied method, the observed compositional changes in VLDL and LDL appear to be metformin-specific (Schneider *et al.*, 1990).


2.4  BLOOD PARAMETERS


Tissue plasminogen activator (t-PA) activity is increased and t-PA antigen decreased (Landin *et al.*, 1991).


2.5  USE AND ADMINISTRATION


Metformin is an antihyperglycaemic agent which can be used to decrease resistance to insulin. It is used in NIDDM when dietary control and sulphonylureas have failed (Clarke and Campbell, 1977; Siitonen *et al.*, 1980). It is sometimes given to patients who no longer respond to sulphonylureas. Overweight NIDDM patients may experience a beneficial weight loss (Bailey, 1992) and this has sometimes been the rationale behind combining insulin and metformin in insulin-dependent diabetes (Gin *et al.*, 1982; Pagano *et al.*, 1983; Bonora *et al.*, 1984).

The administration of metformin at bedtime instead of supper time may improve diabetes control by reducing morning hyperglycaemia (Ravina and Minuchin, 1990). Metformin was not distinguished from tolbutamide in elderly diabetic patients, except in that it was associated with weight loss (Josephkutty and Potter, 1990).


### 2.5.1  Combination with Sulphonylureas


The rationale for this combination is based on the different sites of action of the two kinds of drug and the possibility of obtaining additive or potentiating effects and reduced side effects (see Raptis *et al.*, 1990). The clinical usefulness of chlorpropamide and glyburide in combination with metformin has been demonstrated in some clinical trials. The combination may provide satisfactory glycaemic control for several years, and possibly insulin therapy can be postponed or even avoided. No special safety problems are encountered with the use of the combination other than those attributed to the use of metformin or sulphonylurea alone, i.e. lactacidosis and hypoglycaemia respectively. The lethality risks of these associated conditions are comparable (Hermann, 1979). Low doses of metformin (500 mg twice daily) were administered to 20 diabetic patients, combined with the original sulphonylurea treatment which had become ineffective even at full dosage.

After 1 and 5 weeks, metformin clearly improved glycaemic control by reducing fasting blood glucose (Gregorio et al., 1990); the diurnal blood glucose average fell from 235.33 to 174.66 mg dl$^{-1}$ after 1 week and to 177.65 ± 21.71 mg dl$^{-1}$ after 5 weeks (Gregorio et al., 1990).

## 3 Pharmacokinetics

### 3.1 DOSAGE AND APPLICATION

Treatment with biguanides should begin with a small dose of medication and a progressive build-up over a 1–2-week period (Asmal and Marble, 1984). As far as metformin is concerned, its elimination half-life requires a dosage interval of about 8 h or more (three times or twice a day) which will not induce accumulation when renal function is normal (Pentikäinen et al., 1979).

Metformin is given as a hydrochloride, chlorophenoxyacetate or embonate salt (Martindale, 1989). Therapeutically effective doses are initially 500–850 mg per day which can be increased to about 3000 mg per day (Waldhäusl, 1987). It should preferentially be given two to three times a day (500–850 mg) after meals.

### 3.2 PHARMACOKINETIC PARAMETERS

Metformin is less lipophilic than buformin or phenformin because of its shorter side chain (Table 7).

#### 3.2.1 Absorption

Metformin has an absolute oral bioavailability of about 50–60% of the dose after oral application of a single dose. Deconvolution analysis showed that after a short lag-time, the available remainder of the oral dose was absorbed at an exponential rate over about 6 h (Tucker et al., 1981). The bioavailability of phenformin seems to be more variable but also in the range of about 50% (Beckmann, 1968; Travis and Sayers, 1970). In general, absorption of biguanides is slower than their elimination, hence the plasma levels follow flip–flop kinetics (Pentikäinen et al., 1979).

#### 3.2.2 Plasma Levels

Maximal plasma levels of about 1.5–2.5 mg l$^{-1}$ after a single oral dose of 0.5–1.5 g were reached after 2–4 h (Tucker et al., 1981). The plasma levels

TABLE 7[a]
Pharmacokinetic data of the biguanides

| Compound | | $t_{1/2}$ (h) | Bioavailability (%) | Free plasma fraction (%) | Volume of distribution ($1\,kg^{-1}$) | Fraction excreted unchanged (%) | Total clearance ($ml\,min^{-1}$) |
|---|---|---|---|---|---|---|---|
| Buformin | (e) | 2–6 | – | 80 | – | 100 | 540 |
| | (d) | 1 | – | – | – | – | – |
| Metformin | (e) | 1.5–3 | 60 | 100 | 1 | 100 | 450 |
| | (e)ii | 9 | – | (80) | – | – | – |
| | (b) | 3 | – | – | – | – | – |
| Phenformin | (e) | 9–13 | – | 80 | – | 90 | – |

[a]Taken from Pentikäinen et al. (1979) and Tucker et al. (1981).

$t_{1/2}$ (half-life): e, terminal elimination; (e)ii, second phase of elimination period; d, distribution; b, biological effect.

obtained after continuous application can be predicted from the single-dose kinetics although a discrepancy is seen between the predicted and measured-through levels because of the existence of a slow elimination phase (Tucker et al., 1981). For a daily dose of 1700 mg, a mean plasma level of $0.38\,mg\,l^{-1}$ was obtained, and at 2550 mg per day about $1.04\,mg\,l^{-1}$ (Sirtori et al., 1978).

### 3.2.3 Distribution

Metformin is rapidly distributed, and accumulates in these tissues in which the drug possesses most of its activity (muscles, intestine, liver). For buformin, diffusion in the peripheral compartment is reported to be faster than the rediffusion, leading to an accumulation in the respective tissues (Lintz et al., 1974). Plasma protein binding of the biguanides is only about 20% (Garret et al., 1972) or even undetectable (Rang and Dale, 1991).

### 3.2.4 Elimination and Metabolism

Buformin and metformin undergo glomerular filtration and tubular secretion. In contrast, about one-third of a dose of phenformin is hydroxylated in the liver and partially excreted in the bile. The remainder undergoes renal excretion unchanged (Asmal and Marble, 1984). Nevertheless, for metformin and buformin the urinary recovery of the administered dose is sometimes only about 80%, with no metabolites being detected. Therefore secretion into the intestine in humans was suggested (Lintz *et al.*, 1974). The elimination kinetics is represented by a rapid first phase with a half-life of about 1.7–3 h, which is valid for more than 90% of the absorbed amount, and a slow elimination phase with a half-life of 9–12 h for the remaining 5–10% (Sirtori *et al.*, 1978).

### 3.3 PATHOLOGICAL CHANGES IN THE PHARMACOKINETICS

The elimination of biguanides is correlated with renal function, hence the elimination of metformin follows creatinine clearance. For buformin, the elimination in mild renal failure is unchanged (Held *et al.*, 1970). The elimination half-life of metformin increases with renal failure; at a creatinine clearance of 20–48 ml min$^{-1}$ it is increased to about 5 h because of a decrease in metformin clearance from 450 ml min$^{-1}$ to only 88 ml min$^{-1}$ (Sirtori *et al.*, 1978). Hydroxylation of phenformin is influenced by the genetic polymorphism of the mono-oxygenase. With high circulating amounts of phenformin its metabolism is reduced (Bosisio *et al.*, 1981). Both pathological effects on liver and kidney account for an accumulation of the drug and a related risk of lactacidosis.

## 4 Toxic Effects

Acute poisoning with metformin calls for intensive supportive therapy. Lactacidosis may require treatment with sodium bicarbonate or furosemide, a combination of insulin and glucose or peritoneal dialysis or haemodialysis (Lalau *et al.*, 1989).

## 5 Side Effects

Metformin can cause adverse gastrointestinal effects with anorexia, nausea and vomiting. Patients may experience a metallic taste and there may be weight loss, which in some diabetics could be an advantage. Hypoglycaemia is less of a problem with metformin than with sulphonylureas.

### 5.1 LACTACIDOSIS

This side effect is rare, but dangerous and serious (Misbin, 1977; Korbonen *et al.*, 1979). Lactacidosis, which is fatal in 50% of cases, occurs less with metformin than with phenformin (Cavallo-Perin *et al.*, 1989), usually in patients whose condition contraindicated the use of metformin in the first place. There may be the possibility of a process of adaptation on prolonged treatment (Chandalia and Rangnath, 1990). It was estimated in 1983 that there had only been 28 cases of lactacidosis with metformin; at the time of this estimate the worldwide population receiving metformin was considered to be 650 000 (Lucis, 1983).

Kidney failure requires special attention because of metformin accumulation. Severe lactacidotic coma despite normal renal function has been reported in a 35-year-old diabetic man taking metformin and alcohol (Ryder, 1984). While fasting plasma lactate concentrations remained unaltered after metformin, a rise was noted in response to meals (from $1.4 \pm 0.1$ to $1.8 \pm 0.2$ mM) (Pedersen et al., 1989). Arterial blood gas analysis in one case revealed a pH of 6.76 and a bicarbonate level of 1.6 mM before treatment of lactacidosis. After therapy, which included oxygen, volume expansion and haemodialysis, the patient completely recovered (Gan et al., 1992).

Metformin treatment is associated with less imbalance of intracellular redox state than phenformin, and therefore should be considered advantageous in the long-term treatment of non-insulin-dependent diabetics (Cavallo-Perin et al., 1989). In vitro, the antigluconeogenic effect of $10^{-2}$ M metformin alone is associated with an increased mitochondrial $NADH/NAD^+$ ratio. Thus a reduction in gluconeogenesis caused by high concentrations of metformin may involve changes in redox state. However, therapeutic concentrations of metformin potentiate the antigluconeogenic effect of insulin to a similar extent from a range of substrates, without altering energy status or redox state (Wollen and Bailey, 1988b). Metformin increases glucose utilization, primarily via non-oxidative metabolism; the extra lactate produced is largely extracted by the liver and serves as a substrate to sustain gluconeogenesis (Bailey, 1992).

In order to avoid lactacidosis, it is important to select patients correctly and to ensure that contraindications such as renal involvement, advanced age and chronic alcoholism are observed before treatment with metformin (Lebech and Olesen, 1990). The role of lactic acid in the triggering of panic attacks has been discussed (Gin et al., 1989b).

The risk of lactate accumulation should be appreciated in patients with renal insufficiency, liver dysfunction and after acute illness with hypoxia, when therapy should be stopped. Although metformin is often bracketed with phenformin in the context of lactacidosis, different pharmacodynamics and adherence to prescribing guidelines render such a comparison unwarranted (Bailey and Nattrass, 1988).

5.2  OTHER SIDE EFFECTS

Biguanides are implicated in controversial reports of excessive cardiovascular mortality associated with oral hypoglycaemic therapy (Paterson et al., 1984).

Metformin affects platelet aggregation independently of other metabolic factors (Gin et al., 1989a). Leucopenia and thrombocytopenia are very rare.

Gastrointestinal side effects include loss of appetite, nausea, vomiting and taste disturbances (15–25%). A retrospective survey of diarrhoea episodes in treated diabetic patients was carried out by Dandona et al. (1983). Of 265 patients investigated, 30 reported diarrhoea or alternating diarrhoea and constipation: 11 from 54 taking metformin; 9 from 45 taking metformin with a sulphonylurea; 3 from 53 taking a sulphonylurea only; 5 from 78 on insulin therapy; 2 from 35 on diet alone. Of 150 non-diabetic controls, 12 reported having diarrhoea (Dandona et al., 1983).

## 6  Interactions with Other Drugs

Malabsorption of vitamin $B_{12}$ was observed in 14 of 46 diabetics taking metformin or phenformin (Callaghan et al., 1980; Adams et al., 1983); metformin was more often to blame. Withdrawal of the drug resulted in normal absorption in only 7 of the 14 (Adams et al., 1983).

Tetracyclines increase the danger of biguanide-induced lact-acidosis. Dietary fibre and by-products of some vegetable extracts (guar etc.) are advocated to reduce postprandial hyperglycaemia (see chapter 9). Metformin blood levels showed that when given together with guar there was a reduction in the absorption rate over the first 6 h (Pedersen et al., 1989).

## 7  Clinical Studies

### 7.1  HEALTHY VOLUNTEERS

Biguanides do not affect glycaemia in normal individuals and do not increase insulin output. However, because the liver is the dominant site of action in a physiological in vivo situation, hepatic glucose transport is reduced leading to an increased hepatic insulin sensitivity.

In normal obese hyperinsulinaemic subjects, metformin $3 \times 50$ mg daily influenced insulin binding with increases in insulin receptor capacity (Vigneri et al., 1984), while in normal-weight volunteers no effect on number and affinity of insulin receptors was noted.

Clinical studies indicate a lipid-lowering effect of biguanides (metformin), particularly in patients with hyperlipoproteinaemia type IV (Gustafson et al., 1971; Descovich et al., 1978). A slight reduction in total serum cholesterol was also noted in non-diabetic hyperlipidaemia by Aro et al. (1985). In a double-blind cross-over study of 9 weeks duration with 1 or 2 g metformin, cholesterol was reduced from 328 mg per 100 ml to 313 mg per 100 ml and 294 mg per 100 ml. HDL cholesterol remained unchanged. Metformin, however, is not recommended as the drug of choice in hyperlipoproteinaemia.

In obese NIDDM, metformin tends to promote weight loss. This, however, is felt to be more a "weight-stabilizing effect" than a genuine weight-reducing action. In healthy subjects, biguanides should therefore not be used as anorectic agents.

There have been various reports that metformin increases fibrinolysis, reduces thrombus formation (Weichert and Breddin, 1988) and reduces platelet adhesiveness and aggregation (Holmes et al., 1984). This, however, was mostly felt to be secondary to improved glycaemic control, because similar effects have been reported with sulphonylureas (Vague et al., 1987). In healthy subjects, biguanides should therefore not be used to increase fibrinolytic activity.

## 7.2   TYPE-I DIABETES MELLITUS

Biguanides should not be used for the treatment of IDDM. Biguanides (metformin) have a hypoglycaemic potency which is more of an antihyperglycaemic action since it cannot induce clinical hypoglycaemia. Metformin is not effective via an insulinotropic action. It has, however, an acute insulin-like effect in vitro (Fantus and Brosseau, 1986) and acts in vivo at post-receptor sites without significant effects on insulin-binding capacity (Nosadini et al., 1987). Metformin increases the sensitivity of the liver to insulin and induces a reduction of insulin requirements in Type-I diabetes up to 26% following an additional metformin treatment (2 × 850 mg) for 2 days (Gin et al., 1982). A 25% reduction in insulin was reported by Pagano et al. (1983) following an additional metformin therapy in NIDDM patients as assessed with the artificial pancreas. An increased response to insulin in Type-I diabetics after metformin administration was also noted by Keen et al. (1987).

Metformin might therefore be used to ameliorate the glycaemic profile in Type-I diabetes, with a possible reduction in insulin requirement.

Metformin has also been used occasionally to reduce insulin requirement in cases of true insulin resistance: those requiring more than 200 units a day. In contrast with others (Stowers, 1980), however, we feel that biguanides should not be used at all in gestational diabetes or pregnant Type-I diabetic women.

## 7.3   TYPE-II DIABETES MELLITUS

Biguanides, mainly metformin, are primarily indicated for the treatment of Type-II diabetes, where satisfactory control of blood glucose cannot be obtained by diet alone. The use of metformin in the treatment of diabetes is based on over 30 years of clinical experience. Although still controversial in some respects, metformin is regarded as a valuable drug in the treatment of obese non-ketonic hyperinsulinaemic insulin-resistant Type-II diabetics (Dornan et al., 1988). The main clinical effect of metformin is an antidiabetic action. In addition, metformin has weight-reducing and lipid-lowering properties and effects on fibrinolysis (Campbell, 1990) which could be of additional advantage during treatment of obese diabetics suffering from the metabolic syndrome (Vigneri and Goldfine, 1987).

There are three conditions for the clinical use of metformin as a glucose-lowering agent in patients with NIDDM: (1) as a primary drug, (2) in combination with other oral hypoglycaemic agents such as sulphonylureas and acarbose, and (3) together with insulin after secondary sulphonylurea failure.

Metformin used as monotherapy reduced plasma glucose levels in normal-weight Type-II diabetics considerably (172 to 103 mg per 100 ml), whereas serum insulin was unchanged over a 3 month period (Jackson et al., 1987). The hypoglycaemic action of metformin became fully effective within 2–3 weeks of treatment. Clinical studies point out that gastrointestinal side effects can be avoided if medication is started slowly and taken postprandially (Fig. 25).

More effective blood glucose lowering can be achieved in obese Type-II diabetics where a lowering of fasting blood glucose was noted from 260 to 116 mg per 100 ml and a postprandial drop from 280 to 136 mg per 100 ml (Granovskaja-Svetkova, 1977). In obese Type-II diabetics, Lord et al. (1983) studied the effect of 1500 mg metformin and recorded a decrease in fasting blood glucose from 200 to 160 mg per 100 ml and a reduction of $HbA_1$ from 14.0 to 12.6%.

A reduction in hyperinsulinaemia caused by metformin has been demonstrated in several clinical studies (Schatz et al., 1972; Hausmann and Schubotz, 1975; Ferlito et al., 1983). Sensitivity to insulin was also found to be increased after short-term biguanide treatment with phenformin, buformin and metformin. Biguanides increase both sensitivity to insulin and responsiveness in muscle and to a lesser extent in adipose tissue (Bailey et al., 1984).

A comparison of the blood glucose-lowering effect of metformin and sulphonylureas did not reveal significant differences in their hypoglycaemic–antihyperglycaemic potency or the number of primary or secondary failures in newly diagnosed Type-II diabetics over a 12-month period (Clarke et al., 1967). While sulphonylurea-treated patients gained body weight, metformin therapy induced a weight loss. Similar results were noted in a cross-over trial reported by Clarke and Duncan (1968).

A reduction in hyperinsulinaemia following metformin treatment is the most important argument for the clinical use in obese insulin-resistant Type-II

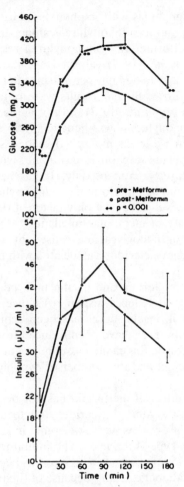

FIG. 25. Mean plasma glucose and plasma insulin responses to oral glucose before
(●) and after (○) 1 week of metformin treatment in NIDDM patients. Plasma glucose
concentrations decreased significantly. (Source: Fantus and Brosseau, 1986.)

diabetics. Despite the controversy about hyperinsulinaemia as an independent risk factor for coronary heart disease, there is no doubt of its relationship
to other risk factors (Campbell, 1990). In contrast to sulphonylureas, the
non-insulinotropic biguanides are therefore the drug of choice (together with
acarbose) for the treatment of dietary failure in obese Type-II diabetes
mellitus. Fasting and postprandial serum insulin after 3 months of metformin
is significantly lower than after treatment with sulphonylureas (McAlpine et
al., 1988).

A combination of biguanides with sulphonylurea can be useful in patients who have failed to respond to sulphonylureas alone. In "secondary failure", the combination of metformin and sulphonylurea responded in more than 50% of cases. Clarke *et al.* (1967) reported a clinical study where blood glucose dropped from 266 to 184 mg per 100 ml after 12 weeks and $HbA_1$ improved from 9.1 to 7.6%. Similar results were obtained by Haupt *et al.* (1989). In contrast, Debry *et al.* (1977) did not agree that the combination of biguanides and sulphonylureas was beneficial. No significant differences were seen in blood glucose levels in Type-II diabetics treated with metformin + sulphonylureas versus sulphonylureas alone, while serum insulin was higher after sulphonylurea treatment only. It has been reported that the choice between metformin and metformin + sulphonylureas does not depend on the age or sex of the subjects. The only factor of therapeutic importance is the degree of intensity of metabolic imbalance.

The mortality risk for hypoglycaemia caused by sulphonylureas is not significantly different from lactacidosis associated with metformin (Campbell, 1984).

The combination of metformin and insulin in Type-II diabetics increases the efficacy of insulin and reduces insulin resistance in obese patients. A considerable reduction in insulin doses has been achieved (Leblanc *et al.*, 1987). Free serum insulin levels have been reduced from 51 to 41 units/ml$^{-1}$ (Stowers, 1980). On mixed biguanide–insulin treatment, the atherogenic effect of hyperinsulinaemia and the number of hypoglycaemic reactions can be reduced.

The hypolipidaemic effect of metformin has not been elucidated satisfactorily. The reduction of serum triglycerides and to a smaller extent total plasma cholesterol, however, is very welcome in the treatment of the metabolic syndrome in Type-II diabetes. The inhibitory effect of metformin on fatty acid oxidation (Schönborn *et al.*, 1975) has been regarded as pivotal in its mechanism of antidiabetic action, because of the interrelations between fatty acid and carbohydrate metabolism.

In conclusion, it can be stated, that biguanides, preferably metformin, have been shown in innumerable clinical trials to be highly effective as antihyperglycaemic drugs. Together with acarbose, they may be the first-choice drug for the treatment of obese hyperinsulinaemic, insulin resistant Type-II diabetics with dietary failure. They help to correct most of the unwanted aspects of the metabolic syndrome, which is felt to contribute most to the high mortality rate of NIDDM patients with heart disease.

# Compounds Acting on Glucose Absorption

## 1 Guar

### 1.1 CHEMISTRY

Guar is derived from the endosperm of the seed *Cyamopsis psoraloides* (*C. tetragonoloba*). It contains more than 66% high-molecular-mass polysaccharides. D-Mannose molecules are 1,4β-connected, and every second mannose is connected to D-galactose in position 6.

1.2 ACTIONS

The postprandial (Jenkins *et al.*, 1977b; Morgan *et al.*, 1979; Torsdottir *et al.*, 1989; Lim *et al.*, 1990; Satchithanandam *et al.*, 1990) increases in blood glucose and insulin concentrations in response to carbohydrate-containing meals are reduced in healthy subjects when they eat test meals containing guar gum, pectin or both (Jenkins *et al.*, 1977b). Even basal plasma glucose may be slightly reduced. Guar postpones the absorption of carbohydrates, but does not avoid it. It is widely accepted that insulin levels fall in parallel (Chuang *et al.*, 1992). Mean urinary glucose excretion falls markedly in diabetics when guar gum is added to their diet (Jenkins *et al.*, 1977a). Guar reduces the rate of amino acid absorption and amino acid-stimulated insulin release (Gulliford *et al.*, 1988a). Modulation of intestinal mechanisms is sufficient to mediate the latter effect (Gulliford *et al.*, 1988b). The reduction in peripheral blood insulin levels caused by guar is not associated with a change in hepatic insulin extraction (Gulliford *et al.*, 1988b).

Postprandial glucose-dependent insulinotropic polypeptide (GIP) levels were lowered in a guar-gum-supplemented meal (Morgan *et al.*, 1990) and may contribute to lower insulin levels. Guar delays intestinal calcium absorption in humans (Gulliford *et al.*, 1988b). The decrease in pancreatic amylase release may simply be a result of diminished insular–exocrine axis.

Optimistic reports about fibre supplementation in the management of diabetes need to be confirmed by careful long-term studies, since there exist negative findings for obese poorly controlled diabetics given guar gum or bran (Cohen and Martin, 1979). A brief review of guar gum concluded that its contribution to the management of diabetic patients remains unproven.

The efficacy of guar is probably dependent mainly on its capacity to hydrate rapidly and thus to increase viscosity in the small intestine postprandially. Measurement of the rate of hydration *in vitro* might therefore be a useful index of the effectiveness of guar formulations. A simple method for monitoring the hydration rate of guar gum has been developed (Ellis and Morris, 1991). Marked differences in hydration rate and ultimate (maximum) viscosity between the different guar samples were observed (Ellis and Morris, 1991). These results may explain why some guar gum preparations are clinically ineffective (Ellis and Morris, 1991).

*1.2.1 Uses and Administration*

Guar gum is used in diabetes mellitus as an adjunct to treatment with diet, insulin or oral hypoglycaemics because it is considered to reduce the peak blood glucose concentrations that occur following meals. It cannot be used instead of other/earlier therapy regimes. It must not be used to reduce obesity. It is given with or immediately before meals in doses of 5 g usually three times daily; each dose should be taken with about 200 ml of water. Guar gum is available in various formulations that attempt to overcome its unpalatability. It is also used to slow gastric emptying in patients with the dumping syndrome and as a thickening agent, emulsion stabilizer and suspending agent as well as a release-retarding material for formulating tablets (Jain *et al.*, 1992).

### 1.2.2   Glucose Metabolism

Guar has no effect on glucose metabolism (Torsdottir *et al.*, 1989).

### 1.2.3   Lipid Metabolism

Many details can be found in numerous papers (Kirsten *et al.*, 1989; Wilson *et al.*, 1989; Lalor *et al.*, 1990; Turner *et al.*, 1990; Uusitupa *et al.*, 1990). Regular intake (15 g for 2 weeks) decreases cholesterol and triglyceride levels by 5–15%, especially LDL. The mechanism is similar to that of cholestyramine (binding of cholic acids) (Todd *et al.*, 1990). Guar gum and its hydrolysate suppresses 3-hydroxy-3-methylglutaryl-coenzyme A (HMG-CoA) reductase activities in the ileum to one-half (Gulliford *et al.*, 1988a). For reducing LDL cholesterol, lovastatin (a HMG-CoA reductase inhibitor) was much more active in combination with cholestyramine than with guar gum (Uusitupa *et al.*, 1991). Guar gum at 6 and 12% in the diet reduces total serum cholesterol by 31 and 51%, respectively, in male sea quail fed on a diet containing 0.5% cholesterol for a period of 1 week (Day, 1991). Plasma cholesterol levels but not triglycerides were significantly lower when soluble gums were consumed for 4 weeks (Behall, 1990).

### 1.2.4   Blood Parameters

Guar has no effect on blood parameters.

### 1.3   PHARMACOKINETICS

### 1.3.1   Dosage and Application

Guar is given with or immediately before meals in doses of 5 g, usually three times daily. Each dose should be taken with about 200–250 ml of liquids (water) (Martindale, 1989).

## 1.3.2   Pharmacokinetic Parameters

Absorption of guar cannot be detected. Its site of action is localized inside the gastrointestinal tract and no absorption is required for effective action. There are no data on absorption, distribution or excretion from plasma.

Excretion from the intestinal tract is accompanied by destruction of the polysaccharides due to microorganisms in the colon (information from the manufacturer).

## 1.4   TOXIC AND SIDE EFFECTS

Guar gum can cause gastrointestinal disturbance with flatulence, diarrhoea or nausea, particularly at the start of the treatment. It should not be used in patients with oesophageal/intestinal obstruction (Opper et al., 1990).

Insufficient data are available on the long-term safety of high-fibre supplements. People at risk of deficiencies, such as postmenopausal women, the elderly, or growing children, may require supplements of calcium and trace minerals. People with upper gastrointestinal dysfunction risk bezoar formation and should be cautioned against a diet high in fibre of the leafy vegetable type. Careful attention must be paid to insulin doses because hypoglycaemia can appear if there is a radical change in fibre intake without appropriate reduction in insulin dose. Care must be exercised in the use of "novel" fibres, including wood celluloses, because little is known of their safety and efficacy.

## 1.5   INTERACTIONS WITH OTHER DRUGS

There is a risk of guar gum affecting the absorption of other drugs. A delay in absorption was observed for sulphonylureas (adapt dose), hormonal contraceptives and oral penicillins (stop guar medication). Guar ingested with glibenclamide did not interfere with its absorption (Uusitupa et al., 1990). Measurement of blood metformin levels showed that, when given together with guar, there was a reduction in the absorption rate over the first 6 h (Gin et al., 1989b). These findings suggest that combination therapy may diminish the antihyperglycaemic action of metformin.

## 1.6   CLINICAL STUDIES

Speculation that fibre-depleted diets may play a role in the development of diabetes has increased the interest in recent studies suggesting that high-fibre diets may be beneficial for treating subjects with diabetes (Anderson et al., 1979).

Dietary fibres have important effects on gastrointestinal physiology and can also therefore be a useful adjunct to the conventional treatment of several metabolic and gastrointestinal diseases.

### 1.6.1 Healthy Volunteers

Clinical studies in healthy subjects demonstrate that the acute addition of the viscous types of dietary fibre such as the gel-forming polysaccharide guar leads to a decrease in postprandial hyperglycaemia by a reduction in gastric-emptying rates and slowing of intestinal carbohydrate absorption.

The **short-term efficacy** of guar on postprandial glucose lowering has been repeatedly shown (Jenkins et al., 1977a, 1978; Johnson and Gee, 1980; Schwartz et al., 1982). The acute effect of guar on carbohydrate and fat metabolism lasts at least 4 h and may result in improved carbohydrate tolerance to subsequent guar-free meals (Jenkins et al., 1980).

Large test meals given to healthy volunteers with fibre supplements clearly induced a postprandial glycaemia, which was significantly less than after a meal alone (Jenkins et al., 1976). A lowering of the postprandial blood glucose response was also seen after consumption of 10 g of guar and 2.5 g of other fibres compared with a placebo without fibres (McIvor et al., 1985). Fibres other than guar, such as gum tragacanth and methylcellulose, reduced hyperglycaemia to a lesser extent, and the effects of bran and cholestyramine were unimpressive (Jenkins et al., 1978).

In other studies, the effects of high-fibre diets on blood glucose levels were generally felt to be rather small (Simpson et al., 1981), and it was noted that postprandial blood glucose levels are influenced only when fibre content is fivefold higher than that of the normal British diet, whereby the effects of the dietary fibre source on carbohydrate metabolism seem to depend on the composition of the source.

No effect of guar gum was seen when hydrolysed non-viscous preparations were used (Jenkins et al., 1978). The viscosity of guar on hydration is of importance in assessing the efficacy of a preparation in clinical use. Addition of guar to a glucose drink had no statistically significant effect on peak blood glucose levels and no effects were seen in patients who had had total gastrectomy (Holt et al., 1979).

It appears that guar must be intimately mixed with the main carbohydrate portion of the meal. When only sprinkled over a meal it remained ineffective (Williams et al., 1980).

**Long-term effects** of plant fibre ingestion on carbohydrate tolerance were examined by Walker et al. (1970) in rural Bantu and urban Caucasian children and African and European students. In groups with high dietary fibre intake the glycaemic and serum insulin response to glucose was always significantly lower. Improved glucose tolerance has also been described in volunteers who had been maintained for extended periods on diets supplemented with fibre (Munoz *et al.*, 1979). These studies suggested, however, that dietary fibre may not only decrease the absorption of carbohydrates but may also have a systemic effect, perhaps by enhancing the peripheral insulin sensitivity and may therefore be beneficial in the management of diabetes mellitus.

### 1.6.2   Type-I Diabetes Mellitus

In patients with Type-I diabetes (IDDM), short-term effects of high-fibre diet resulted in a reduction in postprandial elevation of blood glucose and a reduction in insulin doses. Miranda and Horwitz (1978) fed high-fibre diets to patients with insulin-requiring diabetes for 10 days. The insulin doses were maintained constant and postprandial glucose values were significantly lower than those attained on low-fibre diets. The fact that these patients had more hypoglycaemic reactions was felt to be due to an increased tissue sensitivity to insulin. Increased insulin receptor binding to monocytes and adipocytes has been observed in both insulin- and non-insulin-dependent diabetic patients (Hollund *et al.*, 1983).

An insulin-saving effect was noted after 21 days on a high-carbohydrate high-fibre diet, where the dose was reduced from 25 to 10 units daily (Anderson *et al.*, 1979). In a similar study by Kiehm *et al.* (1976), however, it appeared that the major factor responsible for the improvement in glucose metabolism was more the 75% carbohydrate content than the crude dietary fibre content. Nevertheless, the postprandial glucose levels in labile and stable IDMM patients improved (Monnier *et al.*, 1981), and fasting serum triglycerides were also significantly lower. In addition, insulin requirements were also found to be reduced (Jenkins *et al.*, 1977b).

Since hyperinsulinaemia may be involved in the pathogenesis of macroangiopathy such as coronary heart disease, guar and other similar effective fibres are highly recommended as useful adjuncts to the treatment of diabetes. In **pregnant insulin-dependent diabetic patients**, however, no improvement in metabolic control could be obtained, if the diet was supplemented with guar $(24 \, \text{g day}^{-1})$. Mean blood glucose levels, glucosuria and mean daily insulin dose did not change significantly. The results show that in these patients hospital admission was more favourable for diabetes control than addition of guar gum to the diet (Kühl *et al.*, 1983).

### 1.6.3   Type-II Diabetes Mellitus

Numerous groups have now demonstrated that high plant fibre intake may have a beneficial effect on glucose metabolism in patients with Type-II diabetes mellitus. Atkins *et al.* (1987) noted a significant improvement in

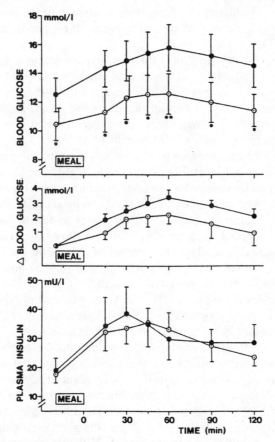

FIG. 26. Blood glucose and plasma insulin levels before and after a standard lunch in Type-II diabetics during supplementation with guar gum (○) or placebo (●). (Source: Aro et al., 1981.)

fasting and postprandial serum glucose and insulin values and a reduction in urinary glucose excretion in non-compliant NIDDM patients. Similar results were obtained in a multicentre study on poorly controlled Type-II diabetics (Laube et al., 1983), where postprandial blood glucose levels in guar-supplemented (3 × 5 g per day) patients were 12% lower than in controls, and urinary glucose excretion could be reduced by 40%.

In another trial, Aro et al. (1981) noted that the mean fasting and postprandial plasma insulin levels were significantly lower in Type-II diabetics after guar supplementation (Fig. 26). A sustained reduction in basal hyperglycaemia, however, was accompanied by only slight reduction in the postprandial increment in blood glucose. The effect described was similar to that found during a high-carbohydrate diet containing natural fibre.

This, however, could not be reproduced when patients were placed on diets containing quantities of uncooked vegetables, seeds, nuts and fruits (Douglass, 1975).

Lowering of fasting and postprandial hyperglycaemia following fibre supplementation resulted in insulin treatment being stopped in 10 Type-II diabetics, treated for an average of 15 months with high-fibre (60 g per day) diet, if less than 30 units of insulin per day were given. However, patients also lost weight and it is debatable whether improvement in metabolism was due to the high-fibre content or to weight loss.

No effect of dietary fibres such as guar was noted if the supplementation was with guar powder (Williams et al., 1980). In 13 maturity-onset non-insulin-dependent diabetics, 10 g of guar failed to decrease significantly the postprandial rise in plasma glucose and insulin seen after a similar meal without supplementation. Only when guar was added to liquid meals or incorporated into foods such as bread, or if dietary fibres had their origin from readily available foods, could metabolic effects be easily identified.

In long-term studies over 1 year, Klimm et al. (1983) noted a reduction in glucosuria up to 70% in the guar-supplemented group, but no effect was seen in the 1 h blood glucose levels. The same was true in NIDDM patients supplemented for 2 months with $2 \times 5$ g guar daily (Jones et al., 1983). Fasting and 1 h postprandial blood glucose did not change but $HbA_1$ fell from 12.0 to 9.4%. It was felt that the blood-glucose monitoring method chosen for that trial was not representative of the whole metabolic situation.

**Serum lipids** can be lowered significantly by plant fibres such as guar gum. In 93 Type-II diabetics, 15 g guar daily lowered the total serum cholesterol from 250 to 225 mg per 100 ml (Laube et al., 1983). Similar effects were reported by Aro et al. (1981). After 3 months guar supplementation LDL cholesterol was significantly lower and LDL/HDL cholesterol ratio was decreased. An impressive improvement in the lipaemic profile was also reported by Tagliaferro et al. (1985) in patients receiving 4 g guar gel in addition to their usual diet for a period of 6 weeks. Guar led to a reduction in total cholesterol (189 versus 169 mg per 100 ml) coupled with an increase in HDL phospholipids.

The effects of guar on serum triglycerides seem less clear and more controversial. A slight decrease in triglycerides was seen in Type-II diabetics following a 15 g guar supplementation for a 4-week period (Laube et al., 1983). No significant lowering of triglycerides was noted by Tagliaferro et al. (1985) and Aro et al. (1981). Similarly, no effects of guar on triglycerides were observed by Atkins et al. (1987) in non-compliant NIDDM fed for 1 month with guar granules. Anderson et al. (1979) called a high-fibre diet ineffective in lowering fasting trigylcerides.

In patients affected by familiar hyperlipidaemia, however, guar gum was highly effective in reducing hyperlipidaemia (Bosello et al., 1984). It therefore appears that the higher the initial cholesterol and triglyceride levels, the

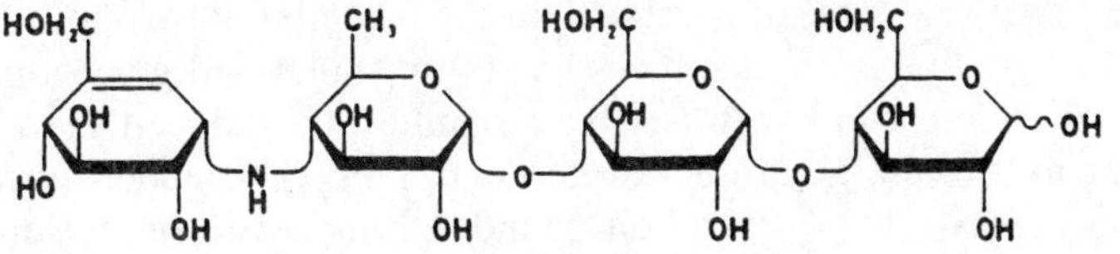

FIG. 27. Chemical structure of acarbose.

greater the decrease after guar supplementation. Improvement in lipaemic profiles in diabetic patients with hyperlipidaemia helps to correct further side effects of the metabolic syndrome in NIDDM by guar gum.

## 2 Acarbose

### 2.1 CHEMISTRY

Acarbose is a pseudotetrasaccharide in which one maltose is exchanged for a pseudomaltose (Fig. 27).

### 2.2 ACTIONS

Many studies have been published (Caspary, 1978; Hillebrand et al., 1979; Sjöström and William-Olsson, 1981; Dimitriadis et al., 1982; Radziuk et al., 1982; Raptis et al., 1982; Aubell et al., 1983; Clissold and Edwards, 1988; Madariaga et al., 1988; Brogard et al., 1989; Reaven et al., 1990). Acarbose decreases alimentary hyperglycaemia and is therefore used in diabetes. It competitively inhibits α-glucosidases, which are important for the degradation of disaccharides during digestion. They are specific for α-connected glucose and digest non-absorbable di-, oligo- and poly-saccharides to absorbable monosaccharides. The affinity of acarbose for saccharase (the enzyme that hydrolyses the dissacharide saccharose to glucose and fructose) is 10 000 to 100 000 times greater than that of saccharose for this enzyme. Because of this the absorption of monosaccharides is delayed. This produces a decrease in the elevated blood glucose levels, $HbA_1$ levels, and postprandial insulin concentrations in diabetics. However, blood glucose cannot be decreased below basal levels, i.e. acarbose is not a hypoglycaemic but an antihyperglycaemic compound. It does not work in the absence of carbohydrates in the meal.

Although the data on $HbA_1$ reduction by about 1% (an indicator of possible late injuries) are contradictory, this may be the major reason to use acarbose. Serum cholesterol, triglycerides and the LDL/HDL ratio are decreased. An oral load of acarbose does not inhibit absorption of glucose; neither does it alter subsequent responses to insulin and glucagon (Richard et al., 1988). Treatment with acarbose significantly reduced the glomerular basement membrane glycation (Cohen et al., 1991). Changes in faecal bile acid and neutral sterol excretion found during acarbose treatment may explain the protective effect of starch malabsorption on colon cancer development (Bartram et al., 1991).

The ability of acarbose to lower plasma glucose concentration was studied in 12 patients with NIDDM who were poorly controlled by diet plus sulphonylurea drugs (Reaven et al., 1990). Neither the plasma insulin response to meals nor insulin-stimulated glucose uptake improved with acarbose therapy, consistent with the view that acarbose improves glycaemic control by delaying glucose absorption. In control obese mice receiving a 10% sucrose-enriched diet, acarbose decreased the gain in body weight, and prevented the rise in glycaemia and insulinaemia (Le-Marchand-Brustel et al., 1990). Insulin receptor autophosphorylation and tyrosine kinase activity were altered in treated and untreated obese mice compared with lean mice (Le-Marchand-Brustel et al., 1990).

Acarbose slows the absorption kinetics of dietary carbohydrates by reversible competitive inhibition of $\alpha$-glucosidase activity, and so reduces the postprandial blood glucose increment and insulin response. For these reasons, the drug has been successfully used not only in the treatment of Type-I and Type-II diabetes, but also in the management of reactive hypoglycaemias and dumping syndrome (McLoughin et al., 1979; Jenkins et al., 1982; Speth et al., 1983). Some results indicate that an $\alpha$-glucosidase inhibitor accelerates mouth to caecum transit time by inducing carbohydrate malabsorption (Ladas et al., 1992).

### 2.2.1 Glycogen Metabolism

The metabolism of skeletal-muscle glycogen is unaffected because of the inability of acarbose to be absorbed (see below) (Calder and Geddes, 1989).

### 2.2.2 Lipid Metabolism

Rabbits fed 30 mg/day acarbose showed reduced levels of plasma cholesterol, intermediate-density lipoprotein (IDL) and LDL (Kritchevsky et al., 1990); sudanophilia was reduced by 23% in rabbits fed 7.5 mg/day acarbose and by 43% in rabbits fed 15 or 30 mg/day (Kritchevsky et al., 1990). The decrease in total cholesterol was shown to be a consequence of a significant reduction in LDL cholesterol. Since HDL cholesterol concentrations remained unaltered, the ratio of HDL/LDL cholesterol changed in a beneficial way (Walter-Sack et al., 1989). Acarbose has been shown to lower serum cholesterol (Kritchevsky et al., 1990; Leonhardt et al., 1991), and to inhibit atherogenesis in rabbits fed 0.2% cholesterol (Kritchevsky et al., 1990). Acarbose decreases cholesterol and fasting triglyceride concentrations, whereas the postprandial increment in triglycerides is not diminished (Walter-Sack et al., 1989). Both the triglyceride- and cholesterol-lowering efficacy were less pronounced with a higher amount of saturated fat than with a lower intake of fat composed mainly of polyunsaturated fatty acids.

### 2.3 USES AND ADMINISTRATION

Acarbose is used in diabetes in addition to other therapeutic regimes in connection with diet. Its clinical usefulness was demonstrated (Hanefeld et al., 1991) but its extent is a matter of controversy. However, a diet is preferable in Type-II diabetes. There are some studies which show the usefulness of its combination with sulphonylureas. Considerable individual variation is noted in the response to acarbose (Reaven et al., 1990). The use of acarbose in patients with NIDDM not well controlled by sulphonylureas appears to have significant clinical benefit (Raptis et al., 1982). One study suggests that it is not an effective substitute for sulphonylureas in non-obese Type-II diabetes uncontrolled by diet alone (Buchanan et al., 1988).

In addition, some data suggest a possible role in the treatment of Type-IV hyperlipidaemia. Nevertheless, the metabolic control of acarbose and placebo groups was not statistically different at the end of the study. The beneficial effect of acarbose appears to be slight (Rodier et al., 1988).

Acarbose has no effect on blood parameters.

### 2.4 PHARMACOKINETICS

The site of action of acarbose is the gut, where it is present almost exclusively.

### 2.4.1 Absorption

Application of single or multiple doses of acarbose (200–300 mg) resulted in an absorption rate of about 0.5 to 1.6% of the ingested dose. Similar values were obtained when the mean urinary recovery of unchanged acarbose was used to calculate its systemic availability (Pütter, 1980; Pütter et al., 1982; Müller and Hillebrand, 1986).

## 2.4.2   Plasma Levels

Administration of a single dose of $^{14}$C-labelled acarbose (200 mg) to volunteers who had received the drug three times daily for 4 weeks revealed that, at steady state, mean $C_{max}$ was 18.4 $\mu g/l$ and $t_{max}$ 2.1 h (Müller and Hillebrand, 1986). The level of radioactivity in blood increased markedly after 6 h, because of the absorption of metabolites formed in the gut.

## 2.4.3   Distribution

After intravenous injection of 0.4 mg/kg in healthy volunteers, plasma acarbose concentrations declined biexponentially and fitted the equation for an open two-compartment model. The volume of distribution of acarbose at steady state following intravenous administration was calculated to be about 0.32 l/kg while the apparent volume of the central compartment was 0.16 l/kg. The mean distribution half-life was found to be approximately 0.5 h after intravenous injection (Pütter et al., 1982) and 3.7 h following oral administration (Müller and Hillebrand, 1986).

## 2.4.4   Half-life

After intravenous administration, the mean elimination half-life was calculated to be 2.7–2.9 h (Pütter, 1980; Pütter et al., 1982), but there was evidence for a third more slowly declining phase (currently below the limits of accurate detection) with a terminal half-life of about 9 h (Müller and Hillebrand, 1986).

## 2.4.5   Metabolism

Acarbose is degraded in the bowel by various amylases which hydrolyse the glucosidic linkages; $\alpha$-amylases (of small intestinal or bacterial origin) produce component-II with three rings (one glucose being liberated) while $\beta$-amylases (usually of plant or fungal origin) produce component-I and leave a maltose residue (Pütter et al., 1982). The metabolites of acarbose are systemically absorbed by 10–30% (Sturm, 1992).

## 2.4.6   Excretion

The faecal excretion of acarbose and component-II was almost complete within 24 h of administration of a single dose of 300 mg orally and amounted to 16% of the ingested dose; only about 5% of the dose was eliminated in the faeces as component-I (Pütter et al., 1982). The total body clearance of acarbose was calculated to be about 600 l/h (Müller and Hillebrand, 1986); this very high value reflects the low systemic availability and rapid degradation of acarbose in the intestinal tract.

## 2.5  TOXIC AND SIDE EFFECTS

Acarbose has no known toxic effects. In contrast, some side effects are known (Clissold and Edwards, 1988), and are more frequent at the beginning. Systemic side effects are not anticipated since only 10–30% of a dose is absorbed and only 2% is "bioavailable". Gastrointestinal disturbances, particularly flatulence and meteorism, may occur and are reported to be due to gases from non-absorbed carbohydrate in the colon.

A finding of renal adenomas in rats given acarbose led to extensive toxicological studies.

Because of the delay in absorption of oligo- and di-saccharides resulting from its administration, a colic bacterial fermentation occurs, accounting for the frequent abdominal discomfort mentioned by the patients. These side effects should be lessened with the second-generation glucosidase inhibitors now being developed.

An increase in osmotic pressure due to retention of unabsorbed carbohydrate in the distal small intestine and proximal colon may explain the acarbose-induced diarrhoea that results from sucrose combined with acarbose (Hayakawa et al., 1989). In cases of hypoglycaemia, glucose has to be preferred over saccharose.

## 2.6  INTERACTION WITH OTHER DRUGS

For a review, see Sachse et al. (1982). Combining acarbose with sulphonylurea or metformin or insulin may lead to hypoglycaemia, although acarbose itself will not produce hypoglycaemia (doses have to be corrected). The effect of acarbose may be reduced by antacids, cholestyramine, pancreatic enzymes and adsorbants. Plasma levels of vitamin $B_6$ increased, and vitamin A concentrations decreased with acarbose (Couet et al., 1989).

## 2.7  CLINICAL STUDIES

### 2.7.1  Healthy Volunteers

It has been understood since the early 1970s (Puls and Kemp, 1973) that carbohydrate absorption might be modified by administration of enzyme inhibitors with meals. Most recent evidence for this came from clinical studies involving acarbose itself. The effect of acarbose in healthy volunteers is characterized by a dose-dependent retardation of the di-, oligo- and poly-saccharide digestion with a prolonged rise in the postprandial blood glucose curve.

Several clinical trials in humans have emphasized the profound effect of acarbose in inhibiting postprandial carbohydrate absorption. Following a 100 g oral sucrose load, 90% of the substrate was digested within 200 min (Radziuk et al., 1982). Following sucrose + acarbose, however, only 62% were resorbed in 400 min. Acarbose appears even more effective if given with a starchy low-sucrose diet in a premeal dosage which may be as low as 50 mg while no effect was seen on glucose absorption.

In normal-weight healthy volunteers a single dose of acarbose (100 mg) added to a standard breakfast induced a marked lowering of the postprandial rise in blood glucose, serum insulin and triglyceride levels (Hillebrand et al., 1979). Similar results were seen when acarbose was added to lunch or dinner.

In moderately obese subjects the reduction in postprandial glucose by acarbose was strictly dose-dependent and accompanied by a striking reduction in serum insulin (Sjöström and William-Olsson, 1982). The mechanism behind the lowered insulin response is a decreased glycaemic and non-glycaemic insulin stimulus (Fölsch et al., 1990). Immunoreactive glucose-induced polypeptide (IR-GIP) response following acarbose was greatly diminished when the glucosidase inhibitor was combined with a liquid mixed meal, which was similar to the effects of dietary fibres.

Acarbose appears also to lower carbohydrate-induced triglyceride over-production in normal subjects (Nestel, 1988). The effects of acarbose on total triglycerides and cholesterol were investigated in healthy male subjects by Walter-Sack et al. (1982). Acarbose was found to reduce fasting total and VLDL triglycerides. In addition, acarbose diminished total and LDL cholesterol, whereas HDL cholesterol remained unchanged. Thus, the HDL/LDL ratio rose markedly.

The duration of treatment may be important for the effect of acarbose upon serum triglycerides. Homma et al. (1982) observed a striking depression of VLDL and triglycerides after 3 weeks acarbose, whereas several others did not see any effect on lipid metabolism after a short-term treatment period.

Several other long-term effects of acarbose were explored in healthy men by Couet et al. (1988). There was an increase in faecal nitrogen excretion, while nitrogen balance decreased. Acarbose also increased the faecal excretion of starch, fat, iron and chromium. Plasma vitamin A decreased following acarbose treatment, while vitamin $B_6$ increased.

The blood ethanol peak was delayed by about 45 min by acarbose, and the fall in blood ethanol was significantly retarded (Jandrain et al., 1988).

In healthy humans, acarbose reduces postprandial hyperglycaemia, hyper-insulinaemia and hypertriglyceridaemia and may therefore be a useful tool for the treatment of diabetic patients and the metabolic syndrome.

## 2.7.2   Type-I Diabetes Mellitus

In Type-I diabetes, insulin is the only drug that can preserve life. Any other drug addition can only be a supportive agent. Clinical trials, however, have shown that acarbose might help to reduce blood glucose fluctuations when given along with insulin (Raptis et al., 1988). This effect could well be quantified by the use of the artificial endocrine pancreas and 24 h blood glucose monitoring. In brittle diabetes, a reduction in mean and maximum blood glucose values was also described (Willms and Sachse, 1982). Following an oral sucrose tolerance test, the insulin requirements could be reduced by 65% when acarbose was given at the same time.

In short-term studies, Petzold et al. (1982) observed a significantly lower postprandial blood glucose level in insulin-dependent diabetics. Urine glucose could be decreased by 80% by acarbose within a 7-day follow-up described by Hillebrand et al. (1982), and by 50% as observed by Aubell et al. (1983). In long-term studies, Raptis et al. (1982) also demonstrated a decrease in insulin requirements following 1 and 6 months acarbose treatment. The findings were confirmed by Beyer et al. (1982) in juvenile diabetics during the day.

In a 1-year study by Aubell et al. (1983) blood sugar lowering was not only seen postprandially but also in a fasting state in Type-I diabetes. A 20% reduction in postprandial hyperglycaemia with decreased insulin require-ments and significantly lower $HbA_1$ following acarbose administration was noted by Schumann et al. (1982). Serum triglycerides, however, did not improve during additional acarbose treatment in Type-I diabetics.

Acarbose reduced the insulin requirements of Type-I diabetics mainly when given immediately before meals, so that no waiting time was necessary. The time relationship between insulin absorption and glucose absorption (delay) is synchronized by acarbose. An additional acarbose treatment in Type-I diabetes should also be applied, when late morning or past-midnight hypoglycaemic reactions cannot be handled sufficiently by diet and changes in insulin application. Under these conditions, acarbose might stabilize blood sugar fluctuations by delaying carbohydrate absorption.

## 2.7.3   Type-II Diabetes Mellitus

In Type-II diabetes, obese patients suffer primarily from a resistance to insulin, which may progress to a final state of insulin deficiency after several years of diabetes duration. Initially, however, insulin resistance in Type-II diabetes is associated with an absolute or relative hyperinsulinaemia often accompanied by obesity, hypertension and hyperlipidaemia, also called metabolic syndrome (Reaven, 1988). In these patients, weight reduction is the most important therapy and near-normoglycaemic control is a reasonable aim.

When diet and education, however, fail to reach the aim, drug treatment must be applied to achieve proper metabolic control, according to the individual treatment goals (Alberti et al., 1988).

No insulinotropic substance should be used as a first-line drug in hyperinsulinaemic insulin-resistant obese Type-II diabetics with dietary failure. The recent pharmacological approach, moreover, has been to delay carbohydrate ingestion by $\alpha$-glucosidase inhibition using acarbose. Probably the most important indication for the use of acarbose is the monotherapy in dietary failure and the beginning of the drug treatment in hyperinsulinaemic obese Type-II diabetics. This effect, however, is not only dose-dependent with respect to acarbose but also with respect to the amount and kind of carbohydrate in the diet. Since di- and oligo-saccharides are the main substrates for acarbose, a marked blood glucose-lowering effect can only be achieved in the presence of a carbohydrate-rich diet. This fits well with the recommendations for a diabetic diet according to most national diabetes associations.

A dose-dependence of starch and/or sucrose has been shown. However, when mono- and di-saccharides were added to a starch meal, the obvious dose-dependence seen with starch alone was lost (Toeller, 1990).

Acarbose induces a significant blood glucose-lowering effect, in particular when given to Type-II diabetics insufficiently controlled by diet alone (Rosenkranz et al., 1982). After breakfast, postprandial blood glucose was reduced by 38 mg per 100 ml and after dinner by 55 mg per 100 ml following $3 \times 100$ mg acarbose compared with diet alone (Laube et al., 1980). A striking dose-dependence was observed in concentrations between 50 and 200 mg per meal (Sachse et al., 1982). Higher doses cause greater inhibition and result in malabsorption of nutrients, fermentation causing flatulence, distension and diarrhoea. A relatively narrow therapeutic range has therefore to be applied (Taylor, 1990b). Therapy should be started with $1 \times 50$ mg (or even 25 mg) in the morning and increased weekly to a final rate of $3 \times 100$ mg daily ("start low – go slow").

In long-term studies of over 6 (Hanefeld et al., 1990, 1991) and 12 months (Aubell et al., 1983), fasting and postprandial blood glucose levels were significantly reduced compared with diet alone (Table 8). $HbA_1$ was lowered from 9.2 to 8.6%. Other investigators reported a decrease of $HbA_1$ from 10.8 to 8.5% following 6 months of treatment with $3 \times 100$ mg acarbose daily. There were no changes noted in the efficacy of acarbose.

Besides the effects on blood glucose, postprandial insulin release was also

TABLE 8[a]

Blood glucose, after fasting and 1 h postprandial (p.p.), and haemoglobin (HbA$_1$) after 24 weeks of treatment with acarbose or placebo

| | Acarbose | Placebo | P |
|---|---|---|---|
| Blood glucose (mg dl$^{-1}$) | | | |
| Fasting | 153 | 172 | <0.01 |
| 1 h p.p. | 189 | 243 | <0.01 |
| HbA$_1$ (%) | 8.68 | 9.29 | <0.01 |

[a]Source: Hanefeld et al. (1990).

markedly reduced, making acarbose the drug of choice for treating the metabolic syndrome after dietary failure (Hanefeld et al., 1990). In long-term trials, acarbose also lowered serum triglycerides and VLDL significantly, while cholesterol levels were not affected (Leonhardt et al., 1991).

The therapeutic effects of acarbose and biguanides have been compared in Type-II diabetics (Pagano and Cavallo-Perin, 1990) and found to be nearly equally effective. The same was true in studies (by Schwedes et al. (1982), who compared acarbose and metformin in poorly controlled NIDDM, while Schöffling et al. (1982) reported that acarbose was even more effective than metformin. Drost et al. (1982) concluded from their studies, however, that there was no basic difference between the hypoglycaemic effects of acarbose and metformin. Petersen (1982) tested the efficacy of acarbose versus buformin in NIDDM. Acarbose was found to reduce postprandial but not fasting blood glucose levels and to be slightly less effective than buformin.

In most countries of the Western world, sulphonylureas are the most widely used oral antidiabetic agents. With the recognition of the metabolic syndrome in many Type-II diabetics, however, it became clear that insulinotropic drugs such as sulphonylureas should no longer be the first choice in the initial treatment of hyperinsulinaemic insulin-resistant diabetics, if other equally effective drugs are available to lower blood glucose levels. For that purpose, several studies were conducted to compare the effect of acarbose and glibenclamide on blood glucose and HbA$_1$ (Fölsch et al., 1990; Spengler et al., 1992). It was found that 3 × 100 mg of acarbose was nearly as effective as 3 × 3.5 mg glibenclamide (Fig. 28). Fasting blood glucose decreased from 8.6 to 6.7 mM following acarbose and from 8.6 to 6.7 mM following glibenclamide. Postprandial blood glucose was lowered from 11.3 to 8.7 versus 11.1 to 8.2 mM. The incidence of hypoglycaemia in sulphonylurea-treated patients was 0.22 per 1000 patient-years, while no hypoglycaemic episodes were reported in acarbose-treated patients (Wiholm and Wester-holm, 1984).

**HbA₁ [%]**
geometric means, 1 s-range

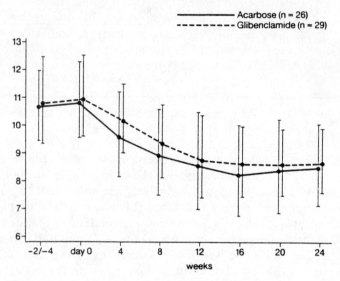

Fig. 28. HbA$_1$ levels during 6 months of treatment with acarbose or glibenclamide. (Source: Fölsch *et al.*, 1990.)

The combination of acarbose and sulphonylureas is mainly used in patients with secondary sulphonylurea failure. Rosak (1990) reported a lowering of fasting blood glucose by 42 mg per 100 ml in diabetics treated with acarbose and sulphonylureas versus 14 mg per 100 ml with only sulphonylureas. Postprandial blood glucose was decreased by 57 mg per 100 ml, while sulphonylureas alone produced an increase of 4 mg per 100 ml in secondary sulphonylurea failure.

The combination of sulphonylureas and acarbose (3 × 100 mg) versus sulphonylureas and phenformin (75 mg) was tested for 3 months by Pagano and Cavallo-Perin (1990), who could not find any significant difference between the two treatments as far as blood glucose, plasma insulin and HbA$_1$ were concerned. However, there was a 20% increase in plasma lactate in the biguanide group and no variation in the acarbose patients.

The treatment with acarbose of Type-II diabetics who had already been transferred to **insulin**, revealed an insulin-saving effect. The total daily insulin dosage was reduced by 10 IU per patient with acarbose, while insulin and placebo increased the daily insulin dosage by 0.7 IU. Blood glucose levels in the acarbose group was lowered (Rosak, 1990) and HbA$_1$ was decreased from 9.1 to 7.5% in 29 Type-II diabetics. Fasting blood glucose was lowered by 0.3 mM, while with insulin only blood glucose increased by 1.1 mM.

In patients with diabetes plus liver cirrhosis, acarbose treatment appears to be favourable because it improves the detoxification of ammonia (Müting, 1984). Acarbose induces an increased growth of lactobacteria, lowers intestinal pH and hyperammonaemia, inducing a beneficial effect on portosystemic encephalopathy. It also reduces lipolysis and ketogenesis in cirrhotic patients (Zillikens *et al.*, 1989), following a late evening meal with 100 mg acarbose.

In conclusion, the best indication for acarbose is in the early stages of NIDDM and in overweight diabetic patients who do not respond well to diet therapy. Acarbose can be used as monotherapy and also in association with sulphonylureas and insulin. It lowers postprandial and fasting blood glucose, decreases hypertriglyceridaemia and hyperinsulinaemia, and improves $HbA_1$. It is therefore justified to expect also a beneficial effect of acarbose on the development of long-term diabetic complications.

# Aldose Reductase Inhibitors as New Antidiabetic Drugs

Increased aldose reductase activity is observed in tissues which are affected by complications of diabetes mellitus. The possible participation of the polyol pathway in the pathogenesis of these complications led to detailed evaluation of the role of this system both to improve the understanding of diabetes mellitus and to open up new therapeutic possibilities in the prevention of complications. The underlying therapeutic idea is to prevent lesions caused by high glucose concentrations. This seems to be possible for those tissues with insulin-independent glucose uptake and high activity of the polyol pathways (for a detailed review on aldose reductase see Sarges, 1989).

## 1   Chemistry

The development of aldose reductase inhibitors began in 1967, when tetramethyleneglutaric acid (TMG) was introduced as the first non-cytotoxic inhibitor of aldose reductase in experimental models (Kinoshita *et al.*, 1968). Of more than a hundred potential aldose reductase inhibitors with *in vitro*

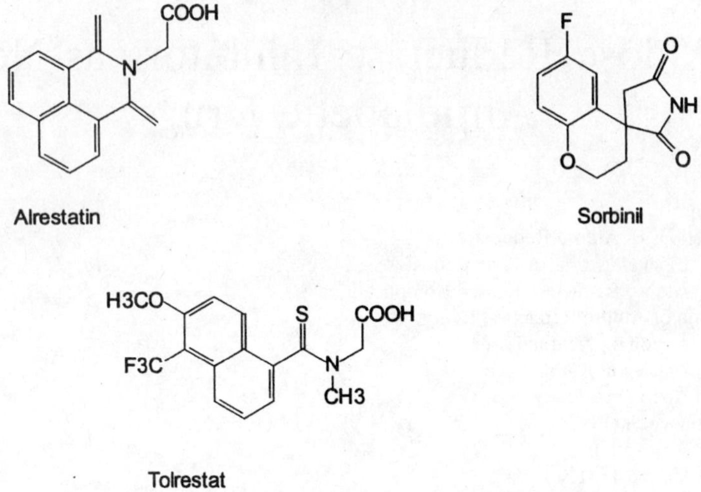

Alrestatin                                              Sorbinil

Tolrestat

FIG. 29. Chemical structure of some aldose reductase inhibitors.

activity, only about half a dozen showed sufficient aldose reductase-inhibiting activity and acceptable toxicity *in vivo* and in man.

Apart from *ad hoc* designed compounds, a number of natural products and their derivatives, predominantly heterocyclic alkanoic acids, are known to inhibit aldose reductase. These are rhodanine derivatives (Tadeo *et al.*, 1982), quinolineacetic acid derivatives (Poulsom and Heath, 1983), phthalazinoneacetic acid (Stribling *et al.*, 1983), furanopropionic acid and synthetic analogues (Okamoto *et al.*, 1984), coumarin-4-acetic acid derivatives (Sarges *et al.*, 1980), benzopyran- and benzothiopyran-carboxylic acids (Belletire, 1980), and a number of natural and synthetic flavones. This wide variety of compounds is representative of the chemical heterogeneity of such inhibitors. Nevertheless, a chromone ring system is common to all aldose reductase inhibitors.

Recent chemical developments are: (1) tetramethyleneglutaric acid (AY-20,037) (Ayerst); (2) alrestatin (Ayerst) (Fig. 29); (3) tolrestat (Ayerst) (Fig. 29); (4) epalrestat (Ono); (5) sorbinil (Pfizer) (Fig. 29); (6) ponalrestat (ICI-128,436) (ICI).

## 2    Functions of Aldose Reductase

### 2.1    BIOCHEMISTRY OF ALDOSE REDUCTASE

Aldose reductase, an aldoketo reductase, is ubiquitous in mammalian tissues. By reducing glucose to sorbitol (the latter being oxidized to fructose) aldose reductase is responsible for the first steps in the polyol cycle. Aldose reductase has a broad substrate specificity including glucose and galactose. Generally, the affinity of aldose reductase for glucose is low, the enzyme operating at low catalytic rates. Its activity increases when hexokinase is saturated and high glucose levels are present. Sorbitol, which is produced under these conditions, accumulates in the cell, thus creating an osmotic effect and thereby tissue hydration. This may underlie, at least in part, certain complications of diabetes.

Although aldose reductase is a widely distributed enzyme system, its general physiological role remains to be convincingly proven. Its only experimentally documented role is its participation in the generation of diabetic complications.

## 2.2    ALDOSE REDUCTASE-RELATED COMPLICATIONS

The participation of aldose reductase in the development of diabetic complications is assumed to be based on a triad of tissue effects: sorbitol accumulation, myo-inositol depletion and decreased activity of Na/K-ATPase. These alterations, first described in the ocular lens, also occur in other tissues like the renal glomerulus, peripheral nerves and the retina. The enhanced activity of aldose reductase may therefore be involved in the development of diabetic neuropathy, diabetic retinopathy and diabetic nephropathy, although it may not be the sole factor underlying these complications.

## 3    Action of Aldose Reductase Inhibitors

Most aldose reductase inhibitors (e.g. sorbinil, alrestatin, tolrestat and ponalrestat) inhibit the enzyme in a non-competitive or uncompetitive way – they compete neither with the substrate nor with the cofactor (NADPH). Therefore, an inhibitory binding site in the enzyme is postulated (Sarges, 1989).

## 3.1    ACTION ON NEURAL TISSUE

Aldose reductase is present in the Schwann cell body but not in the axon. Activation of the polyol pathway depletes myo-inositol and inactivates Na/K-ATPase activity of nerve cells, leading to a reduction in the nerve conduction velocity, at least in diabetic animals.

myo-Inositol is important for the phosphoinositide-mediated regulation of

Na/K-ATPase (Greene *et al.*, 1987a), the inositol phosphate pathway linked to the Na/K-ATPase by a PKC-dependent mechanism (Lattimer *et al.*, 1989). Depletion of inositol phosphates leads to an accumulation of intracellular $Na^+$ and therefore reduced ability to generate action potentials. This effect can be prevented by the use of aldose reductase inhibitors, and is also improved by insulin or the addition of *myo*-inositol. The same mechanism is attributed to structural and morphological lesions in diabetic peripheral nerve disease like swelling of large myelinated nerve fibres at the Ranvier nodes, the axo–glial dysjunction, axonal degeneration and deformity of nerves (Sima *et al.*, 1986). Inhibition of aldose reductase activity can reverse the paranodal swelling in diabetic BB-rats (Greene *et al.*, 1987b), and increases the number of regenerating myelinated nerve fibres in patients with established diabetic neuropathy (Sima *et al.*, 1988).

### 3.2 ACTION ON RETINA

Loss of mural cells (pericytes) in the retinal microcapillaries is a typical event in diabetic retinopathy. These mural cells contain aldose reductase and accumulate sorbitol in experimental hyperglycaemia (Buzney *et al.*, 1977), leading to degenerative changes implying participation of the polyol pathway in cell death.

Use of aldose reductase inhibitors prevents the loss of pericytes in animals maintained on high-galactose diets (Robinson *et al.*, 1989). Also, in streptozocin-diabetic or fructose-fed rats the development of retinopathic changes was prevented by aldose reductase inhibitors (Kojima *et al.*, 1985). In contrast, collagen synthesis by retinal pericytes was unaffected (Li *et al.*, 1985).

The overall accumulation of sorbitol in the retina of diabetic rats seems to be of little significance, but the distribution of the polyols in the different cellular locations could produce osmotic force. In alloxan-diabetic animals the above-mentioned triad of *myo*-inositol depletion, reduced Na/K-ATPase activity and activation of PKC following accumulation of sorbitol is seen and can be prevented by inhibition of aldose reductase (MacGregor and Matschinsky, 1985), although the impact of this system on the generation of diabetic retinopathy remains to be established.

### 3.3 ACTION ON KIDNEY

The presence of aldose reductase in glomerular epithelial and mesangial cells (Corder *et al.*, 1977) and its increased activity in hyperglycaemia (Kikkawa *et al.*, 1987) suggest participation of the polyol cycle in the development of diabetic nephropathy. This is supported by the fact that the above-mentioned triad was found in the renal glomeruli in most studies normalized by aldose reductase inhibitors (Bank *et al.*, 1989).

## 4  Pharmacokinetics

The development of aldose reductase inhibitors as useful drugs is actually at the stage of evaluation of their pharmacodynamic benefit. Data on the pharmacokinetic properties of these drugs are therefore rather scarce. In addition, owing to their chemical heterogeneity, no common principles can be established.

### 4.1  ABSORPTION

Tolrestat is absorbed after oral administration to the extent of about 70% in man. Data on different animal models give higher values (Dvornik *et al.*, 1988).

### 4.2  PLASMA LEVELS

The maximal plasma level after a single oral dose of 100 mg tolrestat is about 5–8 $\mu$g ml$^{-1}$ which is reached after about 2 h. Multiple oral dosing (twice daily) results in a steady state after 6 days, and no unexpected accumulation occurs, yielding linear pharmacokinetics even during chronic dosing (data from Wyeth-Ayerst Int. Inc.).

### 4.3  DISTRIBUTION

The plasma protein binding of tolrestat is very high, only 0.7% of the drug being free in the plasma. No competition exists with warfarin, but to some extent with high concentrations of tolbutamide or salicylate (Moulds *et al.*, 1991).

### 4.4  HALF-LIFE

The plasma half-life of tolrestat after a single dose is about 10–13 h in both healthy and diabetic volunteers (Hicks *et al.*, 1984).

4.5  ELIMINATION

About 70% of tolrestat is eliminated via the kidneys, of which about 60% is unchanged. About one-quarter of a dose can be recovered in the faeces. Tolrestat is metabolized to oxo-tolrestat and sulpho-tolrestat (Wyeth-Ayerst Int. Inc.).

## 5  Pathological Changes in the Pharmacokinetics

Renal dysfunction reduces the clearance of tolrestat, with corresponding increases in the half-life. No effect was reported on the volume of distribution or absorption, suggesting that the dose should be reduced in renal failure (Troy et al., 1992). The fact that one-third of the dose is eliminated by the liver makes it possible to use the drug even in both liver and kidney dysfunction if the possible doubling in the plasma levels is compensated by a reduction in the dosage.

## 6  Toxic and Side Effects

Unsuccessful development is often due to toxicological problems which remain unpublished. Hence little is publicly known about the toxicity of aldose reductase inhibitors.

The presence of aldose reductase in many tissues, which may not be involved in diabetic complications, makes unwanted effects likely, although isozymic differences in the enzyme in different tissues may be possible. Since aldose reductase inhibitors are not yet regularly used and since the effects of long-term inhibition of aldose reductase are not yet known, knowledge on possible unwanted effects is scarce. Information on side effects is therefore based only on individual reports.

The absence of side effects in a 1-year clinical trial with ponalrestat was reported by Ziegler et al. (1991), but in this study no therapeutic efficacy was seen! A 6-month study with ponalrestat to elucidate the effects on kidney function was also free from side effects (Pedersen et al., 1991). Dizziness, possibly based on a blood pressure-lowering effect, was reported for tolrestat. In addition, hepatocyte lesion accompanied by changes in hepatic parameters within the first 3–6 months of treatment was seen (Ryder et al., 1987). For sorbinil, significant hypersensitivity reactions have been reported (Sarges, 1989).

## 7    Interaction with Other Drugs

No report on drug interaction exists as yet. Possible interactions based on plasma protein binding are discussed in the pharmacokinetic section.

## 8    Clinical Trials

### 8.1    INTRODUCTION

The design and interpretation of clinical trials to validate the effects of aldose reductase inhibitors are difficult. The role of aldose reductase in different tissues is quite different, the enzyme appearing typical in the respective tissues and species. Furthermore, since the activity of the enzyme is high only in the presence of high glucose concentrations, it will be very difficult if not impossible to design appropriate studies with untreated control patients, especially when taking into account the long-lasting and irreversible development of diabetic complications (Kirchhain and Rendell, 1990; Stribling, 1990). Problems also arise from the safety and efficacy of the different compounds being developed by different companies. The lack of clear relationships between structure and action for this class of drugs implies that the failure or benefit of one compound may probably not be valid for another. Therefore, missing data cannot be taken as proof or lack of usefulness.

### 8.2    EFFECT ON NEUROPATHY

Because the development of diabetic neuropathy has a point of irreversibility, the benefit of aldose reductase inhibitors is restricted to the early stages of this process (Masson and Boulton, 1990).

Tolrestat was able to stop the progression of neuropathy in a 1-year placebo-controlled clinical trial (Giugliano et al., 1993), and even a reversal of mild forms of autonomic and peripheral neuropathy was observed. Boulton et al. (1990) have also been able to show improvement in nerve conduction velocity by tolrestat. Ponalrestat was unable to improve the signs of peripheral neuropathy although it was effective on autonomic neuropathy (Sundkvist et al., 1992). In another study, the absence of any curing effect of ponalrestat was reported (Ziegler et al., 1991).

### 8.3    EFFECT ON DIABETIC RETINOPATHY

A lack of effect on the course of minimal diabetic retinopathy of ponalrestat was reported by Tromp et al. (1991). For sorbinil, there was no preventive effect on retinopathy in a 41-month trial (Sorbinil Retinopathy Trial Research Group, 1990).

## 8.4   EFFECT ON DIABETIC NEPHROPATHY

No conclusive trials on possible benefits on diabetic nephropathy have yet been published.

# Conclusions

The use of present and future antidiabetic drugs in Type-I and Type-II diabetes mellitus must be based on the pathophysiological and molecular aspects of these diseases.

In Type-I diabetes, which is due to the loss of insulin-producing cells as a consequence of autoimmune disorders, substitution of insulin is the most important measure. However, merely to inject one daily dose is not an adequate therapy. Here, the objective is to mimic the daily variations in plasma insulin which are closely related to food intake. One such attempt which has improved microvascular complications is intensified insulino-therapy through multiple daily injections of insulin. Another approach is to develop techniques of islet transplantation and using a bioartificial pancreas. In the case of islet transplantation, tissues will not only respond to changes in blood glucose levels but also to hormones of the entero–insular axis.

Prevention of Type-I diabetes mellitus is also an important target. Here, methods must be improved for the detection of relevant markers appearing in the blood before the destruction of B-cells by the immune system. In this connection, further development of immunosuppressive agents with minimal side effects and high specifity against B-cell destruction is necessary.

Since Type-II diabetes mellitus is quite different from Type-I in its pathophysiology, other therapeutic concepts (except the administration of insulin) must be envisaged. Diet, weight control and education of the patient take place before any antidiabetic drug is used. If we accept the following chain of events, namely insulin resistance $\rightarrow$ hyperglycaemia $\rightarrow$ hyper-insulinaemia $\rightarrow$ exhaustion of the secretory mechanism $\rightarrow$ defective insulin secretion and, in addition, increased glucose production in the liver, the following strategies are reasonable.

The first aim is to lower blood sugar levels by retarding glucose absorption. This is the goal of compounds that inhibit glucose absorption. In fact, acarbose has not only been shown to lower postprandial glucose and insulin levels but also to improve $HbA_{1c}$ values. However, there are still no data indicating a long-term protecting effect against diabetic complications.

A second possibility for lowering blood glucose without the help of B-cells are compounds that improve peripheral glucose utilization by a direct effect. Here, biguanides are effective. They have been shown to lower blood glucose, body weight and $HbA_{1c}$ values. However, for biguanides also, no proof of prevention of diabetic complications is yet available. Nevertheless, the development of agents that improve peripheral glucose uptake/utilization and/or the sensitization of tissues to insulin should be encouraged. A possible target could be the insulin receptor tyrosine kinase. Such compounds could probably protect B-cells first from overstimulation and second from exhaustion of the secretory mechanism. If hyperglycaemia is the consequence of defective secretory machinery, the use of sulphonylureas is justified. If it is true, as recently suggested, that "glucose toxicity" inhibits GLUT-2 and glucokinase expression, then it must be assumed that glucose metabolism in the B-cell does not provide sufficient signal metabolites in order to initiate and modulate insulin secretion. Here, sulphonylureas that trigger insulin release directly via closure of $K_{ATP}$ channels are a pharmacological alternative for the provision of insulin. The lowering effect on blood glucose and $HbA_{1c}$ by sulphonylureas is well known, although in this case also a protective effect against diabetic complications has yet to be proven. It should, however, not be forgotten that treatment of Type-II diabetics with antidiabetic drugs will improve acute symptoms of this disease. In theory, improvement of insulin release could also be achieved by compounds that enhance glucose metabolism of the B-cell or increase the positive modulating effects of adenylate cyclase and/or PLC.

The mechanism by which glucose production in the liver is elevated in Type-II diabetes is unclear. It is conceivable that it is the result of decreased sensitivity to insulin. Nevertheless, compounds that inhibit hepatic glucose production/output may also be potential antidiabetic drugs.

# References

Abbott, A. M., Bueno, R., Pedrini, M. T., Murray, J. M. and Smith, R. J. (1992). *J. Biol. Chem.* **267**, 10759–10763.

Abrahamson, H., Berggren, P.-O. and Rorsman, P. (1985). *FEBS Lett.* **190**, 21–23.

Adams, J. F., Clark, J. S., Ireland, J. T., Kesson, C. M. and Watson, W. S. (1983). *Diabetologia* **24**, 16–18.

Adamson, U. (1981). *Eur. J. Clin. Invest.* **11**, 115–119.

Adir, J., Miller, A. K. and Vestal, R. E. (1982). *Clin. Pharmacol. Ther.* **31**, 488–493.

Ahrén, B., Taborsky, G. J. and Porte, D., Jr. (1986). *Diabetologia* **29**, 827–836.

Ahrén, B., Östenson, C.-G. and Efendic, S. (1991). *In* "The Endocrine Pancreas" (E. Samols, ed.), pp. 153–173. Raven Press, New York.

Aicardi, G., Pollo, A., Sher, E. and Carbone, E. (1991). *FEBS Lett.* **281**, 201–204.

Akanuma, Y., Kosaka, K., Kanazawa, Y., Kasuga, M., Fukuda, M. and Aoki, S. (1988). *Diabetes Res. Clin. Pract.* **5**, 81–90.

Akhtar, M. S., Verspohl, E. J., Hegner, D. and Ammon, H. P. T. (1977). *Diabetes* **26**, 857–863.

Alberti, K. G. M., Gries, F. A. and the European NIDDM Policy Group (1988). *Diabetic Med.* **5**, 275–281.

Alemany, S., Mato, J. M. and Stralfors, P. (1987). *Nature* **330**, 77–79.

Altman, J. J., Pehuet, M., Slama, G. and Tchobroutsky, C. (letter) (1983). *Lancet* **ii**, 524.

Amiel, S., Tamborlane, W., Simonson, D. and Sherwin, R. (1987). *N. Engl. J. Med.* **316**, 1376–1983.

Amiranoff, B., Servin, A. L., Rouyer-Fessard, C., Couvineau, A., Tatemoto, K. and Laburthe, M. (1987). *Endocrinology* **121**, 284–289.

Ämmälä, C., Ashcroft, F. M. and Rorsman, P. (1993). *Nature* **363**, 356–358.

Ammon, H. P. T. (1975). *Naunyn-Schmiedeberg's Arch. Pharmacol.* **290**, 251–264.

Ammon, H. P. T. and Abdel-Hamid, M. (1981). *Naunyn-Schmiedeberg's Arch. Pharmacol.* **317**, 262–267.

Ammon, H. P. T. and Mark, M. (1985). *Cell Biochem. Funct.* **3**, 157–171.

Ammon, H. P. T. and Verspohl, E. J. (1976). *Endocrinology* **99**, 1469–1476.

Ammon, H. P. T. and Verspohl, E. J. (1979). *Diabetologia* **17**, 41–44.

Ammon, H. P. T. and Wahl, M. A. (1989). *Exp. Clin. Endocrinol.* **93**, 136–142.

Ammon, H. P. T. and Wahl, M. A. (1994). *In* "Frontiers of Insulin Secretion and Pancreatic B-Cell Research" (P. R. Flatt and S. Lenzen, eds), pp. 113–122. Smith-Gordon Co., London.

Ammon, H. P. T., Akhtar, M. S., Niklas, H. and Hegner, D. (1977). *Mol. Pharmacol.* **13**, 598–605.

Ammon, H. P. T., Akhtar, M. S., Grimm, A. and Niklas, H. (1979a). *Naunyn-Schmiedeberg's Arch. Pharmacol.* **307**, 91–96.

Ammon, H. P. T., Hoppe, E., Akhtar, M. S. and Niklas, H. (1979b). *Diabetes* **28**, 593–599.

Ammon, H. P. T., Grimm, A., Lutz, S., Wagner-Teschner, D., Händel, M. and Hagenloh, I. (1980). *Diabetes* **29**, 830–834.

Ammon, H. P. T., Hoppe, E., Eujen, R. and Lutz, S. (1981). *Horm. Metab. Res.* **13**, 60–61.

Ammon, H. P. T., Amm, U., Eujen, R., Hoppe, E., Trier, G. and Verspohl, E. J. (1983a). *Life Sci.* **34**, 247–257.

Ammon, H. P. T., Hägele, R., Youssif, N., Eujen, R. and El-Amri, N. (1983b). *Endocrinology* **112**, 720–726.

Ammon, H. P. T., Abdel-Hamid, M., Rao, G. and Enz, G. (1984). *Diabetes* **33**, 251–257.

Ammon, H. P. T., Kuehner, W. and Youssif, N. (1986). *Cell Calcium* **7**, 221–231.

Ammon, H. P. T., Reiber, C., Verspohl, E. J. (1991). *J. Endocrinol.* **128**, 27–34.

Amoroso, S., Schmid-Antomarchi, H., Fosset, M. and Lazdunski, M. (1990). *Science* **247**, 852–854.

Andersen, D. K., Elahi, D., Brown, J. C., Tobin, J. D. and Andres, R. (1978). *J. Clin. Invest.* **62**, 152–161.

Anderson, J. A. and Adkinson, N. F. (1987). *J. Am. Med. Assoc.* **258**, 2891–2899.

Anderson, J. W., Midgley, W. R. and Wedman, B. (1979). *Diabetes Care* **2**, 369–379.

Anderson, S. K., Gibbs, C. P., Tanaka, A., Kung, H. and Fujita, D. J. (1985). *Mol. Cell. Biol.* **5**, 1122–1129.

Anderssen, T., Berggren, P. O., Gylfe, E. and Hellman, B. (1982). *Acta Physiol. Scand.* **114**, 235–241.

Andreasen, P. B., Simonsen, K., Brocks, K., Dimo, B. and Bouchelouche, P. (1981). *Br. J. Clin. Pharmacol.* **12**, 581–583.

Anjaneyulu, K., Anjaneyulu, R., Sener, A. and Malaisse, W. J. (1982). *Biochimie* **64**, 29–36.

Anonymous (1985). *Lancet* **2**, 759–760.

Arias, P., Kerner, W., Zier, H., Navascues, I. and Pfeiffer, E. F. (1985). *Diabetes Care* **8**, 134–140.

Arkins, J. A., Enghieing, N. H. and Lennon, E. J. (1926). *Allergy* **33**, 69–74.

Aro, A., Uusitupa, M., Voutilainen, E., Hersio, K., Korhonen, T. and Siitonen, O. (1981). *Diabetologia* **21**, 29–31.

Aro, A., Voutilainen, E., Pentikainen, P., Uusitupa, M. and Penttilä, I. (1985). *Diabetes Res. Clin. Pract.*, Abstr. 62, pp. 24.

Ashcroft, F. M. (1988). *Annu. Rev. Neurosci.* **11**, 97–118.

Ashcroft, F. M. and Rorsman, P. (1989) *Prog. Biophys. Mol. Biol.* **54**, 87–143.

Ashcroft, S. J. H., Weerasingh, L. C. C., Basset, J. M. and Randle, P. J. (1972). *Biochem. J.* **126**, 525–532.

Ashcroft, F. M., Ashcroft, S. J. H. and Harrison, D. E. (1988). *J. Physiol.* **400**, 501–527.

Ashcroft, F. M., Rorsman, P. and Trube, G. (1989). *Ann. N.Y. Acad. Sci.* **560**, 410–412.

Asherov, J., Mimouni, M., Varsano, J., Lubin, E. and Laron, Z. (1979). *Arch. Dis. Childh.* **54**, 148–149.

Asmal, A. C. and Marble, A. (1984). *Drugs* **28**, 62–78.

Asplund, K., Wiholm, B. E. and Lithner, F. (1983). *Diabetologia* **24**, 412–417.

Atkins, T. W., Al-Hussary, N. A. and Taylor, K. G. (1987). *Diabetes Res. Clin. Pract.* **3**, 153–159.

Attvall, S., Fowelin, J., von Schenck, H. and Smith, U. (1987). *Diabetologia* **30**, 691–697.

Aubell, R., Boehme, K., Berchtold, P. (1983). *Arzneimittelforschung (Drug Res.)* **33**, 1314–1318.

Auger, K. R., Serunian, L. A., Soltoff, S. P., Libby, P. and Cantley, L. C. (1989). *Cell* **57**, 167–175.

Augustine, J. A., Schlager, J. W. and Abraham, R. T. (1990). *Biochim. Biophys. Acta* **1052**, 313–322.

Axen, K. V., Schubart, U. K., Blake, A. D. and Fleischer, N. (1983). *J. Clin. Invest.* **72**, 13–21.

Backer, J., Shoelson, S. E., Häring, E. and White, M. F. (1991a). *J. Cell. Biol.* **115**, 1535–1545.

Backer, J. M., Schroeder, G. G., Cahill, D. A., Ullrich, A., Siddle, K. and White, M. F. (1991b). *Biochemistry* **30**, 6366–6372.

Backer, J. M., Myers, Jr., M. G., Shoelson, S. E., Chin, D. J., Sun, X. J., Miralpeix, M.,

Hu, P., Margolis, B., Skolnik, E. Y., Schlessinger, J. and White, M. F. (1992). *EMBO J.* **11**, 3469–3479.

Bailey, C. J. (1992). *Diabetes Care* **15**, 755–772.

Bailey, C. J. and Nattrass, M. (1988). *Baillieres Clin. Endocrinol. Metab.* **2**, 455–476.

Bailey, C. J., Lord, J. M. and Atkins, T. W. (1984). *In* "Recent Advances in Diabetes" (M. Nattrass and J. Santiago, eds), pp. 27–44. Churchill, Livingstone, Edinburgh.

Bailyes, E. M., Guest, P. C. and Hutton, J. (1993). *In* "Insulin" (F. M. Ashcroft and S. J. H. Ashcroft, eds), pp. 64–96. IRL Press, Oxford.

Ballagi-Pordany, G., Koszeghy, A., Koltai, M. Z., Arayi, Z. and Pogatsa, G. (1989). *Diabetes Res.* **12**, 193–197.

Ballagi-Pordany, G., Koltai, M. Z., Aranyi, Z. and Pogatsa, G. (1991). *Diabetes Res. Clin. Pract.* **11**, 47–52.

Ballou, L. M. and Fisher, E. H. (1986). *In* "The Enzymes" 17 (P. D. Boyer and E. G. Krebs, eds), pp. 311–361. Academic Press, Inc., Orlando, FL.

Baltensperger, K., Lewis, R. E., Woon, C. W., Vissavajjhala, P. and Ross, A. H. (1992). *Proc. Natl Acad. Sci. USA* **89**, 7885–7889.

Baltensperger, K., Kozma, L. M., Cherniack, A. D., Klarlund, J. K., Chawla, A., Banerjee, U. and Czech, M. P. (1993). *Science* **260**, 1950–1952.

Band, A. M., Jones, P. M. and Howell, S. L. (1992). *J. Mol. Endocrinol.* **8**, 95–101.

Bank, N., Mower, P., Aynedjian, H., Wilkes, B. M., Silverman, S. (1989). *Am. J. Physiol.* **256**, F1000–F1006.

Banting, F. G., Best, C. B., Collip, J. B., Cambell, W. R. and Fletcher, A. A. (1922). *Med. Assoc. J.* **2**, 141–146.

Barnes, A. J., Garbien, K. J. T., Crowley, M. F. and Bloom, A. (1974). *Lancet* **ii**, 69–72.

Barron, E. S. G. (1951). *Adv. Enzymol. Relat. Subj. Biochem.* **11**, 201.

Bartram, H. P., Scheppach, W., Heid, C., Fabian, C. and Kasper, H. (1991). *Cancer Res.* **51**, 4238–4242.

Basudev, H., Jones, P. M., Persaud, S. J. and Howell, S. L. (1992). *FEBS Lett.* **296**, 69–72.

Beckmann, R. (1968). *Ann. N.Y. Acad. Sci.* **148**, 820–832.

Beck-Nielsen, H. (1988). *Diabetic Med.* **5**, 613–620.

Beck-Nielsen, H. (1991). *In* "Pharmacology of Diabetes: Present Practice and Future Perspectives" (C. E. Mogensen and E. Standl, eds), pp. 75–92. De Gruyter, Berlin and New York.

Behall, K. M. (1990). *Adv. Exp. Med. Biol.* **270**, 7–16.

Bell, G. I., Kayano, T., Buse, J. B., Burant, C. F., Takeda, J., Lin, D., Fukumoto, H. and Seino, S. (1990). *Diabetes Care* **13**, 198–208.

Belletire, J. L. (1980). US Patent 4,210,663.

Benakis, A. and Glasson, B. (1980). *In* "Gliclazide and the Treatment of Diabetes", International Congress and Symposium Series No. 20, pp. 57–69. Academic Press and Royal Society of Medicine, London.

Benecke, H., Flier, J. S. and Moller, D. E. (1992). *J. Clin. Invest.* **89**, 2066–2070.

Bennett, P. H. (1990). *In* "Diabetes Mellitus" (H. Rifkin and D. Porte, eds), pp. 357–377. Elsevier, New York.

Benson, E. A., Healy, L. A. and Barron, E. J. (1985). *Am. J. Med.* **78**, 857–860.

Bergenstal, R., Polonsky, K., Pons, G., Jaspan, J. and Rubenstein, A. (1983). *Diabetes* **32**, 398–402.

Berger, M., Cüppers, H. J., Hegner, H., Jörgens, V. and Berchthold, P. (1982). *Diabetes Care,* **5**, 77–91.

Berger, W. (1971). *Schweiz. Med. Wochenschr.* **101**, 1013–1022.

Berger, W., Caduff, F., Pasquel, M. and Rump, A. (1986). *Schweiz. Med. Wochenschr.* **116**, 145–151.

184     ANTIDIABETIC AGENTS

Berggren, P.-O., Arkhammar, P. and Nilsson, T. (1989). *Biochem. Biophys. Res. Commun.* **165**, 416–421.

Berggren, P.-O., Rorsman, P., Efendic, S., Ostenson, C.-G., Flatt, P. R., Nilsson, T., Arkhammar, P. and Juntti-Berggren, L. (1992). *In* "Nutrient Regulation of Insulin Secretion" (P. R. Flatt, ed.), pp. 289–318. Portland Press, London and Chapel Hill.

Bergmann, L., Kroncke, K. D., Suschek, C., Kolb, H. and Kolb-Bachofern, V. (1992). *FEBS Lett.* **299**, 103–106.

Bergsten, P. and Hellman, B. (1984). *Endocrinology* **114**, 1854–1859.

Bernier, M., Laird, D. M. and Lane, D. M. (1987). *Proc. Natl Acad. Sci. USA* **84**, 1844–1848.

Berthoud, H. R. (1984). *Metab. Clin. Exp.* **33**, 18–25.

Berti, L., Mosthaf, L., Kroder, G., Kellerer, M., Tippmer, S., Mushack, J., Seffer, E., Seedorf, K. and Häring, H. U. (1994). *J. Biol. Chem.* **269**, 3381–3386.

Bertrand, G., Petit, P., Bozem, M. and Henquin, J.-C. (1989). *Am. J. Physiol.* **257**, E473–E478.

Besedovsky, H. and Del Rey, A. (1987). *J. Neurosci. Res.* **18**, 172–178.

Besedovsky, H. and Del Rey, A. (1989). *Horm. Res.* **31**, 94–99.

Best, L. (1992). *In* "Nutrient Regulation of Insulin Secretion" (P. R. Flatt, ed.), pp. 157–171. Portland Press, London and Chapel Hill.

Beyer, J., Cordes, U., Krall, H., Sell, G. and Schöffling, K. (1972). *Arzneimittel-Forsch.* **22**, 2167–2172.

Beyer, J., Schulz, G., Jäger, H., Krause, U. and Cordes, U. (1982). *In* "Proceedings of the First International Symposium on Acarbose" (W. Creutzfeld, ed.), pp. 427–432. Excerpta Medica, Amsterdam.

Bilous, R. W. and Alberti, K. G. (1990). *In* "New Antidiabetic Drugs" (C. J. Bailey and R. P. Flatt, eds), pp. 19–31. Smith-Gordon, London.

Binder, C. and Bendtson, I. 24 (1992). *Baillieres Clin. Endocrinol. Metab.* **6**, 23–39.

Birkitt, D. J. (1982). *Br. J. Clin. Pharmacol.* **14**, 574–578.

Birnbaum, M. J. (1989). *Cell* **57**, 305–315.

Birnbaum, M. J., Haspel, H. C. and Rosen, O. M. (1986). *Proc. Natl Acad. Sci. USA* **83**, 5784–5788.

Blackshear, P. J., Rotner, H. E., Kriauciunas, K. A. M. and Kahn, C. R. (1983). *Ann. Int. Med.* **99**, 182–184.

Bleach, N. R., Dunn, P. J., Khalafalla, M. E. and McConkey, B. (1979). *Br. Med. J.* **2**, 177–178.

Boden, G., Reichard, G., Heldtke, R., Rezwani, I., Owen, O. (1981). *N. Engl. J. Med.* **305**, 1200–1205.

Bogardus, C., Lillioja, A., Stone, K. and Mott, D. (1984). *J. Clin. Invest.* **73**, 1185–1190.

Bolinger, R. E., Morris, J. H., McKnight, P. G. and Diederich, D. A. (1964). *N. Engl. J. Med.* **270**, 767–770.

Bolli, G. and Periello, G. (1990). *Horm. Metab. Res.* (Suppl. 14), 87–96.

Bolli, G., De Feo, P., De Cosmo, S., Periello, G., Angeletti, G., Ventura, M., Santeusanio, F., Brunetti, B. and Gerich, J. (1984b). *Diabetes* **33**, 394–400.

Bolli, G., Tsalikian, E., Haymond, M., Cryer, P., Gerich, J. (1984c). *J. Clin. Invest.* **73**, 1532–1541.

Bolli, G. B. and Gerich, J. E. (1984). *N. Engl. J. Med.* **310**, 746–750.

Bolli, G. B., Gottesman, I. S., Campbell, M. W., Haymond, M. W., Cryer, P. E. and Gerich, J. E. (1984a). *N. Engl. J. Med.* **311**, 1214–1219.

Bonner-Weir, S. (1991). Anatomy of the islet of Langerhans in the endocrine pancreas. *In* "The Endocrine Pancreas" (E. Samols, ed.), pp. 15–27. Raven Press, New York.

Bonora, E., Cigolini, M., Bosello, O., Zancanaro, C., Capretti, L., Zavaroni, I., Coscelli, C. and Butturini, V. (1984). *Curr. Med. Res. Opin.* **9**, 47–51.

Boschero, A. C. and Malaisse, W. J. (1979). *Am. J. Physiol.* **236**, E139–146.

Bosello, O., Cominacini, L., Zocca, I., Garbin, U., Ferrari, F. and Davoli, A. (1984). *Am. J. Clin. Nutr.* **40**, 1165–1174.

Bosisio, E., Galli Kienle, M., Galli, G., Ciconali, M., Negri, A., Sessa, A., Morosati, S. and Sirtori, C. R. (1981). *Diabetes* **30**, 644–649.

Bottazzo, G. F., Dean, B. M., McNally, J. M., MacKay, E. H., Swift, P. G. and Gable, D. R. (1985). *N. Engl. J. Med.* **313**, 353–360.

Bottermann, P., Gyaram, H., Wahl, K., Ermler, R. and Lebender, A. (1981). *Diabetes Care* **4**, 168–169.

Boulton, A. J., Levin, S. and Comstock, J. (1990). *Diabetologia* **33**, 431–437.

Bouman, P. R. and Goorenstroom, J. H. (1961). *Metabolism* **10**, 1095–1099.

Boyd, A. E. III and Huynh, T. Q. (1990). *Contemp. Intern. Med.* **2**, 13–33.

Brambilla, P., Artavia-Loria, E., Chaussain, J. L. and Bougneres, P. F. (1987). *Diabetes Care* **10**, 44–48.

Brange, J. (1987). "Galenics of Insulin." Springer Verlag, Berlin, Heidelberg, New York, London, Paris, Tokyo.

Brange, J., Owen, D. R., Kang, S. and Volund, A. (1990). *Diabetes Care* **13**, 923–954.

Bratusch-Marrain, P. R. (1983). *Diabetologia* **24**, 74–79.

Bratusch-Marrain, P. R., Komjati, M. and Waldhäusl, W. K. (1986). *Diabetes* **35**, 922–926.

Briggs, M. S. and Gierasch, L. M. (1986). *Adv. Protein Chem.* **38**, 109–180.

Brindle, N. P., Tavare, J. M., Dickens, M., Whittaker, J. and Siddle, K. (1990). *Biochem. J.* **268**, 615–620.

Brink, S. J. and Steward, C. (1986). *J. Am. Med. Assoc.* **255**, 617–621.

Brismar, K., Grill, V., Efendic, S. and Hall, K. (1991). *Metabolism* **40**, 728–732.

Brocklehurst, K. W. and Hutton, J. C. (1983). *Biochem. J.* **210**, 533–539.

Brogard, J. M., Willemin, B., Blickle, J. F., Lamalle, A. M. and Stahl, A. (1989). *Rev. Med. Interne* **10**, 365–74.

Brown, J. C., Dryburgh, J. R., Ross, S. A. and Dupré, J. (1975). *Recent Prog. Horm. Res.* **31**, 487–532.

Bruce, D., Storlien, L. H., Furler, S. M. and Chisholm, D. J. (1987). *Metabolism* **36**, 721–725.

Brunetti, P., Bueti, A., Antonella, M. A., Calabrese, G., Fabietti, P. G., Santeusiano, F. and Massi-Benedetti, M. (1984). *Exp. Clin. Endocrinol.* **83**, 130–135.

Buchanan, D. R., Collier, A., Rodrigues, E., Millar, A. M., Gray, R. S. and Clarke, B. F. (1988). *Eur. J. Clin. Pharmacol.* **34**, 51–53.

Burke, B. J., Hartog, M., Waterfield, M. R. (1984). *Acta Endocrinol.* **107**, 70–77.

Buysschaert, M., Marchnad, E., Ketelslegers, J. M. and Lambert, A. E. (1983). *Diabetes Care* **6**, 1–5.

Buzney, S. M., Frank, R. N. and Varma, S. D. (1977). *Invest. Ophthalmol. Vis. Sci.* **16**, 392–393.

Calder, P. C. and Geddes, R. (1989). *Carbohydr. Res.* **191**, 71–78.

Callaghan, T. S., Hadden, D. R. and Tomkin, G. H. (1980). *Br. Med. J.* **280**, 1214–1215.

Camerini-Davalos, R. A., Velasco, C. A., Glasser, M. and Bloodworth, J. M. (1988). *Diabetes Res. Clin. Pract.* **5**, 113–123.

Campbell, I. W. (1984). *Br. Med. J.* **289**, 289.

Campbell, I. W. (1985). *Horm. Metab. Res.* **15** (Suppl. 1), 105–111.

Campbell, I. W. (1990). *In* "New Antidiabetic Drugs" (C. J. Bailey and P. R. Flatt, eds), pp. 33–51. Smith-Gordon, London.

Campbell, P. J., Bolli, G. B., Cryer, P. E. and Gerich, J. E. (1985). *N. Engl. J. Med.* **312**, 1473–1479.

Cantley, L. C., Auger, K. R., Carpenter, C., Duckworth, B., Graziani, A., Kapeller, R. and Soltoff, S. (1991). *Cell* **64**, 281–302.

Carafoli, E. (1987). *Annu. Rev. Biochem.* **56**, 395–433.

Caraty, A., Grino, M., Locatelli, A., Guillaime, V., Boudouresque, F., Conte-Devolx, B. and Oliver, C. (1990). *J. Clin. Invest.* **85**, 1716–1721.

Carini, C., Brostoff, J. and Kurtz, A. B. (1982). *Diabetologia* **22**, 324–326.

Carrascosa, J. M., Schleicher, E., Maier, R., Hackenberg, C. and Wieland, O. H. (1988). *Biochim. Biophys. Acta Ser. Mol. Cell. Res.* **971**, 170–178.

Carrascosa, J. M., Vogt, B., Ullrich, A. and Häring, H. U. (1991). *Biochem. Biophys. Res. Commun.* **174**, 123–127.

Carveth-Johnson, A. O., Mylvaganam, K. and Child, D. F. (letter) (1982). *Lancet* **ii**, 1287.

Casner, P. R. (1988). *Clin. Pharmacol. Ther.* **44**, 594–603.

Caspary, W. F. (1978). *Lancet* **i**, 1231–1233.

Cavallo-Perin, P., Aluffi, E., Estivi, P., Bruno, A., Carta, Q., Pagano, G. and Lenti, G. (1989). *Riv. Eur. Sci. Med. Farmacol.* **11**, 45–49.

Chaikoff, I. L. and Forker, L. L. (1950) *Endocrinology* **46**, 319–327.

Chandalia, H. B. and Rangnath, M. (1990). *J. Assoc. Physicians India* **38**, 620–622.

Charles, M. A., Lawecki, J., Pictet, R. and Grodsky, G. M. (1975). *J. Biol. Chem.* **250**, 6134–6140.

Charron, M. C., Brosius, F. C., Alper, S. and Lodish, H. F. (1989). *Proc. Natl Acad. Sci. USA* **86**, 2535–2539.

Chou, C. K., Dull, T. J., Russell, D. S., Gherzi, R., Lebwohl, D., Ullrich, A. and Rosen, O. (1987). *J. Biol. Chem.* **262**, 1842–1847.

Christensen, L. K. and Skovsted, L. (1969). *Lancet* **ii**, 1397–1399.

Christie, M. R. and Ashcroft, S. J. H. (1984). *Biochem. J.* **218**, 87–99.

Chuang, L. M., Jou, T. S., Yang, W. S., Wu, H. P., Huang, S. H., Tai, T. Y. and Lin, B. J. (1992). *Taiwan I Hsueh Hui Tsa Chih.* **91**, 15–19.

Clark, A., Cooper, G. J. S., Lewis, C. E., Morris, J. F., Willis, A. C., Reid, K. B. M. and Turner, R. C. (1987). *Lancet* **ii**, 231–234.

Clarke, B. F. and Campbell, I. W. (1977). *Br. Med. J.* **2**, 1576–1578.

Clarke, B. F. and Duncan, J. P. (1968). *Lancet* **i**, 123–126.

Clarke, B. F., Marshall, A., McGill, R. C., McCuish, A. C. and Duncan, J. P. (1967). *In* "Tolbutamide – After Ten Years" (J. H. Butterfield and W. van Westerring, eds), pp. 312–322. Excerpta Medica, Amsterdam.

Clarke, W. L., Melton, T. W. and Bright, G. M. (1983). *Acta Endocrinol.* **102**, 557–560.

Clissold, S. P. and Edwards, C. (1988). *Drugs* **35**, 214–243.

Cohen, D. R., Matteson, R., Parsey, V. and Sala, S. (1990). *Biophys. J.* **57**, 509A.

Cohen, M. and Martin, F. I. R. (letter) (1979). *Br. Med. J.* **1**, 616.

Cohen, M. P., Klepser, H. and Wu, V. Y. (1991). *Gen. Pharmacol.* **22**, 515–519.

Colca, J. R., Kotagal, N., Lacy, P. E. and McDaniel, M. L. (1983a). *Biochim. Biophys. Acta* **729**, 176–184.

Colca, J. R., Kotagal, N., Lacy, P. E. and McDaniel, M. L. (1983b). *Biochem. J.* **212**, 113–121.

Colca, J. R., Brooks, C. L., Landt, M. and McDaniel, M. L. (1983c). *Biochem. J.* **212**, 819–827.

Conlon, J. M. (1988). *Diabetologia* **31**, 563–566.

Cook, D. L. and Hales, C. N. (1984). *Nature* **311**, 271–273.

Cooper, D. R., Ishizuka, T., Dao, M. L., Watson, J. E., Standaert, M. L. and Farese, R. V. (1990a). *Biochim. Biophys. Acta* **1054**, 95–102.

Cooper, D. R., Vila, M. C., Watson, J. E., Nair, G., Pollet, R. J., Standaert, M. and Farese, R. V. (1990b). *Diabetes* **39**, 1399–1407.

Corbett, J. A., Lancaster, J. R., Jr., Sweetland, M. A. and McDaniel, M. L. (1991). *J. Biol. Chem.* **266**, 21351–21354.

Corder, C. N., Collins, J. G., Brannan, T. S. and Sharma, J. (1977). *J. Histochem. Cytochem.* **25**, 1–8.

Cormont, M., Tanti, J. F., Gremeaux, T., Van Obberghen, E. and LeMarchand-Brustel, Y. (1991). *Endocrinology* **129**, 3342–3350.

Couet, C., Ulmer, M., Hamdaoui, M. and Derby, G. (1988). *In* "Acarbose for the Treatment of Diabetes Mellitus" (W. Creutzfeldt, ed.), pp. 69. Springer Verlag, Berlin, Heidelberg.

Couet, C., Ulmer, M., Hamdaoui, M., Bau H. M. and Debry, G. (1989). *Eur. J. Clin. Nutr.* **43**, 187–196.

Crooks, M. J. and Brown, K. F. (1975). *Biochem. Pharmacol.* **24**, 298–299.

Cryer, P. E. (1983) *Adv. Metab. Disord.* **10**, 469–483.

Cryer, P. E. and Gerich, J. E. (1985). *N. Engl. J. Med.* **313**, 232–241.

Cuatrecasas, P. (1971). *Proc. Natl Acad. Sci. USA* **68**, 1264–1268.

Cüppers, H. J., Berchtold, P. and Berger, M. (letter) (1980). *Br. Med. J.* **281**, 307.

Cüppers, H. J., Franzke, D., Esken, P., Jörgens, V. and Berger, M. (1982). *Akt. Endokrinol. Stoffwechsel* **3**, 102–108.

Cushman, S. W. and Wardzala, L. J. (1980). *J. Biol. Chem.* **255**, 4758–4762.

Czech, M. P. (1985). *Annu. Rev. Physiol.* **47**, 357–381.

Dahl-Jörgensen, K. (1987). *Acta Endocrinol.* **284** (Suppl.), 1–38.

Dahl-Jörgensen, K., Brinchmann-Hansen, O., Hanssen, K. F., Sandvik, L. and Aagenaes, O. (1985). *Brit. Med. J.* **290**, 811–815.

Damsbo, P., Vaag, A., Hother-Nielsen, O. and Beck-Nielsen, H. (1991). *Diabetologia* **34**, 239–245.

Dandona, P., Hooke, D. and Bell, J. (1978). *Br. Med. J.* **1**, 479–480.

Dandona, P., Fonseca, V., Mier, A. and Beckett, A. G. (1983). *Diabetes Care* **6**, 472–474.

Davidson, M. B. (1992). *Postgrad. Med.* **92**, 69–70, 73–76, 79–85.

Davidson, M. B. and Sladen, G. (1987). *Metabolism* **36**, 925–930.

Davies, I. B. (1984). *Br. J. Clin. Pharmacol.* **17**, 622 P.

Day, C. E. (1991). *Artery* **18**, 107–114.

DCC-Trial (1993). *N. Engl. J. Med.* **329**, 977–986.

Debant, A., Clauser, D. O., Morgan, M., Edery, R. A. and Roth, W. I. (1988). *Proc. Natl Acad. Sci. USA* **85**, 8032–8036.

Debant, A., Ponzio, G., Clauser, E., Contreres, J. O. and Rossi, B. (1989). *Biochemistry* **28**, 14–17.

Debry, G., Martin, J. M., Pointel, J. P. and Drouin, P. (1977). *In* "Part Played by the Biguanides in the Treatment of Diabetes", *Int. Symp.* Moscow (E. A. Babaian, E. A. Vasiukova and N. K. Shagako, eds), pp. 15–20.

DeFronzo, R. A. (1988). *Diabetes* **37**, 667–687.

DeFronzo, R. A. and Simonson, D. C. (1984). *Diabetes Care* **7** (Suppl. 1), 72–80.

Deleers, M., Lebrun, P. and Malaisse, W. J. (1983). *FEBS Lett.* **154**, 97–100.

DeMeyts, P., Gu, J. L., Shymko, R. M., Bell, G. and Whittaker, J. (1988). *Diabetologia* **31**, 484A.

DeMeyts, P., Gu, J. L., Katuria, S., Shymko, R. M., Kaplan, B. and Smal, J. (1989). *Diabetes* **38**, A3.

Dent, P., Lavionne, A., Nakielny, S., Candwell, F. B., Watt, P. and Cohen, P. (1990). *Nature* **348**, 302–308.

Descovich, G., Montaguti, U., Ceredi, C., Cocuzza, E. and Sirtori, C. R. (1978). *Artery* **4**, 348–359.

De Silva, N. E. and Tumbridge, W. M. G (1981). *Lancet* **i**, 128–131.

Deutsch, P. S., Wan, C. F., Rosen, O. M. and Rubin, C. S. (1983). *Proc. Natl Acad. Sci. USA* **80**, 133–136.

Devlin, J. G. (letter) (1984). *Am. Intern. Med.* **2**, 237.

Dey, N. G., Castleden, C. M., Ward, J., Cornhill, J. and McBurney, A. (1983). *Br. J. Clin. Pharmacol.* **16**, 438–440.

Diabetes Control and Complication Trial Research Group (1993). *N. Engl. J. Med.* **329**, 977–986.

Dimitriadis, G., Tessari, P. and Go, V. (1982). *In* "Proceedings of the First International Symposium on Acarbose" (W. Creutzfeld, ed), pp. 216–222. Excerpta Medica, Amsterdam.

DiPaolo, S. (1992). *Acta Endocrinol.* **126**, 117–123.

Dixon, K., Exon, P. D. and Malins, J. M. (1985). *Q.J. Med.* **44**, 543–555.

Dockray, G. F. (1987). *In* "Physiology of the Gastrointestinal Tract" (L. R. Johnson, ed.), Vol. 1, pp. 41–66. Raven Press, New York.

Dornan, T. L., Heller, S. R., Peck, G., Gregory, R. and Tattersall, R. B. (1988). *Diabetic Med.* **5** (Suppl. 2), A17.

Dornan, T. L., Heller, S. R., Peck, G. M. and Tattersall, R. B. (1991). *Diabetes Care* **14**, 342–344.

Douglass, J. M. (1975). *Ann. Int. Med.* **82**, 61–62.

Drejer, K., Vaag, A., Bech, K., Hansen, P. E., Sorensen, A. R. and Mygind, N. (1990). *Diabetologia* **33** (Suppl.), A61.

Drost, H., Hillebrand, I., Koschinsky, T., Voegle-Bohringer, M., Gries, F. A. (1982). *In* "Proceedings of the First International Symposium on Acarbose" (W. Creutzfeldt, ed.), pp. 330–334. Excerpta Medica, Amsterdam.

Drucker, D. J., Philippe, J., Mojsov, S., Chick, W. L. and Habener, J. F. (1987). *Proc. Natl Acad. Sci. USA* **84**, 3434–3438.

Drug Information: Glucotard, Boehringer, Mannheim, FRG.

Dunlop, M. E. and Larkins, R. G. (1988). *Biochem. J.* **253**, 67–72.

Dunlop, M. E. and Malaisse, W. J. (1986). *Arch. Biochem. Biophys.* **244**, 421–429.

Dunning, B. E., Ahrén, B., Veith, R. C., Böttcher, G., Sundler, F. V. and Taborsky, G. J., Jr. (1986). *Am. J. Physiol.* **251**, E127–E133.

Dvornik, D., Millen, J., Hicks, D., Cayen, M. and Sredy, J. (1988). *In* "Polyol Pathway and its Role in Diabetic Complications" (N. Sakamoto, J. H. Kinoshita, P. F. Kador and N. Hotta, eds), pp. 61–71. Elsevier Science Publishers BV, Amsterdam.

Easom, R. A., Hughes, J. H., Landt, M., Wolf, B. A., Turk, J. and McDaniel, M. L. (1989). *Biochem. J.* **264**, 27–33.

Ebert, R. and Creutzfeldt, W. (1982). *Endocrinology* **111**, 1601–1606.

Ebina, Y., Ellis, L., Jarnagin, K., Edery, M., Graf, L., Clauser, E., Ou, J., Masiar, F., Kan, Y. W., Goldfine, I. D., Roth, R. A. and Rutter, W. J. (1985). *Cell* **40**, 747–758.

Ebina, Y., Araki, E., Taira, M., Shimada, F., Craik, C. S., Siddle, K., Pierce, S. B., Roth, R. A. and Rutter, W. J. (1987). *Proc. Natl Acad. Sci. USA* **84**, 704–708.

Eckel, R. H., Fujimoto, W. J. and Brunzell, J. D. (1978). *Diabetes* **28**, 1141–1142.

Egan, J. J., Saltis, J., Wek, S. A., Simpson, I. A. and Londos, C. (1990). *Proc. Natl Acad. Sci. USA* **87**, 1052–1056.

Egan, S. E., Giddings, B. W., Brooks, M. W., Buday, L., Sizeland, A. M. and Weinberg, R. A. (1993). *Nature* **363**, 45–51.

Egger, M. and Smith, G. D. (letter) (1992). *Lancet* **340**, 301.

Egger, M., Smith, G. D. and Teuscher, A. (1992). *Br. Med. J.* **305**, 351–355.

Eizirik, D. L., Bendtzen, K. and Sandler, S. (1991a). *Endocrinology* **128**, 1611–1616.

Eizirik, D. L., Tracey, D. E., Bendtzen, K. and Sandler, S. (1991b). *Diabetologia* **34**, 445–448.

Elahi, D., Meneilly, G. S., Hinaker, K. L., Rowe, J. W. and Andersen, D. K. (1986). *In* "Proc. 6th Int. Conf. Gastrointestinal Hormones", Vancouver, BC, p. 18. National Research Council of Canadian Research Journals, Ottawa.

Ellis, L., Clauser, D. O., Morgan, M., Edery, R. A. and Roth, W. I. (1986). *Cell* **45**, 721–732.

Ellis, P. R. and Morris, E. R. (1991). *Diabetic. Med.* **8**, 378–381.

Elrick, H., Stimmler, L., Hlad, C. J. and Arai, Y. (1964). *J. Clin. Endocrinol. Metab.* **24**, 1076–1082.

Elvander-Stahl, E., Melander, A. and Wahlin-Boll, E. (1984). *Br. J. Clin. Pharmacol.* **18**, 773–778.

Endemann, G., Yonezawa, K. and Roth, R. A. (1990). *J. Biol. Chem.* **265**, 396–400.

Eriksson, J., Franssila-Kallunki, A., Ekstrand, A., Saloranta, C., Widen, E., Schalin, C. and Groop, L. (1989). *N. Engl. J. Med.* **321**, 337–343.

Escobedo, J. A., Kaplan, D. R., Kavanaugh, W. M., Turck, C. W. and Williams, L. T. (1991). *Mol. Cell. Biol.* **11**, 1125–1132.

Evans, M. H., Pace, C. S. and Clements, R. S. (1983). *Diabetes* **32**, 509–515.

Exton, J. H., Taylor, S. J., Augert, G. and Bocckino, S. B. (1991). *Mol. Cell Biochem.* **104**, 81–86.

Faber, O. K., Beck-Nielsen, H., Binder, C., Butzer, P., Damsgaard, E. M. and Froland, F. (1990). *Diabetes Care* **13** (Suppl. 3), 26–31.

Falck, J. R., Manna, S., Moltz, J., Chacos, N. and Capdevirla, J. (1983). *Res. Commun. Chem. Pathol. Pharmacol.* **114**, 743–749.

Falko, J. M. and Osei, K. (1985). *Am. J. Med.* **79**, 91–101.

Fantus, I. G. and Brosseau, R. (1986). *J. Clin. Endocrinol. Metab.* **63**, 898–905.

Farese, R. V., Ishizuka, T., Standaert, M. L. and Cooper, D. R. (1991). *Metabolism* **40**, 196–200.

Federlin, K., Laube, H. and Velcovsky, H. G. (1981). *Diabetes Care* **4**, 170–174.

Feely, J., and Peden N. (1983). *Br. J. Clin. Pharmacol.* **15**, 607 P.

Fehlmann, M., Carpentier, J. L., VanObberghen, E., Freychet, P., Thamm, P., Saunders, D., Brandenburg, D. and Orci, L. (1982). *Proc. Natl Acad. Sci. USA* **79**, 5921–5925.

Fehmann, H.-C., Göke, R., Göke, M. E., Trautmann, M. E. and Arnold, G. (1989). *FEBS Lett.* **252**, 109–112.

Fehmann, H.-C., Göke, R., Göke, B., Bachle, R., Wagner, B. and Arnold, R. (1991). *Biochim. Biophys. Acta* **1091**, 356–363.

Feinglos, M. N. and Jegasothy, B. V. (1979). *Lancet* i, 122–124.

Feldmann, J. M. (1985). *Pharmacotherapy* **5**, 43–62.

Ferlito, S., Del Campo, F., Di Vincenzo, S., Damante, G. and Coco, R. (1983). *Farmaco (Sci.)* **38**, 248–254.

Ferner, R. E. (1988). *Med. Clin. North Am.* **72**, 1323–1335.

Ferner, R. E. and Chaplin, S. (1987). *Clin. Pharmacokinet.* **12**, 379–401.

Ferrari, C., Frezzati, S., Testori, G. P. and Bertazzoni, A. (1976). *N. Engl. J. Med.* **294**, 1184.

Field, J. B. (1979). *In* "Endocrinology" (L. J. de Groot, ed.), Vol. 7, pp. 1069–1074. Grune & Stratton, New York.

Findlay, L., Ashcroft, F. M., Kelly, R. P., Rorsman, P., Petersen, O. H. and Trube, G. (1989). *Ann. N.Y. Acad. Sci.* **560**, 403–409.

Fineberg, S. E., Galloway, J. A., Fineberg, N. S., Rathbun, M. J. and Hufferd, S. (1983). *Diabetologia* **25**, 465–469.

Fisher, B. M., Gillen, G., Hepburn, D. A., Dargie, H. J. and Frier, B. M. (1990). *Am. J. Physiol.* **258**, H1775–1179.

Fleig, W. E., Noether-Fleig, G., Fußgänger, R. and Ditschuneit, H. (1984). *Diabetes* **33**, 285–289.

Flores, D., Arcais, A., Morandi, F., Beccari, L., Meschi, F. and Chiumello, G. (1984). *Horm. Res.* **19**, 65–69.

Flores-Riveros, J. R., Sibley, E., Kastelic, T. and Lane, M. D. (1989). *J. Biol. Chem.* **264**, 21557–21572.

Florholmen, J., Malm, D., Vonen, B. and Burhol, P. G. (1989). *Am. J. Physiol.* **257**, G865–870.

Folling, I. and Norman, N. (1972). *Diabetes* **21**, 814–826.

Fölsch, U. R., Bert, R. and Creutzfeldt, W. (1981). *Scand. J. Gastroenterol.* **16**, 629–663.

Fölsch, U. R., Spengler, M., Boehme, K. and Sommerauer, B. (1990). *Diabetes Nutr. Metab.* (Suppl. 1), 63–68.

Fox, J. A., Soliz, N. M. and Saltiel, A. R. (1987). *Proc. Natl Acad. Sci. USA* **84**, 2663–2667.

Frank, H. J. L., Donohoe, M. T. and Morris, W. L. (1985). *Am. J. Med.* **79** (Suppl. 3B), 53–58.

Frankland, A. W. (letter) (1982). *Lancet* **ii**, 1468.

Frattali, A. L., Treadway, J. L. and Pessin, J. E. (1992). *J. Cell. Biochem.* **48**, 43–50.

Frauman, A. G., Cooper, M. E., Parsons, B. J., Jerums, G. and Louis, W. J. (1987). *Diabetes Care* **10**, 573–578.

Freychet, P., Kahn, C. R., Jarret, D. B. and Roth, J. (1971). *Proc. Natl Acad. Sci USA* **68**, 1833–1837.

Freymond, D., Bogardus, C., Okubo, M., Sotne, K. and Mott, D. (1988). *J. Clin. Invest.* **82**, 1503–1509.

Frias, I. and Waugh, S. M. (1989). *Diabetes* **38**, A238.

Fridolf, T., Karlsson, S. and Ahrén, B. (1988). *Biochem. Biophys. Res. Commun.* **184**, 878–882.

Friedman, J. E., Pories, W. J., Legget-Frazier, N., Roy, L. L., Long, S. D., Caro, J. F. and Dohm, G. L. (1991). *Diabetes* **40**, A630.

Froesch, E. R. and Zapf, J. (1985). *Diabetologia* **28**, 485–493.

Fuhrmann, K. (1986). *Acta Endocrinol.* **277** (Suppl.), 74–76.

Fui, S. N. T., Keen, H., Jarrett, R. J., Straleosch, C., Murrells, T. and Marsden, P. (1983). *Br. Med. J.* **287**, 1509–1512.

Fukumoto, H., Seino, S., Imura, H., Seino, Y., Eddy, R. L., Fukishima, Y., Byers, M. G., Shows, T. B. and Bell, G. I. (1988). *Proc. Natl Acad. Sci. USA* **85**, 5434–5438.

Fukumoto, H., Kayano, T., Buse, J. B., Edwards, Y., Pilch, P., Bell, G. I. and Seino, S. (1989). *J. Biol. Chem.* **264**, 7776–7779.

Gachályi, B., Tornyossy, A., Vas, A. and Káldor, A. (1980). *Int. J. Clin. Pharmacol.* **18**, 133–135.

Gaines, K. L., Hamilton, S. and Boyd, A. E. III (1988). *J. Biol. Chem.* **263**, 2589–2592.

Gan, S. C., Barr, J., Arieff, A. I. and Pearl R. G. (1992). *Arch. Intern. Med.* **152**, 2333–2336.

Ganz, M. A., Unterman, T., Roberts, M., Uy, R., Sahgal, S., Samter, M. and Grammer, L. C. (1990). *J. Allergy Clin. Immunol.* **86**, 45–51.

Garcia de Herreros, A. and Birnbaum, M. (1989). *J. Biol. Chem.* **264**, 9885–9890.

Garcia-Ortega, P., Knobel, H. and Mirada, A. (1984). *Brit. Med. J.* **288**, 1271.

Garret, E. R., Tsau, J. and Hinderling, P. H. (1972). *J. Pharm. Sci.* **61**, 1411–1418.

Garrino, M. G., Schmeer, W., Nenquin, M., Meissner, H. P. and Henquin, J. C. (1985). *Diabetologia* **28**, 697–703, 1985.

Garvey, W. T., Hueckstaedt, T. P., Matthaei, S. and Olefsky, J. M. (1988). *J. Clin. Invest.* **81**, 1528–1536.

Gaulton, G. N. (1991). *Diabetes* **40**, 1297–1304.

Gawler, D., Milligan, G., Spiegel, A. M., Unson, L. G. and Houslay, M. D. (1987). *Nature* **327**, 229–232.

Gawler, D., Milligan, G. and Houslay, M. D. (1988). *Biochem. J.* **249**, 537–542.

Gawler, D. J., Wilson, A. and Houslay, M. D. (1989). *J. Endocrinol.* **122**, 207–212.

Geisen, K., Hitzel, V., Ökomonopoulos, R., Pünter, J., Weyer, R. and Summ, H. D. (1985). *Drug Res.* **35**, 707–712.

Gerich, J. (1985). *Mayo Clin. Proc.* **60**, 434–439.

Gerich, J. (1988). *Diabetes* **37**, 1608–1617.

Gerich, J., Langlois, M., Noacco, C., Karam, J., Forsham, P. (1973). *Science* **182**, 171–173.

Gerich, J., Davis, J., Lorenzi, M., Rizza, R., Karam, J., Lewis, S., Kaplan, R., Schultz, T. and Cryer, P. (1979). *Am. J. Physiol.* **236**, E380–385.

Gerich, J. E. (1989). *N. Engl. J. Med.* **321**, 1231–1245.

Gerich, J. E., Mitrakou, A., Kelley, D., Veneman, T., Jenssen, T., Pangburn, T. and Reilly, Y. (1990). *Diabetes* **39**, 211–216.

German, M. S. (1993). *Proc. Natl Acad. Sci. USA* **90**, 1781–1785.

Gherzi, R., Sesti, G., Andraghetti, G., De Pirro, R., Lauro, Adezati, J. and Cordera, R. (1989). *J. Biol. Chem.* **264**, 8627–8635.

Gill, V. G. (1991). *In* "Textbook of Diabetes" (J. C. Pickup and G. Williams, eds), pp. 24–29. Blackwell Sci. Publications, Oxford.

Gilon, P. and Henquin, J.-C. (1992). *J. Biol. Chem.* **267**, 20713–20720.

Gin, H., Slama, G., Weissbrodt, P., Poynard, T., Vexiau, P., Klein, J. C. and Tchobroutsky, G. (1982). *Diabetologia* **23**, 34–36.

Gin, H., Viala, R., Rigal, F., Morlat, P., Beauvieux, J. M. and Aubertin, J. (1989a). *Rev. Med. Interne.* **10**, 361–363.

Gin, H., Orgerie, M. B. and Aubertin, J. (1989b). *Horm. Metab. Res.* **21**, 81–83.

Giroix, M.-H., Sener, A. and Malaisse, W. J. (1985). *FEBS Lett.* **185**, 1–3.

Giugliano, D., Marfella, R., Quatraro, A., De-Rosa, N., Salvatore, T., Cozzolino, D., Ceriello, A. and Torella, R. (1993). *Ann. Intern. Med.* **118**, 7–11.

Golay, A., DeFronzo, R. A., Ferrannini, E., Simonson, D. C., Thorin, D., Acheson, K., Thiebaud, D., Curchod, B., Jequiem, B. and Felber, J. P. (1988). *Diabetologia* **31**, 585–591.

Goldberg, R. B., Reeves, M. L., Seigler, D. E., Ryan, E. A., Miller, N., Hsia, S. L. and Skyler, J. S. (1985). *Acta Diabetol. Lat.* **22**, 93–101.

Goldfine, I. D. (1987). *Endocr. Rev.* **8**, 235–255.

Goldgewicht, C., Slama, G., Papoz, I. and Tchobroutsky, G. (1983). *Diabetologia* **24**, 95–99.

Goldman, J., Baldwin, D., Rubenstein, A. H., Klink, D. D., Blackard, W. G., Fisher, L. K., Roe, T. F. and Schnure, J. J. (1979). *J. Clin. Invest.* **63**, 1050–1059.

Goldstein, B. J. (1992). *J. Cell Biochem.* **48**, 33–42.

Goodner, C. J., Koerker, D. J., Stagner, J. I. and Samols, E. (1991). *Am. J. Physiol.* **260**, E422–E429.

Gopalakrishnan, M. and Triggle, D. J. (1992). *Biochem. Pharmacol.* **44**, 1843–1847.

Goren, H. J., White, M. F. and Kahn, C. R. (1987). *Biochemistry* **26**, 2374–2382.

Gorus, F. K., Schuit, F. C., In't Veld, P. A., Gepts, W. and Pipeleers, D. G. (1988). *Diabetes* **37**, 1090–1095.

Grammer, L. C., Metzger, B. E. and Patterson, R. (1984). *J. Am. Med. Assoc.* **251**, 1459–1460.

Granovskaja-Svetkova, A.M. (1977). *In* "Part Played by the Biguanides in the Treatment of Diabetes", *Int. Symp.*, Moscow (E. A. Babaian, E. A. Vasiukova and N. K. Shagako, eds), p. 14.

Gray, R. S., Cowan, P., di Mario, U., Elton, R. A., Clarke, B. F. and Duncan, L. J. P. (1985). *Br. Med. J.* **290**, 1687–1691.

Green, A., Borch-Johnsen, K., Kragh Andersen, P., Keiding, N., Kreiner, S. and Deckert, T. (1985) *Diabetologia* **28**, 389–342

Greene, D. A., Lattimer, S. A. and Sima, A. A. (1987a). *N. Engl. J. Med.* **316**, 599–606.

Greene, D. A., Chakrabarti, S., Lattimer, S. A. and Sima, A. A. (1987b). *J. Clin. Invest.* **79**, 1479–1485.

Greenfeld, M. S., Doberne, L., Rosenthal, M., Vreman, H. J. and Reaven, G. M. (1982). *Arch. Intern. Med.* **142**, 1498–1500.

Gregorio, F., Filipponi, P., Ambrosi, F., Christallini, S., Marchetti, P., Calafiore, R., Navalesi, R. and Brunetti, P. (1989). *Diabete Metab.* **15**, 111–117.

Gregorio, F., Ambrosi, F., Marchetti, P., Christallini, S., Navalesi, R., Brunetti, P. and Filipponi, P. (1990). *Acta Diabetol. Lat.* **27**, 139–155.

Griffith, O. W. and Meister, A. (1979). *J. Biol. Chem.* **254**, 7558–7560.

Grill, V. and Cerasi, E. (1976). *Biochim. Biophys. Acta* **437**, 36–50.

Groop, L., Harno, K. and Tolppanen, E. M. (1984). *Acta Endocrinol.* **106**, 97–101.

Groop, L., Harno, K., Nikkila, E. A., Pelkonen, R. and Tolppanen, E. M. (1985). *Acta Med. Scand.* **217**, 33–39.

Groop, L., Schalin, C., Franssila-Kallunki, A., Widen, E., Ekstrand, A. and Eriksson, J. (1989). *Am. J. Med.* **87**, 183–190.

Gu, X. H., Kurose, T., Kato, S., Masuda, K., Tsuda, K., Ishida, H. and Seino, Y. (1993). *Life Sci.* **52**, 687–694.

Gulliford, M. C., Bicknell, E. J. and Scarpello, J. H. (1988a). *Eur. J. Clin. Nutr.* **42**, 871–876.

Gulliford, M. C., Pover, G. G., Bicknell, E. J., and Scarpello, J. H. (1988b). *Eur. J. Clin. Nutr.* **42**, 451–454.

Gunderson, K., Crim, J. A., Bryant, D. D. and Hearron, A. E. (1975). "Micronase, Pharmacological and Clinical Evaluation". *Int. Symp.* Series 382, pp. 216–224. Excerpta Medica, Amsterdam.

Gustafson, A., Björntorp, P. and Fahlen, M. (1971). *Acta Med. Scand.* **190**, 491–494.

Gyimesi, A. and Ivanyi, J. (1989). *Orv. Hetil.* **130**, 2751–2752.

Gylfe, E., Hellmann, B., Sehlin, J., Täljedal, I.-B. (1984). *Experientia* **40**, 1126–1133.

Hampton, S. M., Morgan, L. M., Tredger, J. A., Cramb, R. and Marks, V. (1986). *Diabetes* **35**, 612–616.

Handberg, A., Vaag, A., Damsbo, P., Beck-Nielsen, H. and Vinten, J. (1990). *Diabetologia* **33**, 625–627.

Hanefeld, M., Fischer, S., Schulze, J., Lüthke, C. and Spengler, M. (1990). *Diabetes Nutr. Metab.* (Suppl. 1), 51–57.

Hanefeld, M., Fischer, S., Schulze, J., Spengler, M., Wargenau, M., Schollberg, K. and Fucker, K. (1991). *Diabetes Care* **14**, 732–737.

Hansen, B. C., Jen, K. L., Pek, S. B. and Wolfe, R. A. (1982). *J. Clin. Endocrinol. Metab.* **54**, 785–792.

Hansen, T., Bjorback, C., Vestergaard, H., Bak, J. F. and Pedersen, O. (1992). *Diabetologia* **35**, 76A.

Hanssen, K. F. (1991). In "Textbook of Diabetes" (J. C. Pickup and G. Williams, eds), pp. 519–525. Blackwell Sci. Publications, Oxford.

Häring, H. U. (1991). *Diabetologia* **34**, 848–861.

Häring, H. U. and Mehnert, H. (1993). *Diabetologia* **36**, 176–182.

Häring, H. U., Biermann, E. and Kemmler, W. (1981). *Am. J. Physiol.* **240**, E556–E565.

Häring, H. U., Biermann, E. and Kemmler, W. (1982a). *Am. J. Physiol.* **242**, E234–E240.

Häring, H. U., Kasuga, M. and Kahn, C. R. (1982b). *Biochem. Biophys. Res. Commun.* **108**, 1538–1545.

Häring, H. U., Kasuga, M., White, M. F., Crettaz, M. and Kahn, C. R. (1984). *Biochemistry* **23**, 3298–3306.

Häring, H. U., White, M. F., Kahn, C. R., Ahmad, Z., DePaoli-Roach, A. A. and Roach, P. J. (1985). *J. Cell. Biochem.* **28**, 171–182.

Häring, H. U., Kirsch, D., Obermaier, B., Ermel, B. and Machicao, F. (1986a). *Biochem. J.* **234**, 59–66.

Häring, H. U., Kirsch, D., Obermaier, B., Ermel, B. and Machicao, F. (1986b). *Biochem. J.* **261**, 3869–3875.

Häring, H. U., White, M. F., Machicao, F., Ermel, B., Schleicher, E. and Obermaier, B. (1987). *Proc. Natl Acad. Sci. USA* **84**, 113–117.

Harris, E. L. (1971). *Br. Med. J.* **3**, 29–30.

Harrison, D. E. and Ashcroft, S. J. H. (1982). *Biochim. Biophys. Acta* **714**, 313–319.

Harrower, A. D. (1985). *Curr. Med. Res.* **9**, 676–680.

Harrower, A. D. and Wong, C. (1990). *Diabetes Res.* **13**, 19–21.

Hartling, S. G., Faber, O. K., Wegmann, M. L., Wahlin-Boll, E. and Melander, A. (1987). *Diabetes Care* **10**, 683–686.

Hartman, H., Ebert, R. and Creutzfeldt, W. (1986). *Diabetologia* **29**, 112–114.

Hasselblatt, A. (1989). *In* "Diabetes and the Kidney" (A. Heidland, K. M. Koch and E. Heidbreder, eds) Vol. 73, pp. 139–146. S. Karger Verlag, Basel.

Hatao, K., Kaku, K., Matsuda, M., Tsuchiya, M. and Kaneko, T. (1985). *Diabetes Res. Clin. Pract.* **1**, 49–53.

Haupt, E., Putschky, F. and Schöffling, K. (1984). *Deutsche Med. Wo. Schr.* **109**, 210–213.

Haupt, E., Knick, B., Koschinsky, T., Liebermeister, H., Schneider, J. and Hirsche, H. (1989) *Med. Welt* **40**, 118–123.

Hausmann, L., Schubotz, R. (1975). *Arzneimittel-Forschung/Drug Res.* **25**, 668–675.

Hayakawa, T., Kondo, T., Okumura, N., Nagai, K., Shibata, T. and Kitagawa, M. (1989). *Am. J. Gastroenterol.* **84**, 523–526.

Hedeskov, C. J. (1980). *Physiol. Rev.* **60**, 442–509.

Hedo, J. A., Kasuga, M., Vanobberghen, E., Roth J. and Kahn, C. R. (1981). *Proc. Natl Acad. Sci.* **78**, 4791–4795.

Hedo, J. A., Kahn, C. R., Hayashi, M., Yamada, K. M. and Kasuga, M. (1983). *J. Biol. Chem.* **259**, 9913–9921.

Held, H., Kaminsky, B. and v. Oldershausen, H. F. (1970). *Diabetologia* **6**, 386–391.

Hellman, B. (1981). *Mol. Pharmacol.* **20**, 83–88.

Hellman, B. (1986). *Diabetes/Metab. Rev.* **2**, 215–241.

Hellman, B. (1988). *In* "Pathology of the Endocrine Pancreas" (P. J. Lefebvre and D. G. Pipeleers, eds), pp. 249–268. Springer Verlag, Heidelberg.

Hellman, B. and Gylfe, E. (1986). *In* "Calcium and Cell Function" (W. E. Cheung, ed.) Vol. VI, pp. 253–326. Academic Press, Orlando.

Hellman, B., Idahl, L.-Å. and Danielsson, Å. (1969). *Diabetes* **18**, 509–516.

Hellman, B., Idahl, L., Lernmark, A., Sehlin, J. and Täljedal, I. B. (1975). *Biochim. Biophys. Acta* **392**, 101–109.

Hellman, B., Sehlin, J., Täljedal, I.-B. (1984). *Acta Endocrinol. Copen.* **105**, 385–390.

Hellman, B., Gylfe, E., Grapeugiesser, E., Lund, P.-E. and Marcström, A. (1992). *In* "Nutrient Regulation of Insulin Secretion" (P. R. Flatt, ed.), pp. 213–246. Portland Press, London and Chapel Hill.

Henquin, J.-C. (1980a). *Biochem. J.* **186**, 541–550.

Henquin, J.-C. (1980b). *Diabetologia* **18**, 151–160.

Henquin, J.-C. (1985). *In* "The Diabetes Annual I" (K. G. F. M. M. Alberti and J. P. Krall, eds), pp. 389–405. Elsevier Science Publishers B.V., Amsterdam.

Henquin, J.-C. and Meissner, H. P. (1982). *Biochem. Pharmacol.* **31**, 1407–1415.

Henquin, J.-C. and Meissner, H. P. (1983). *Biochem. Biophys. Res. Commun.* **112**, 614–620.

Henquin, J.-C. and Meissner, H. P. (1984). *Experientia* **40**, 1043–1052.

Henquin, J.-C., Schmeer, W. and Meissner, H. P. (1983). *Endocrinology* **112**, 2218–2220.

Henquin, J.-C., Debuyser, A., Drews, G. and Plant, T. D. (1992). *In* "Nutrient Regulation of Insulin Secretion" (P. R. Flatt, ed.), pp. 173–191. Portland Press, London and Chapel Hill.

Hermann, L. S. (1979). *Diabetes Metab.* **3**, 233–245.

Hermansen, K. (1983). *Endocrinology* **113**, 1149–1154.

Hermansen, K. (1984). *Endocrinology* **114**, 1770–1775.

Hermansen, K. and Ahrén, B. (1990). *Acta Physiol. Scand.* **138**, 175–179.

Herrera, R., Lebwohl, D., Garcia de Herreros, A., Kallen, R. G. and Rosen, O. M. (1988). *J. Biol. Chem.* **263**, 5560–5568.

Heurich, R. O., Friderich, G. and Ammon, H. P. T. (1992). *Diabetologia* **35** (Suppl. 1), A112.

Heyworth, C. M. and Houslay, M. D. (1983). *Biochem. J.* **214**, 547–552.

Heyworth, C. M., Whetton, A. D., Wong, S., Martin, B. R. and Houslay, M. D. (1985). *Biochem. J.* **228**, 593–603.

Hicks, D. R., Kraml, M., Cayen, M. N., Dubuc, J., Ryder, S. and Dvornik, D. (1984). *Clin. Pharmacol. Ther.* **36**, 493–499.

Hillaire-Buys, D., Bertrand, G., Gross, R. and Loubatieres-Mariani, M. M. (1987). *Eur. J. Pharmacol.* **136**, 109–112.

Hillebrand, I., Boehme, K., Frank, G., Fink, H. and Berchtold, P. (1979). *Res. Exp. Med.* **175**, 81–86.

Hillebrand, I., Reis, H. E., Boehme, K. and Jahnke, K. (1982). *In* "Proceedings of the First International Symposium on Acarbose" (W. Creutzfeldt, ed.), pp. 482–485. Excerpta Medica, Amsterdam.

Hirata, Y., Tominaga, M., Ito, J. I. and Noguchi, A. (1974). *Ann. Intern. Med.* **81**, 214–218.

Hoffmann, R. D., Flores-Riveros, J. R., Liao, K., Laird, D. M. and Lane, M. D. (1988). *Proc. Natl Acad. Sci. USA* **85**, 8835–8839.

Hoich, R. I. and Ng, F. M. (1986). *Pharmacol. Res. Commun.* **18**, 419–430.

Holdaway, I. M. and Wilson, J. D. (1984). *Br. Med. J.* **289**, 1565–1566.

Holloszy, J. O., Constable, S. H. and Young, D. A. (1986). *Diabetes Metab. Rev.* **1**, 409–424.

Hollund, E., Pedersen, O., Richelsen, B., Beck-Nielsen, H. and Schwarz-Sörensen, N. (1983). *Metabolism* **32**, 1067–1075.

Holman, R. R. and Steemson, J. (1989). *Diabetic Med.* **6** (Suppl. 1), A41.

Holman, R. R., Dornan, T. L., Mayon-White, V., Howard-Williams, J., Orde-Peckar, C., Jenkins, L. and Steemson, J. (1983). *Lancet* i, 204–208.

Holman, R. R., Steemson, J., Turner, R. C. (1987). *Diabetic Med.* **4**, 457–462.

Holmes, B., Heel, R. C., Brodgen, R. N., Speight, T. M. and Avery, G. S. (1984). *Drugs* **27**, 301–327.

Holst, J. J. (1992). *In* "Nutrient Regulation of Insulin Secretion" (P. R. Flatt, ed.), pp. 23–39. Portland Press, London and Chapel Hill.

Holst, J. J., Fahrenkrug, J., Knuhtsen, S., Jensen, S. L., Poulsen, S. S. and Nielsen, O. V. (1984). *Regul. Pept.* **8**, 245–259.

Holst, J. J., Fahrenkrug, J., Knuhtsen, S. L., Nielsen, O. V., Lundberg, J. M. and Hökfelt, T. (1987). *Am. J. Physiol.* **252**, G182–189.

Holt, S., Heading, R. C., Carter, D. C., Prescott, L. F. and Tothill, P. (1979). *Lancet* ii, 636–639.

Homma, Y., Irie, N., Yano, Y., Nakaya, N. and Goto, Y. (1982). *Tokai J. Exp. Clin. Med.* **7**, 393–396.

Hother-Nielsen, O., Schmitz, O., Andersen, P. H., Beck-Nielsen, H. and Pedersen, O. (1989). *Acta Endocrinol. Copenh.* **120**, 257–265.

Housley, M. D. (1991). *Eur. J. Biochem.* **195**, 9–27.

Hsu, W. H., Xiang, H. D., Rajan, A. S., Kunze, D. L. and Boyd, A. E. (1991). *J. Biol. Chem.* **266**, 837–843.

Hughes, S. J. and Ashcroft, S. J. H. (1992). *In* "Nutrient Regulation of Insulin Secretion" (P. R. Flatt, ed.), pp. 271–288. Portland Press, London and Chapel Hill.

Hundal, H. S., Ramlal, T., Reyes, R., Leiter, L. A. and Klip, A. (1992). *Endocrinology* **131**, 1165–1173.

Husband, D. J. and Gill, G. V. (letter) (1984). *Lancet* ii, 1477.

Hutton, J. C., Penn, E. J. and Peshavaria, M. (1983). *Biochem. J.* **210**, 297.

Ichihara, K., Shima, K., Saito, Y., Noraka, K., Tarui, S. and Nishikawa, M. (1977). *Diabetes* **26**, 500–506.

Ipp, E. and Unger, R. H. (1979). *Endocrinol. Res. Commun.* **6**, 37–42.

Ipp, E., Dobbs, R. and Unger, R. H. (1978). *Nature* **276**, 190–191.

Issekutz, B. (1980). *Diabetes* **29**, 629–635.

Ivy, J. and Holloszy, J. O. (1981) *Am. J. Physiol.* **241**, C200–203.

Izumi, T., White, M. F., Kadowaki, T., Takaku, F., Akanuma, Y. and Kasuga, M. (1987). *J. Biol. Chem.* **262**, 1282–1287.

Jackson, J. E. and Bressler, R. (1981). *Drugs* **22**, 211–245, 295–320.

Jackson, R. A., Hawa, M. I., Jaspan, J. B., Sim, B. M., Disilvio, L., Featherbe, D. and Krutz, A. B. (1987). *Diabetes* **36**, 632–640.

Jacob, R., Barrett, E., Plewe, G., Fagin, K. D. and Sherwin, R. S. (1989). *J. Clin. Invest.* **83**, 1717–1723.

Jacobs, D. B. and Jung, C. Y. (1985). *J. Biol. Chem.* **260**, 2593–2596.

Jacobs, S. and Cuatrecasas, P. (1981). *Endocrinol. Rev.* **2**, 251–263.

Jacobs, S., Sahyoun, N. E., Saltiel, A. R. and Cuatrecasas, P. (1983). *Proc. Natl Acad. Sci. USA* **80**, 6211–6213.

Jain, A. K., Ryan, J. R., McMahon, F. G. (1975). *N. Engl. J. Med.* **293**, 1283–1286.

Jain, N. K., Kulkarni, K. and Talwar, N. (1992). *Pharmazie* **47**, 277–278.

James, D. E., Brown, R., Navarro, J. and Pilch P. F. (1988). Nature **333**, 183–185.

James, D. E., Strube, M. and Mueckler, M. (1989). *Nature* **338**, 83–87.

Janbon, M., Chaptal, J., Vedel, A. and Schaap, J. (1942a). *Montpellier Med.* **21–22**, 441.

Janbon, M., Lazergbes, P. and Metropolitansky, J. H. (1942b). *Montpellier Med.* **21–22**, 489.

Jandrain, B., Gerard, J., Verdin, E. and Leferbvre, P. J. (1988). *In* "Acarbose for the Treatment of Diabetes Mellitus" (W. Creutzfeldt, ed.), pp. 66. Springer Verlag, Heidelberg, Berlin.

Jarret, R. J. (1991). *In* "Textbook of Diabetes" (J. C. Pickup and G. Williams, eds), pp. 47–56. Blackwell Sci. Publications, Oxford.

Jarrett, A. M. (1986). *Diabetic Med.* **3**, 552–556.

Jenkins, D. J., Leeds, A. R., Gassull, M. A., Wolever, T. M., Goff, D. V., Alberti, K. G. and Hockaday, T. D. (1976), *Lancet* ii, 172–174.

Jenkins, D. J. A., Hockaday, T. D. R., Howarth, R., Apling, E. C., Wolever, T. M. S., Leeds, A. R., Bacon, S. and Dilawari, J. (1977a). *Lancet* ii, 779–780.

Jenkins, D. J., Leeds, A. R., Gassull, M. A., Cochet, B. and Alberti, K. G. (1977b). *Ann. Intern. Med.* **86**, 20–23.

Jenkins, D. J., Wolever, T. M., Leeds, A. R., Gassull, M. A., Haisman, P., Dilawari, J., Goff, D. V., Metz, G. L., Alberti, K. G. (1978). *Br. Med. J.* **1**, 1392–1394.

Jenkins, D. J., Wolever, T. M., Nineham, R., Sarson, D. L., Bloom, S. R., Ahern, J., Alberti, K. G. and Hockaday, T. D. (1980). *Diabetologia* **19**, 21–24.

Jenkins, D. J. A., Barker, H. M., Taylor, R. H. and Fielden, H. (letter) (1982). *Lancet* i, 109.

Jensen, S. L., Fahrenkrug, J., Holst, J. J., Nielsen, O. V. and Schaffalitzky de Muckadell, O. B. (1978). *Am. J. Physiol.* **235**, E387–E391.

Jerums, G., Murray, R. M., Seeman, E., Cooper, M. E., Edgley, S., Marwick, K., Larkins, R. G. and Martin, T. J. (1987). *Diabetes Res. Clin. Pract.* **3**, 71–80.

Jo, H., Davis, H. W. and McDonald, J. M. (1990). *Diabetes* **39** (Suppl. 1), 1A.

Johnson, I. T. and Gee, M. J. (1980). *Proc. Nutr. Soc.* **39**, 52A.

Johnson, J. D., Wong, M. L. and Rutter, W. J. (1988). *Proc. Natl Acad. Sci. USA* **85**, 7516–7520.

Johnston, D. G. and Alberti, K. G. (1982). *J. Clin. Endocrinol. Metab.* **11**, 329–361.

Jones, D. B., Slaughter, P., Lousley, S., Carter, R. D., Jelfs, D., Fischer, K. and Mann, J. I. (1983). In "Pflanzenfasern – Neue Wege in der Stoffwechseltherapie" (S. Karger, ed.), pp. 216–221. S. Karger Verlag, Basel.

Jones, I. R., Owens, D. R., Moody, A. J., Luzio, S. D., Morris, T. and Hayes, T. M. (1987). *Diabetologia* **30**, 707–712.

Jones, P. M., Stutchfield, J. and Howell, S. L. (1985). *FEBS Lett.* **191**, 102–106.

Jones, P. M., Persaud, S. J. and Howell, S. L. (1992) *Life Sci.* **50**, 761–767.

Joost, H. G. (1985). *Trends Pharmacol. Sci.* **6**, 239–241.

Joost, H. G., Weber, T. M., Cushman, S. W. and Simpson, I. A. (1986). *J. Biol. Chem.* **261**, 10017–10020.

Joost, H. G., Weber, T. M., Cushman, S. W. and Simpson, I. A. (1988). *Biochem. J.* **249**, 155–161.

Jörgensen, S. and Drejer, K. (1990). In "New Antidiabetic Drugs" (C. J. Baily and R. P. Flatt, eds), pp. 83–92. Smith-Gordon, London.

Josephkutty, S. and Potter, J. M. (1990). *Diabetic Med.* **7**, 510–514.

Judis, J. (1973). *J. Pharm. Sci.* **62**, 232–237.

Kabachi, U. M. and Birkenholz, M. R. (1988). *Arch. Intern. Med.* **148**, 1745–1749.

Kadowaki, T., Koyasu, S., Nishida, E., Tobe, K., Izumi, T., Takaku, F., Sakai, H., Yahara, J. and Kasuga, M. (1987). *J. Biol. Chem.* **262**, 7342–7350.

Kadowaki, H., Kadowaki, T., Marcus-Samuels, B., Cama, A., Rovira, A. and Taylor, S. (1989). *Diabetes* **38**, A8.

Kaestner, K. H., Christy, R. J., McLenithan, J. C., Braiterman, L. T., Cornelius, P., Pekala, P. H. and Lane, M. D. (1989). *Proc. Natl Acad. Sci. USA* **86**, 3150–3154.

Kahn, B. B. and Cushman, S. W. (1987). *J. Biol. Chem.* **262**, 5118–5124.

Kahn, C. R. (1985). *Annu. Rev. Med.* **36**, 429–451.

Kahn, C. R. and Schechter, Y. (1990). *In* "Goodman and Gilman's The Pharmacological Basis of Therapeutics", 8th edition (A. Goodman Gilman, T. W. Rall, A. S. Nies and P. Taylor, eds), pp. 1463–1495. Pergamon Press, New York, Oxford.

Kahn, C. R., White, M. F., Shoelson, S. E., Backer, J. M., Araki, E., Cheatham, B., Csermely, P., Folli, F., Goldstein, B. J. and Huertas, P. (1993). *Recent Prog. Horm. Res.* **48**, 291–339.

Kaiser, N., Tur Sinal, A. and Cerasi, E. (1983). *Isr. J. Med. Sci.* **19**, 304.

Kanefsky, T. M. and Medoff, S. J. (1980). *Arch. Intern. Med.* **140**, 1543.

Kang, S., Owen, D. R., Vora, J. P. and Brange, J. (1990). *Lancet* **335**, 303–306.

Kannisto, H. and Neuvonen, P. J. (1984). *J. Pharm. Sci.* **73**, 253–256.

Kaplan, D. R., Whitman, M., Schaffhausen, B., Pallas, D. C., White, M. F., Cantley, L. and Roberts, M. (1987). *Cell* **50**, 1021–1029.

Karnieli, E., Armoni, M., Cohen, P., Kanter, Y. and Rafaeloff, R. (1987). *Diabetes* **36**, 925–931.

Karsh, J. (1990). *Drug Saf.* **5**, 317–327.

Kasanicki, M. A. and Pilch, P. F. (1990). *Diabetes Care* **13**, 219–227.

Kasuga, M., Karlsson, F. A. and Kahn, C. R. (1982a). *Science* **215**, 185–187.

Kasuga, M., Zick, M., Blithe, D. L., Karlsson, F. A., Häring, H. U. and Kahn, C. R. (1982b). *J. Biol. Chem.* **257**, 9891–9894.

Kaubisch, N., Hammer, R., Wollheim, C., Renold, A. E. and Offord, R. E. (1982). *Biochem. Pharmacol.* **31**, 1171–1174.

Kawahara, D. J., Everts, M., Buckingham, B., Sandborg, C. and Berman, M. (1991). *J. Immunother.* **10**, 182–188.

Kawazu, S., Sener, A., Couturier, E. and Malaisse, W. J. (1980). *Naunyn-Schmiedebergs Arch. Pharmacol.* **312**, 277–283.

Kayano, T., Fukumoto, H., Eddy, R. L., Fan, Y. S., Byers, M. G., Shows, T. B. and Bell, G. I. (1988). *J. Biol. Chem.* **263**, 15245–15248.

Keen, H., Collins, C. G. and Bending, J. J (1987). *Diabetologia* **30**, 538A (Abstr.)

Kellerer, M., Seffer, E., Mushack, J., Obermaier-Kusser, B. and Häring, H. U. (1990). *Biochem. Biophys. Res. Commun.* **172**, 446–454.

Kellerer, M., Machicao, F., Seffer, E., Mushack, J., Ullrich, A. and Häring, H. U. (1991a). *Biochem. Biophys. Res. Commun.* **181**, 566–572.

Kellerer, M., Obermaier-Kusser, B., Pröfrock, A., Schleicher, E., Seffer, E., Mushack, J.,

Ermel, B. and Häring, H. U. (1991b). *Biochem. J.* **276**, 103–108.

Kellerer, M., Lammers, R., Ermel, B., Ullrich, A. and Häring, H. U. (1992). *Biochemistry* **31**, 4588–4596.

Kellerer, M., Sesti, G., Seffer, E., Obermaier-Kusser, B., Pongratz, D. E., Mosthaf, L. and Häring, H. U. (1993a). *Diabetologia* **36**, 628–632.

Kellerer, M., Mühlhöfer, A., Zierath, J., Henriksson-Wallberg, H. and Häring, H. U. (1993b). *Diabetologia* **36**, A53.

Kellerer, M., Machicao, F., Berti, L., Sixt, B., Mushack, J., Seffer, E., Mosthaf, L., Ullrich, A., Häring, H. U. (1993c). *Biochem. J.* **295**, 699–704.

Kelly, K. L., Mato, J. M. and Jarrett, L. (1986). *FEBS Lett.* **209**, 238–242.

Kelly, K. L., Mato, J. M., Merida, J. and Jarrett, L. (1987). *Proc. Natl Acad. Sci. USA* **84**, 6404–6407.

Kemmer, F. W., Sonnenberg, G. E., Cüppers, H. J. and Berger, M. (1983). *Münch. Med. Wochenschr.* **125**, Suppl. 1, 85.

Kern, W., Lieb, K., Kerner, W., Born, J. and Feha, H. L. (1990). *Diabetes* **39**, 1091–1098.

Kida, Y., Esposito-Del Puente, A., Bogardus, C. and Mott, D. M. (1990). *J. Clin. Invest.* **85**, 476–481.

Kida, Y., Raz, I., Maeda, R., Nyomba, B. L., Stone, K., Bogardus, C., Sommercorn, J. and Mott, D. M. (1992). *J. Clin. Invest.* **89**, 610–617.

Kiehm, T. G., Anderson, J. W. and Ward, K. W. (1976). *Am. J. Clin. Nutr.* **29**, 895–899.

Kikkawa, R., Umemura, K., Haneda, M., Arimura, T., Ebata, K. and Shigeta, Y. (1987). *Diabetes* **36**, 240–243.

King, G. L. and Kahn, C. R. (1984). *In* "Growth and Maturation Factors" (G. Geeroff, ed.) Vol. 2, pp. 224–265. John Wiley & Sons, New York.

Kinoshita, J. H., Dvornik, D., Kraml, M. and Gabbay, K. H. (1968). *Biochim. Biophys. Acta* **158**, 472–475.

Kirchhain, W. R. and Rendell, M. S. (1990). *Pharmacotherapy* **10**, 326–336.

Kirsten, R., Doming, B., Nelson, K., Nemeth, K., Oremek, G., Hubner-Steiner, U. and Speck, U. (1989). *Eur. J. Clin. Pharmacol.* **37**, 117–120.

Klaff, L. J., Vinik, A. I., Jackson, W. P. U., Malan, E., Kernoff, L. and Jacobs, P. (1979). *S. Afr. Med.* **56**, 247–250.

Klimm, H. D., Vollmar, J. and Bräuning, C. (1983). *In* "Pflanzenfasern – Neue Wege in der Stoffwechseltherapie" (S. Karger, ed.), pp. 206–215. S. Karger Verlag, Basel.

Klip, A. and Leiter, L. A. (1990). *Diabetes Care* **13**, 696–704.

Klip, A., Ramlal, T., Young, D. A. and Holloszy, J. O. (1987). *FEBS Lett.* **224**, 224–230.

Klumpp, S. and Ammon, H. P. T. (1988). *Akt. Endokrin. Stoffw.* **9**, 88, 1988.

Knuhtsen, S., Holst, J. J., Schwartz, T. W., Jensen, S. L. and Nielsen, O. V. (1986). *Regul. Pept.* **17**, 169–176.

Koepfer-Hobelsberger, B. and Wieland, O. H. (1984). *Mol. Cell. Endocrinol.* **36**, 123–129.

Koivisto, V. A. (1980a). *Br. Med. J.* **280**, 1411–1413.

Koivisto, V. A. (letter) (1980b). *Br. Med. J.* **281**, 621–622.

Koivisto, V. A. and Felig, P. (1978). *N. Engl. J. Med.* **298**, 79–83.

Kojima, K., Matsubara, H., Harada, T., Mizuno, K., Suzuki, M., Hotta, N., Kakuta, H. and Sakamoto, N. (1985). *Jpn. J. Ophthalmol.* **29**, 99–109.

Kollind, M. (1988). *Acta Med. Scand.* (Suppl.) **727**, 1–56.

Kollind, M., Adamson, U., Lins, P. E. and Efendic, S. (1987). *Horm. Metab. Res.* **19**, 156–169.

Kolterman, O. G. and Olefsky, J. M. (1984). *Diabetes Care* **7** (Suppl. 1), 81–88.

Kono, T. and Barham, F. W. (1971). *J. Biol. Chem.* **246**, 6210–6216.

Kono, T., Suzuki, K., Dansey, L. E., Robinson, F. W. and Blevins, T. L. (1981). *J. Biol. Chem.* **256**, 6400–6407.

Konrad, R. J., Jolly, Y. C., Major, C. and Wolf, B. A. (1992a). *Biochem. J.* **287**, 283–290.

Konrad, R. J., Jolly, Y. C., Major, C. and Wolf, B. A. (1992b). *Biochim. Biophys. Acta.* **1135**, 215–220.

Konrad, R. J., Jolly, Y. C., Major, C. and Wolf, B. A. (1993). *Mol. Cell. Endocrinol.* **92**, 135–140.

Koranyi, L., James, D. E., Kraegen, E. W. and Permutt, M. A. (1992). *J. Clin. Invest.* **89**, 432–436.

Korbonen, T., Idänpään-Heikkilä, J. and Aro, A. (1979). *Eur. J. Clin. Pharmacol.* **15**, 407–410.

Kosower, E. M. and Kanety-Londner, H. (1976). *J. Am. Chem. Soc.* **98**, 3001–3007.

Kosower, N. S., Kosower, E. M., Wertheim, B. and Correa, W. S. (1969). *Biochem. Biophys. Res. Commun.* **37**, 593–596.

Koss, F. W., Kopitar, Z. and Hammer, R. (1976). *Diabetes Croat.* **5**, 355–371.

Krall, L. (1984). *Clin. Ther.* **6**, 746, 762.

Krarup, T. (1988). *Endocr. Rev.* **9**, 122–134.

Kreymann, B., Yiangou, Y., Kanse, S., Williams, G., Ghatei, M. A. and Bloom, S. R. (1988). *FEBS Lett.* **242**, 167–170.

Kristensen, J. S., Falholt, K. and Jensen, J. (letter) (1984). *Br. Med. J.* **289**, 1382.

Kritchevsky, D., Tepper, S. A., Davidson, L. M. and Klurfeld, D. M. (1990). *Artery* **17**, 170–175.

KROC-Study Group (1988). *J. Am. Med. Assoc.* **260**, 37–41.

Krupinski, J., Rajaram, R., Lakonishok, M., Benovic, J. L. and Cerione, R. A. (1988). *J. Biol. Chem.* **263**, 12333–12341.

Kühl, C., Molsted-Pedersen, L. and Horness, P. J. (1983). *Diabetes Care* **6**, 152–154.

Kurtz, A. (1986). *J. Annu. Diabétol. Hotel Dieu* pp. 145–154.

Kwasowski, P., Flatt, P. R., Bailey, C. J. and Marks, V. (1985). *Biosci. Rep.* **5**, 701–705.

Ladas, S. D., Frydas, A., Papadopoulos, A. and Raptis, S. A. (1992). *Gut* **33**, 1246–1248.

Lager, I., Lonnroth, P., v. Schenck, H. and Smith, U. (1983). *Br. Med. J. (Clin. Res.)* **287**, 1661–1664.

Lalau, J. D., Andrejak, M., Moriniere, P., Coevoet, B., Debussche, X., Westeel, P. F., Fournier, A. and Quichaud, J. (1989). *Int. J. Clin. Pharmacol. Ther. Toxicol.* **27**, 285–288.

Lalor, B. C., Bhatnagar, D., Winocour, P. H., Ishola, M., Arral, S., Brading, M. and Durrington, P. N. (1990). *Diabetic Med.* **7**, 242–245.

Lambert, A. E., Kanazawa, Y., Burr, I. M., Orci, L. and Renold, A. E. (1971). *Ann. N.Y. Acad. Sci.* **185**, 232–244.

Landin, K., Tengborn, L. and Smith, U. (1991). *J. Intern. Med.* **229**, 181–187.

Larkins, R. G., Jerums, G., Taft, J. L., Godfrey, H., Smith, I. L. and Martin, T. J. (1988). *Diabetes Res. Clin. Pract.* **4**, 81–87.

Larner, J. (1983). *Am. J. Med.* **17**, 38–51.

Lattimer, S. A., Sima, A. F. and Greene, D. A. (1989). *Am. J. Physiol.* **256**, E264–E269.

Laube, H., Fouladfar, M., Aubell, R. and Schmitz, H. (1980). *Arzneimittelforschung/Drug Res.* **30**, 1154–1157.

Laube, H., Federlin, K., Knick, B., Irsigler, K., Najemnik, C., Wahl, P., Klimm, H. D., Vollmar, J. and Bräuning, C. (1983). In "Pflanzenfasern – Neue Wege in der Stoffwechseltherapie" (S. Karger, ed.), pp. 177–194. S. Karger Verlag, Basel.

Laurino, J. P., Colca, J. R., Pearson, J. D., De Wald, D. B. and McDonald, J. M. (1988). *Arch. Biochem. Biophys.* **265**, 8–21.

Lavoinne, A., Erikson, E., Moller, J. L., Price, D. J., Avruch, J. and Cohen, P. (1991). *Eur. J. Biochem.* **199**, 723–728.

Lawrence, J. R. and Dunnigan M. G. (letter) (1979). *Br. Med. J.* **2**, 445.

Layschock, S. G. (1982). *Cell Calcium* **3**, 43–54.

Layschock, S. G. (1983). *Biochem. J.* **216**, 101–106.

Layschock, S. G. and Bilgin, S. (1989). *Biochem. Pharmacol.* **38**, 2511–2520.

Lazner, J. (1970). *Med. J. Aust.* **1**, 327–330.

Lebech, M. and Olesen, L. L. (1990). *Ugeskr. Laeger* **152**, 2511–2512.

Leblanc, H., Marre, M., Billault, B. and Passa, P. (1987). *Diabetes Metab.* **13**, 613–617.

Le-Marchand-Brustel, Y., Rochet, N., Gremeaux, T., Marot, I. and Van Obberghen, E. (1990). *Diabetologia* **33**, 24–30.

Leonhardt, W., Hanefeld, M., Fischer, S., Schulze, J., Spengler, M. (1991). *Arzneimittelforschung/Drug Res.* **41**, 735–738.

Leslie, R. D. G. and Pyke, D. A. (1978). *Br. Med. J.* **2**, 1519–1521.

Lev, J. D., Zeidler, A. and Kumar, D. (1987). *Diabetes Care* **10**, 679–682.

Lewis, R. E., Perregaux, D. G. and Perregaux, S. B. (1989). *Diabetes* **38**, A4.

Lewis, R. E., Wu, G. P., MacDonald, R. G. and Czech, M. P. (1990). *J. Biol. Chem.* **265**, 947–954.

Lewitt, M. S., Yu, V. K., Rennie, G. C., Carter, J. N., Marel, G. M., Yue, D. K. and Hopper, M. J. (1989). *Diabetes Care* **12**, 379–383.

Li, N., Batzer, A., Daly, R., Vajnik, V., Skolnik, E., Chardin, P., Bar-Sagi, D., Margolis, B. and Schlessinger, J. (1993). *Nature* **363**, 85–88.

Li, W., Khatami, M. and Rockey, J. H. (1985). *Exp. Eye Res.* **40**, 439–444.

Lightman, J. M., Townsend, J. C. and Selvin, G. J. (1989). *J. Am. Optom. Assoc.* **60**, 849–53.

Lim, H. S., Ee, C. H. and Aw, T. C. (1990). *Ann. Acad. Med. Singapore* **19**, 455–458.

Lindskog, S., Ahrén, B., Dunning, B. E. and Sundler, F. (1991). *Cell Tissue Res.* **264**, 363–368.

Lindskog, S., Skoglund, G. and Ahrén, B. (1992). *Diabetes Res.* **19**, 119–123.

Lindström, P. and Sehlin, J. (1984). *Biochem. J.* **218**, 887–892.

Lintz, W., Berger, W., Aenishaenslin, W., Kutova, V., Baerlocher, Ch., Kapp, J. P. and Beckmann, R. (1974). *Eur. J. Clin. Pharmacol.* **7**, 433–448.

Lockwood, D. H., Maloff, B. L., Nowak, S. M. and McCaleb, M. L. (1983). *Am. J. Med.* **74**, 102–108.

Longo, E. A., Tornheim, K., Deeney, J. T., Varnum, B. A., Tillotson, D., Prentki, M. and Corkey, B. E. (1991). *J. Biol. Chem.* **266**, 9314–9319.

Lopez-Alarcon, L., Marcos, M. L., Guijarro, M. C. and Felin, J. E. (1986). *IRCS Med. Sci.* **14**, 457–458.

Lord, J. M., White, S. J., Bailey, C. J., Atkins, T. W, Fletcher, R. F. and Taylor, K. G. (1983). *Br. Med. J.* **286**, 830–831.

Lotz, N., Bachmann, W., Ladik, T. and Mehnert, H. (1988). *Klin. Wochenschr.* **66**, 1079–1084.

Loubatieres, A. (1944). *Compt. Rend.* **138**, 766–767.

Loubatieres, A. (1957). *Ann. N.Y. Acad. Sci.* **71**, 4–11.

Loud, F. B., Holst, J. J., Christiansen, J. and Rehfeld, J. F. (1988). *Dig. Dis. Sci.* **33**, 405–408.

Lucis, O. J. (1983). *Can. Med. Assoc. J.* **128**, 24–26.

Lupo, B. and Bataille, D. (1987). *Eur. J. Pharmacol.* **140**, 157–169.

Lyn, P. C. W. (letter) (1985). *Br. Med. J.* **291**, 1047.

MacDonald, M. J. and Kowluru, A. (1982). *Diabetes* **31**, 566–570.

MacGregor, L. C. and Matschinsky, O. H. (1985). *J. Clin. Invest.* **76**, 887–889.

Machicao, F. and Wieland, O. H. (1984). *FEBS Lett.* **175**, 113–116.

Machicao, F., Häring, H. U., White, M. F., Carrascosa, J. M., Obermaier, B. and Wieland, O. H. (1987). *Biochem. J.* **243**, 797–801.

Machicao, F., Mushack, J., Seffer, E., Ermel, B. and Häring, H. U. (1990). *Biochem. J.* **266**, 909–916.

MacWalter, R. S., ElDebani, A. H., Feels, J. and Stevenson, J. H. (1985). *Br. J. Clin. Pharmacol.* **19**, 121P–122P.

Madariaga, H., Lee, P. C., Heitlinger, L. A. and Lebenthal, E. (1988). *Dig. Dis. Sci.* **33**, 1020–1024.

Maddux, B. A. and Goldfine, I. D. (1990). *J. Biol. Chem.* **266**, 6731–6736.

Madoff, D. H., Martensen, T. M. and Lane, D. M. (1988). *Biochem. J.* **252**, 7–15.

Maegawa, H., McClain, D. A., Freidenberg, G., Olefsky, J. M., Napier, M., Lipari, T., Dull, T. J., Lee, J. and Ullrich, A. (1988). *J. Biol. Chem.* **263**, 8912–8917.

Malaisse, W. J. (1992). In "Nutrient Regulation of Insulin Secretion" (P. R. Flatt, ed.), pp. 83–100. Portland Press, London and Chapel Hill.

Malaisse, W. J. and Malaisse-Lagae, F. (1984). *Experientia* **40**, 1068–1075.

Malaisse, W. J. and Sener, A. (1987). *Biochim. Biophys. Acta* **927**, 190–195.

Malaisse, W. J., Malaisse-Lagae, F. and Sener, A. (1982). *Diabetes* **31**, 90–93.

Malaisse, W. J., Dufrane, S. P., Mathias, P. C. F., Carpinelli, A. R., Malaisse-Lagae, F., Garcia-Morales, P., Valverde, I. and Sener, A. (1985a). *Biochim. Biophys. Acta* **844**, 256–264.

Malaisse, W. J., Dunlop, M. E., Mathias, P. C. F., Malaisse-Lagae, F. and Sener, A. (1985b). *Eur. J. Biochem.* **149**, 23–27.

Maloff, B. L. and Lockwood, D. H. (1981). *J. Clin. Invest.* **68**, 85–90.

Mandarino, L. J., Wright, K. S., Verity, L. S., Nichols, J., Bell, J. M., Kolterman, O. G. and Beck-Nielsen, H. (1987). *J. Clin. Invest.* **80**, 655–663.

Marble, A. and Camerini-Davalos, R. W. (1961). In "Proc. 4th Congr. Diabetes Fed." (Ed. Medicine et Hygiene, Geneva), pp. 751–752.

Marfaing, P., Ktorza, A., Berthault, M. F., Predine, J., Picon, L. and Penicaud, L. (1991). *Diabete Metab.* **17**, 55–60.

Margolis, R. N., Taylor, S. I., Seminara, D. and Hubbard, A. L. (1988). *Proc. Natl Acad. Sci. USA* **85**, 7256–7259.

Marks, V., Tan, K. S., Stagner, J. I. and Samols, E. (1990). *Biochem. Soc. Trans.* **18**, 103–104.

Marks, V., Samols, E. and Stagner, J. (1992). In "Nutrient Regulation of Insulin Secretion" (P. R. Flatt, ed.), pp. 41–57. Portland Press, London and Chapel Hill.

Markussen, J., Diers, I., Hougaard, P., Langkjaer, L., Norris, K., Snel, L., Sorensen, A. R., Sorensen, E. and Voigt, H. O. (1988). *Protein Eng.* **2**, 157–166.

Marshall, S. M., Home, P. D., Taylor, R. and Alberti, K. G. (1987). *Diabetic Med.* **4**, 521–525.

Martindale (1989). "The Extra Pharmacopeia, 29th Edition" pp. 386–399. The Pharmaceutical Press, London.

Martindale, R., Levin, S. and Alfin-Slater, R. (1982). *Regul. Pept.* **3**, 313–324.

Martz, A., Mookerjee, B. K. and Jung, C. Y. (1986). *J. Biol. Chem.* **261**, 13606–13609.

Martz, A., Jo, I. and Jung, C. Y. (1989). *J. Biol. Chem.* **264**, 13672–13678.

Massague, J. and Czech, M. P. (1982). *J. Biol. Chem.* **257**, 5038–5045.

Masson, E. A. and Boulton, A. J. (1990). *Drugs* **39**, 190–202.

Masuda, A., Shibasaki, T., Hotta, M., Yamauchi, N., Ling, N., Demura, H. and Shizume, K. (1990). *Regul. Pept.* **31**, 53–64.

Mato, J. M. (1989). *Cell. Signal.* **1**, 143–146.

Mato, J. M., Kelly, K. L., Abler, A. and Jarrett, L. (1987). *J. Biol. Chem.* **262**, 2131–2137.

Matsushime, H., Wang, L. and Shibuya, M. (1986). *Mol. Cell. Biol.* **6**, 3000–3004.

Matsutani, A., Kaku, K. and Kaneko, T. (1984). *Diabetes* **33**, 495–498.

Matthaei, S., Garvey, W. T., Horuk, R., Hueckstaedt, T. P. and Olefsky, J. M. (1987). *J. Clin. Invest.* **79**, 703–709.

Matthaei, S., Hamann, A., Klein, H. H., Benecke, H., Kreymann, G., Flier, J. S. and Greten, H. (1991). *Diabetes* **40**, 850–857.

Matthews, E. K. and Dean, P. M. (1970). *Postgrad. Med. J.* **46** (Suppl. 1), 21–23.

McAlpine, L. G., McAlpine, C. H., Waclawski, E. R., Storer, A. M., Kay, J. W. and Frier, B. M. (1988). *Eur. J. Clin. Pharmacol.* **34**, 129–132.

McCaleb, M. L. and Myres, R. D. (1982). *Am. J. Physiol.* **242**, R596–R601.

McClain, D. A. (1991). *Mol. Endocrinol.* **5**, 734–739.

McClain, D. A., Maegawa, H., Levy, J., Hueckstaedt, T., Dull, T. J., Lee, J., Ullrich, A. and Olefsky, J. M. (1988). *J. Biol. Chem.* **263**, 8904–8911.

McGuinness, O. P., Green, D. R. and Cherrington, A. D. (1987). *Diabetes* **36**, 472–476.

McGuire, M. C., Fields, R. M., Nyomba, B. L., Raz, I., Bogardus, C., Tonks, N. K. and Sommercorn, J. (1991). *Diabetes* **40**, 939–942.

McIntyre, N., Holdsworth, D. and Turner, D. S. (1964). *Lancet* **ii**, 20–21.

McIvor, M. E., Cummings, C. C., Leo, T. A. and Medeloff, A. I. (1985). *Diabetes Care* **8**, 274–278.

McLoughin, J. C., Buchanan, K. D. and Alam, M. J. (1979). *Lancet* **ii**, 603–605.

McNally, P. G., Jowett, N. I., Kurinczuk, J. J., Peck, R. W. and Hearnshaw, J. R. (1988). *Postgrad. Med. J.* **64**, 850–853.

Meissner, H. P. and Atwater, I. J. (1976). *Horm. Metab. Res.* **8**, 11–16.

Meissner, H. P., Henquin, J.-C. and Preissler, M. (1978). *FEBS Lett.* **94**, 87–89.

Meissner, H. P., Preissler, M. and Henquin, J.-C. (1979). *Excerpta Med. Int. Congr. Ser.* **500**, 166–171.

Melander, A., Bitzen, P. O., Faber, O. and Gropp, L. (1989). *Drugs* **37**, 58–72.

Melander, A., Lebovitz, H. E. and Faber, O. K. (1990). *Diabetes Care* **13** (Suppl. 3), 18–25.

v. Mering, J., Minkowski, O. (1889). *Naunyn-Schmiedeberg's Arch.* **26**, 371–378.

Metz, S., van Rollins, M., Strife, R., Fujimoto, W. and Robertson, R. P. (1983). *J. Clin. Invest.* **71**, 1191–1295.

Meuli, C. and Froesch, E. R. (1977). *Biochem. Biophys. Res. Commun.* **75**, 689–695.

Meurice, J. C., Lecomte, P., Renard, J. P. and Girard, J. J. (1983). *Presse Méd.* **12**, 1670.

Mezitis, N. H. E., Heshka, S., Saitas, V., Bailey, T. S., Costa, R. and Pisunyer, F. S. (1992). *Diabetes Care* **15**, 265–269.

Miller, E. R. and Ullrey, D. E. (1987). *Annu. Rev. Nutr.* **7**, 361–382.

Miller, R. E. (1981). *Endocr. Rev.* **4**, 471–494.

Miners, J. O., Wing, L. M., Lillywhite, K. J. and Smith, K. J. (1984). *Br. J. Clin. Pharmacol.* **18**, 853–860.

Miranda, P. M. and Horwitz, D. L. (1978). *Ann. Intern. Med.* **88**, 482–486.

Misbin, R. I. (1977). *Ann. Intern. Med.* **87**, 591–595.

Misler, D. S., Falke, L. C., Gillis, K. and McDaniel, M. L. (1986). *Proc. Natl Acad. Sci. USA* **83**, 7119–7123.

Mojsov, S., Weir, G. C. and Habener, J. F. (1987). *J. Clin. Invest.* **79**, 616–619.

Moller, D. E., Yokota, A., Caro, J. F. and Flier, J. S. (1989). *Mol. Endocrinol.* **3**, 1263–1269.

Momomura, K., Topa, K., Seyama, Y., Takaku, F., Kasuga, M. (1988). *Biochem. Biophys. Res. Commun.* **155**, 1181–1186.

Monge, L., Ortega, J. L., Cabello, M. A. and Felin, J. E. (1985). Additive effect of chlorpropamide and insulin on gluconeogenesis and on fructose 2,6-biphosphate levels in isolated rat hepatocytes. Abstract International Diabetes Federation, Spain.

Monnier, L. H., Blotman, M. J., Volette, C., Monnier, M. P. and Mirouze, J. (1981). *Diabetologia* **20**, 12–17.

Montague, W. and Howell, S. L. (1972). *Biochem. J.* **129**, 551–560.

Mooradian, A. D. (1987). *Diabetologia* **30**, 120–121.

Moore, M. R. and McColl, K. E. L. (1987). Porphyrias Drug Lists. Porphyria Research Unit, University of Glasgow, Glasgow.

Morgan, L. M. (1992). *In* "Nutrient Regulation of Insulin Secretion" (P. R. Flatt, ed.), pp. 1–22. Portland Press, London and Chapel Hill.

Morgan, L. M., Goulder, T. J., Tsiolakis, D., Marks, V. and Alberti, K. G. M. M. (1979). *Diabetologia* **17**, 85–89.

Morgan, L. M., Tredger, J. A., Wright, J. and Marks, V. (1990). *Br. J. Nutr.* **64**, 103–110.

Morgan, N. G. and Montague, W. (1992). *In* "Nutrient Regulation of Insulin Secretion" (P. R. Flatt, ed.), pp. 125–155. Portland Press, London and Chapel Hill.

Mosbacher, E. M. (1992). *Naunyn-Schmiedeberg's Arch. Pharmacol.* **345** (Suppl.) A360.

Moses, A. C., Gordon, G. S., Carey, M. C. and Flier, J. S. (1983). *Diabetes* **32**, 1040–1047.

Moses, A. M., Howanitz, J. and Miller, M. (1973). *Ann. Intern. Med.* **78**, 541–544.

Moses, R. G., Hubert, P. A. and Lewis-Driver, D. J. (1985). *Med. J. Aust.* **142**, 294–296.

Mosthaf, L., Grako, K., Dull, T. J., Coussens, L., Ullrich, A. and McClain, D. A. (1990). *EMBO J.* **9**: 2409–2414.

Mosthaf, L., Vogt, B. and Häring, H. U. (1991). *Proc. Natl Acad. Sci. USA* **88**, 4728–4730.

Mosthaf, L., Eriksson, J., Häring, H. U., Groop, L., Widen, E. and Ullrich, A. (1993). *Proc. Natl Acad. Sci. USA* **90**, 2633–2635.

Moulds, R. F., Fullinfaw, R. O., Bury, R. W., Plehwe, W. E., Jacka, N., McGrath, K. M. and Martin, F. I. (1991). *Br. J. Clin. Pharmacol.* **31**, 715–718.

Moxham, C. P. and Jacobs, S. (1992). *J. Cell. Biochem.* **48**, 136–140.

Moxham, C. P., Duronio, V. and Jacobs, S. (1989). *Biol. C hem.* **264**, 13238–13244.

Mueckler, M. (1990). *Diabetes* **39**, 6–11.

Mueckler, M., Caruso, C., Baldwin, S. A., Panico, M., Blench, I., Morris, H. R., Allard, W. J., Lienhard, G. E. and Lodish, H. F. (1985). *Science* **229**, 941–945.

Mühlbacher, C., Karnieli, E., Schaff, P., Obermaier, B., Mushack, J., Rattenhuber, E. and Häring, H. U. (1988). *Biochem. J.* **249**, 865–870.

Mühlhauser, I., Bruckner, I., Berger, M., Cheta, D., Jörgens, V., Ionescu-Tirgoviste, C., Scholz, V. and Mincu, I. (1987). *Diabetologia* **30**, 681–690.

Müller, F. O. and Hillebrand, I. (1986). *Acta Pharmacol. Toxicol.* **59** (Suppl. V), 303.

Müller, H., Kellerer, M., Ermel, B., Mühlhöfer, A., Obermaier-Kusser, B., Vogt, B. and Häring, H. U. (1991). *Diabetes* **40**, 1440–1448.

Munoz, J. M., Sandstead, H. H. and Jacob, R. A. (1979). *Diabetes* **28**, 496–502.

Müting, D. (1984). *Therapiewoche* **34**, 2566–2572.

Myers, M. G., Jr., Sun, X. J., Chetaham, B., Jachna, B. R., Glasheen, E. M., Backer, J. M. and White, M. F. (1993). *Endocrinology* **132**, 1421–1430.

Nathan, D. M., Singer, D. E., Gadine, J. E. and Perlmutter, L. C. (1986). *Am. J. Med.* **81**, 837–842.

Nathan, M. H. and Pek, S. B. (1990). *Prostaglandins Leukot. Essent. Fatty Acids* **40**, 21–25.

Nauck, M., Stockmann, F., Ebert, R. and Creutzfeldt, W. (1986). *Diabetologia* **29**, 46–52.

Nelson, D. A., Aguilar-Bryan, L., Raef, H. and Boyd A. E., III (1992). *In* "Nutrient Regulation of Insulin Secretion" (P. R. Flatt, ed.), pp. 319–339. Portland Press, London and Chapel Hill.

Nelson, E. (1964). *Am. J. Med. Sci.* **248**, 657–659.

Nelson, T. Y., Gaines, K. L., Rajan, A. S., Berg, M. and Boyd, A. E., III (1987). *J. Biol. Chem.* **262**, 2608–2612.

Nestel, P. J. (1988). *In* "Acarbose for the Treatment of Diabetes Mellitus" (W. Creutzfeld, ed.), pp. 68. Springer Verlag, Berlin, Heidelberg.

Neuvonen, P. J. and Kärkkäinen, S. (1983). *Clin. Pharmacol. Ther.* **33**, 386–393.

Neuvonen, P. J., Kannisto, H. and Hirvisalo, E. L. (1983). *Eur. J. Clin. Pharmacol.* **24**, 243–246.

Niki, I., Kelly, R. P., Ashcroft, S. J. H. and Ashcroft, F. M. (1989). *Pfluegers Arch.* **415**, 47–55.

Niki, I., Nicks, J. L. and Ashcroft, S. J. H. (1990). *Biochem. J.* **268**, 713–718.

Nishi, S., Seino, Y., Ishida, H., Seino, M., Taminato, T., Sakurai, H. and Imura, H. (1987). *J. Clin. Invest.* **79**, 1191–1196.

Nishizuka, Y. (1988). *Nature* **334**, 661–665.

Nong, E. C. C., Eacks, D. B., Laurino, J. F. and McDonald, J. M. (1988). *Endocrinology* **123**, 1830–1836.

Nosadini, R., Avogaro, A. and Trevisan, R. (1987). *Diabetes Care* **10**, 62–67.

Nyomba, B. L., Freymond, D., Raz, I., Stone, K., Mott, D. M. and Bogardus, C. (1990). *Metabolism* **39**, 1204–1210.

Oben, J., Morgan, L., Fletcher, J. and Marks, V. (1991). *J. Endocrinol.* **130**, 267–272.

Obermaier, B., Ermel, B., Kirsch, D., Mushack, J., Rattenhuber, E., Biemer, E., Machicao, F. and Häring, H. U. (1987). *Diabetologia* **30**, 93–99.

Obermaier-Kusser, B., Ermel, B., Mühlbacher, C. and Häring, H. U. (1988a). *Diabetes Res. Clin. Pract.* **60** (Suppl. 1), 67–93.

Obermaier-Kusser, B., Mühlbacher, C., Mushack, J., Rattenhuber, E., Fehlmann, M. and Häring, H. U. (1988b). *Biochem. J.* **256**, 515–520.

Obermaier-Kusser, B., Mühlbacher, C., Mushack, J., Seffer, E., Ermel, B., Machicao, F., Schnidt, F. and Häring, H. U. (1989). *Biochem. J.* **261**, 699–705.

O'Brian, R. M., Houslay, M. D., Milligan, G. and Siddle, K. (1987). *FEBS Lett.* **212**, 281–288.

Odawara, M., Yamamoto, R., Kadowaki, T., Shiba, T., Shibasaki, Y., Mikami, Y., Matsuura, N., Takaku, F., Taylor, S. I. and Kasuga, M. (1989). *Diabetes* **38**, A66.

O'Hare, T. and Pilch, P. F. (1988). *Biochemistry* **27**, 5693–5700.

Ohno, M., Ito, K., Saito, S., Kageyama, S., Ikeda, Y., Tanese, T. and Abe, M. (1983). *Tohoku J. Exp. Med.* **141** (Suppl.), 723–732.

Okabayashi, Y., Otsuki, M., Ohki, A., Sakamoto, C. and Baba, S. (1983). *Endocrinology* **113**, 2210–2215.

Okamoto, M., Uchida, I., Umehara, K., Kohsaka, M. and Imanaka, H. (1984). European Patent 099,692.

Olefsky, J. M. and Reaven, G. M. (1976). *Am. J. Med.* **60**, 89–95.

Onoda, K., Hagiwara, M., Hachiya, T., Usuda, N., Nagata, T. and Hidaka, H. (1990). *Endocrinology* **126**, 1235–1240.

Opper, F. H., Isacs, K. L. and Warshauer, D. M. (1990). *J. Clin. Gastroenterol.* **12**, 667–669.

O'Rahilly, S. P., Nugent, Z. and Rudenski, A. S. (1986). *Lancet* **ii**, 360–364.

O'Rahilly, S., Choi, W. H., Patel, P., Turner, R. C., Flier, J. S. and Moller, D. E. (1991). *Diabetes* **40**, 777–782.

Orlander, P. (letter) (1985). *N. Engl. J. Med.* **312**, 444.

Owens, D. R., Vora, J. P., Heding, L. G., Luzio, S., Ryder, R. E. J., Atiea, J. and Hayes, T. M. (1986). *Diabetic Med.* **3**, 326–329.

Pagano, G. and Cavallo-Perin, P. (1990). *Diabetes Nutr. Metab.* **3** (Suppl. 1), 69–76.

Pagano, G., Tagliaferro, V., Carta, Q., Caselle, M. T., Bozzo, C., Vitelli, F., Trovati, M. and Cocuzza, E. (1983). *Diabetologia*, **24**, 351–354.

Paice, B. J., Paterson, K. R. and Lawson, D. H. (1985). *Adverse Drug React. Ac. Pois. Rev.* **4**, 23–26.

Palmberg, P., Smith, M. and Waltman, S. (1981). *Ophthalmology* **88**, 613–618.

Panten, U. (1987). *Naunyn-Schmiedeberg's Arch. Pharmacol.* **335** (Suppl.), R73.

Panten, U. and Christians, J. (1973). *Naunyn-Schmiedeberg's Arch. Pharmacol.* **276**: 55–62.

Panten, U., Burgfeld, J., Goerke, F., Rennicke, M., Schwanstecher, M., Wallasch, A., Zuenkler, B. J. and Lenzen, S. (1989). *Biochem. Pharmacol.* **38**, 1217–1229.

Panten, U., Schwanstecher, M. and Schwanstecher, C. (1992) *Horm. Metab. Res.* **24**, 549–554.

Parr, J. H., Abraham, R. R., Davie, M. W. J., Dornhorst, A. and Wynn, V. (letter) (1982). *Lancet* **ii**, 831.

Patel, Y. C., Papachristou, D. N., Zingg, H. H. and Farkas, E. M. (1991). *Endocrinology* **128**, 1754–1762.

Paterson, K. R., Paice, B. J. and Lawson, D. H. (1984). *Adverse Drug React. Ac. Pois. Rev.* **3**, 173–183.

Patterson, R., Roberts, M. and Grammer, L. C. (1990). *Ann. Allergy* **64**, 459–462.

Peacock, I., Tattersall, R. B. (1984). *Br. Med. (Clin. Res.)* **288**, 1956–1959.

Pedersen, M. M., Christiansen, J. S. and Mogensen, C. E. (1991). *Diabetes* **40**, 527–531.

Pedersen, O., Nielsen, O., Bak, J., Richelsen, B., Beck-Nielsen, H. and Sorensen, N. (1989). *Diabetic Med.* **6**, 249–256.

Pedersen, O., Bak, J. F., Andersen, P. H., Lund, S., Moller, D. E., Flier, J. S. and Kahn, B. B. (1990). *Diabetes* **39**, 865–870.

Pelkonen, R., Koivisto, V. and Mustajoki, P. (1985). *Acta Endocrinol.* **272** (Suppl.), 49–55.

Pendergast, B. D. (1984). *Clin. Pharmacol.* **3**, 473–485.

Penman, E., Wass, J. A. H., Medback, S., Morgan, L. M., Lewis, J., Besser, G. M. and Rees, L. H. (1981). *Gastroenterology* **81**, 692–699.

Penn, E. J., Bracklehurst, K. W., Sopwith, A. M., Hales, C. N. and Hutton, J. C. (1982). *FEBS Lett.* **139**, 4–8, 1982.

Pentikäinen, P. J., Neuvonen, P. J. and Penttilä, A. (1979). *Eur. J. Clin. Pharmacol.* **16**, 195–202.

Pentikäinen, P. J., Voutilainen, E., Aro, A., Uusitupa, M., Penttilä, I. and Vapaatalo, H. (1990). *Ann. Med.* **22**, 307–312.

Persaud, S. J., Jones, P. M., Sugden, D. and Howell, S. L. (1989a). *FEBS Lett.* **245**, 80–84.

Persaud, S. J., Jones, P. M., Sugden, D. and Howell, S. L. (1989b). *Biochem. J.* **264**, 753–758.

Persaud, S. J., Jones, P. M. and Howell, S. L. (1992). In "Nutrient Regulation of Insulin Secretion" (P. R. Flatt, ed.), pp. 247–269. Portland Press, London and Chapel Hill.

Peter-Reisch, B., Fathi, M., Schlegel, W. and Wollheim, C. B. (1988). *J. Clin. Invest.* **81**, 1154–1161.

Petersen, K. G. (1982). In "Proceedings of the First International Symposium on Acarbose" (W. Creutzfeld, ed.), pp. 325–329. Excerpta Medica, Amsterdam.

Petersen, K. G., Khalaf, A., Naithani, V., Gattner, H. and Kerp, L. (1989). *Diabetes Res. Clin. Pract.* **7**, 41–46.

Petersen, O. H. and Findlay, I. (1987). *Physiol. Rev.* **67**, 1054–1116.

Petzold, R., Vrahimis, J., Finck, H. D. and Sauer, H. (1982). In "Proceedings of the First International Symposium on Acarbose" (W. Creutzfeld, ed.), pp. 427–432. Excerpta Medica, Amsterdam.

Pfeifer, M. A., Halter, J. B., Judzewitsch, R. G., Beard, J. C., Best, J. D., Ward, W. K. and Porte, D. (1984). *Diabetes Care* **7** (Suppl. 1), 25–34.

Pfeiffer, E. F., Thum, C. and Clemens, A. H. (1974). *Horm. Metab. Res.* **6**, 339–342.

Phillips, M., Simpson, R. W., Holmann, R. R. and Turner, R. L. (1979). *Q.J. Med.* (new series) **48**, 493–506.

Pickup, J. (1986). *Br. Med. J.* **292**, 155–157.

Pipeleers, D. G. (1987). *Diabetologia* **30**, 277–290.

Pipeleers, D. G., In't Veld, P., Maes, E. and van de Winkel, M. (1982). *Proc. Natl Acad. Sci. USA* **70**, 7322–7325.

Plant, T. D. (1988). *J. Physiol.* **404**, 731–747.

Pogatsa, G., Koltai, M. Z., Balkanyi, I., Devai, I., Kiss, V. and Koszeghy, A. (1988). *Acta Physiol. Hung.* **71**, 243–250.

Poggi, C., LeMarchand-Brustel, Y., Zapf, J., Froesch, E. R. and Freychet, P. (1979). *Endocrinology* **105**, 723–730.

Pontiroli, A. E., Alberetto, M., Capra, F. and Pozza, G. (1990). *J. Endocrinol. Invest.* **13**, 241–245.

Popiela, H. and Moore, W. (1991). *Pancreas* **6**, 464–469.

Popovic, V., Micic, D., Damjanovic, S., Petakov, M., Manojilovic, D. and Micic, J. (1990). *Endicrinol. Exp.* **24**, 167–173.

Potter, J., Clarke, P., Gale, E. A. M., Dave, S. H. and Tattersall, R. B. (1982). *Br. Med. J.* **285**, 1180–1182.

Poulsen, J. E. and Deckert, T. (1976). *Acta Med. Scand.* **601** (Suppl.), 197–245.

Poulsom, R. and Heath, H. (1983). *Biochem. Pharmacol.* **32**, 1495–1499.

Pralong, W. F., Bartley, C. and Wollheim, C. B. (1990). *EMBO J.* **9**, 53–60.

Pramming, S., Thorsteinsson, B., Bendtson, I. and Ronn, B. (1985). *Br. Med. J.* **291**, 376–379.

Prentki, M. and Matschinsky, F. M. (1987). *Physiol. Rev.* **67**, 1185–1248.

Prentki, M. and Wollheim, C. B. (1984). *Experientia* **40**, 1052–1060.

Prentki, M., Janjic, D. and Wollheim, C. D. (1983). *J. Biol. Chem.* **258**, 7597–7602.

Prentki, M., Janjic, D., Biden, T. J., Blondel, B. and Wollheim, C. B. (1984a). *J. Biol. Chem.* **259**, 10118–10123.

Prentki, M., Biden, T. J., Janjic, D., Irvine, R. F., Berridge, M. J. and Wollheim, C. B. (1984b). *Nature* **309**, 562–564.

Prigent, S. A., Stanley, K. K. and Siddle, K. (1990). *J. Biol. Chem.* **265**, 9970–9971.

Prince, M. J. and Olefsky, J. M. (1980). *J. Clin. Invest.* **66**, 608–611.

Puls, W. Kemp, U. (1973). *Diabetologia* **9**, 97–101.

Putnam, W. S., Andersen, D. K., Jones, R. S. and Lebovitz, H. E. (1981). *J. Clin. Invest.* **67**, 1016–1023.

Pütter, J. (1980). *In* "Enzyme Inhibitors" (U. Brodbeck, ed.), pp. 139–151. Verlag Chemie, Weinheim.

Pütter, J., Keup, U., Krause, H. P., Müller, L. and Weber, H. (1982). *In* "Pharmacokinetics of Acarbose" (W. Creutzfeldt, ed), pp. 38–44. Excerpta Medica, Amsterdam.

Pyke, D. A. (1979). *Diabetologia* **17**, 333–343.

Pyke, D. A. and Leslie, R. D. (1978). *Br. Med. J.* **2**, 1521–1522.

Pyke, D. A. and Nelson, P. G. (1976). *In* "The Genetics of Diabetes Mellitus" (W. Creutzfeldt, J. Köbberling and J. V. Neel eds), pp. 194–202. Springer Verlag, Berlin.

Quatraro, A., Consoli, G., Ceriello, A. and Giugliano, D. (1986). *Diabetes Metab.* **12**, 315–318.

Radziuk, J., Kemmer, F., Berchtold, P., Vranik, M. (1982). In "Proceedings of the First International Symposium on Acarbose" (W. Creutzfeld, ed.), pp. 113–122. Excerpta Medica, Amsterdam.

Rafaeloff, R., Patel, R. G., Yip, C. C. and Hawley, D. M. (1989). *Diabetes* **38**, A2.

Raffle, P. A. B. (1981). *Prescribers' J.* **21**, 197–200.

Rains, S. G., Wilson, G. A., Richmond, W. and Elkeles, R. S. (1988). *Diabetic Med.* **5**, 653–658.

Rains, S. G., Wilson, G. A., Richmond, W. and Elkeles, R. S. (1989). *R. Soc. Med.* **82**, 93–94.

Ramanadham, S., Gross, R. and Turk, J. (1992). *Biochem. Biophys. Res. Commun.* **184**, 647–653.

Randle, P., Garland, P., Hales, C. and Newsholm, E. (1963). *Lancet* **i**, 785–789.

Rang, H. P. and Dale, M. M. (1991). "Pharmacology" 2nd ed. Churchill Livingstone, Edinburgh, London, Melbourne, New York, Tokyo and Madrid.

Raptis, A. E., Tountas, N., Yalouris, A. G., Hadjidakis, D., Zaharis, A., Miras, K. and Raptis, S. A. (1990). *Acta Diabetol. Lat.* **27**, 11–22.

Raptis, S., Dimitriadis, G., Karaiskos, C., Diamantopoulos, E., Hadjidakis, D., Souvatzoglou, A. Moulopoulos, S. (1982). *In* "Proceedings of the First International Symposium on Acarbose" (W. Creutzfeld, ed.), pp. 393–401. Excerpta Medica, Amsterdam.

Raptis, S., Dimitriadis, G., Hadjidakis, D. (1988). *In* "Acarbose for the Treatment of Diabetes Mellitus, 2nd International Symposium on Acarbose" (W. Creutzfeld, ed.), pp. 141–152. Springer Verlag, Berlin, Heidelberg.

Ratner, E. E., Phillips, T. M. and Steiner, M. (1990). *Diabetes* **39**, 728–733.

Ravina, A. and Minuchin, O. (1990). *Harefuah*, **119** (7-B), 200–203.

Rayman, G., Santo, M., Salomon, F., Almog, S., Paradinas, F. J., Pinkhas, J., Reynolds, K. W. and Wise, P. H. (1984). *J. Clin. Pathol.* **37**, 651–654.

Reaven, G. M. (1988). *Diabetes* **37**, 1595–1607.

Reaven, G. M. and Dray, J. (1967). *Diabetes* **16**, 487–492.

Reaven, G. M., Lardinois, C. K., Greenfield, M. S., Schwartz, H. C. and Vreman, H. J. (1990). *Diabetes Care* (Suppl. 3), 32–36.

Rees-Jones, R. and Taylor, S. (1985). *J. Biol. Chem.* **227**, 887–892.

Reichlin, S. (1983). *N. Engl. J. Med.* **309**, 1495–1501.

Reimers, J., Nauck, M., Creutzfeldt, W., Strietzel, J., Ebert, R., Cantor, P. and Hoffman, G. (1988). *Diabetologia* **14**, 271–280.

Richard, J. L., Rodier, M., Monnier, L., Orsetti, A. and Mirouze, J. (1988). *Diabete Metab.* **14**, 114–118.

Riedel, H., Dull, T. J., Schlessinger, J. and Ullrich, A. (1986). *Nature* **324**, 68–70.

Rinderknecht, E. and Humbel, R. E. (1978). *J. Biol. Chem.* **353**, 2769–2776.

Rinninger, F., Kirsch, D., Häring, H. K. and Kemmler, W. (1984). *Diabetologia* **26**, 462–465.

Robertson, R. P. (1981). *Med. Clin. North Am.* **65**, 759–771.

Robinson, W. G., Nagata, M., Laver, W. (1989). *Invest. Ophthalmol. Vis. Sci.* **30**, 2285–2287

Rodier, M., Richard, J. L., Monnier, L. and Mirouze, J. (1988). *Diabete Metab.* **14**, 12–14.

Rohner-Jeanrenaud, F., Bobbioni, E., Ionescu, E., Sauter, J.-F. and Jeanrenaud, B. (1983). *Adv. Metab. Disord.* **10**, 193–220.

Rönfeldt, M., Safayhi, H., Ammon, H. P. T. (1992). *Naunyn-Schmiedeberg's Arch. Pharmacol.* **346**, 527–531.

Ronnett, G. V., Knutson, V. P., Kohansky, R. A., Simpson, T. L and Lane, M. D. (1984). *J. Biol. Chem.* **259**, 4566–4575.

Rorsman, P. and Trube, G. (1985). *Pfluegers Arch.* **405**, 305–309.

Rorsman, P. and Trube, G. (1990). In "Potassium Channels: Structure Function and Therapeutic Potential" (N. S. Cook, ed.), pp. 300–326. Ellis Horwood, Chichester.

Rorsman, P., Bokvist, K., Åmmälä, C., Arkhammar, P., Berggren, P.-O., Larsson, O. and Wåhlander, K. (1991). *Nature* **349**, 74–77.

Rosak, C. (1990). *Diabetes Nutr. Metab.* **3** (Suppl. 1), 59–62.

Rosenkranz, R., Hillebrand, I., Boehme, K., Bach, I. and Daweke, H. (1982). In "Proceedings of the First International Symposium on Acarbose" (W. Creutzfeld, ed.), pp. 305–308. Excerpta Medica, Amsterdam.

Rosetti, L., Frontoni, S., Dimarchi, R., DeFronzo, R. A. and Giaccari, A. (1991). *Diabetes* **40**, 444–448.

Rothenberg, P. L. and Kahn, C. R. (1988). *J. Biol. Chem.* **263**, 15546–15552.

Rothenberg, D. L., Shulman, R. G. and Shulman, G. I. (1992) *J. Clin. Invest.* **89**, 1069–1075.

Rothmann, D. L., Shulman, R. G. and Shulman, G. I. (1992). *J. Clin. Invest.* **89**, 1069–1075.

Rousseau-Migneron, S., Turcotte, L. and Tancrede, G. (1988). *Diabetes Res.* **9**, 97–100.

Ruderman, N., Kapeller, R., White, M. F. and Cantley, L. C. (1990). *Proc. Natl Acad. Sci. USA* **87**, 1411–1415.

Rushakoff, R. J., Goldfine, I. D., Carter, J. D. and Liddle, R. A. (1987). *J. Clin. Endocrinol. Metabol.* **65**, 395–401.

Ryder, R. E. J. (1984). *Br. J. Clin. Pract.* **38**, 229–232.

Ryder, S., Sarokhan, B., Shand, D. G. and Mullane, J. F. (1987). *Drug Dev. Res.* **11**, 131–143.

Sachse, G., Mäser, E. and Laube, H. (1982) *In* "Proceedings of the First International Symposium on Acarbose" (W. Creutzfeld, ed.), pp. 298–304. Excerpta Medica, Amsterdam.

Safayhi, H., Koopmann, I., Ammon, H. P. T. (1993). *Mol. Cell. Endocrinol.* **91**, 143–148.

Sale, J., Fujita-Yamaguchi, Y. and Kahn, C. R. (1986). *Eur. J. Biochem.* **155**, 345–352.

Saltiel, A. R. (1987). *Endocrinology* **120**, 967–972.

Saltiel, A. R. and Cuatrecasas, P. (1986). *Proc. Natl Acad. Sci. USA* **83**, 5793–5797.

Saltiel, A. R., Fox, J. A., Sherkine, P. and Cuatrecasas, P. (1986). *Science* **233**, 967–972.

Samanta, A., Jones, G. R., Burden, A. C. and Shakir, I. (1984). *Br. J. Clin. Pharmacol.* **18**, 647–648.

Samanta, A., Burden, A. C. and Kinghorn, H. A. (1987). *Diabetes Res.* **4**, 183–185.

Samols, E. (1983). *In* "Handbook of Experimental Pharmacology" (P. J. Lefebvre, ed.) Vol. 66/I, pp. 485–518. Springer-Verlag, Berlin.

Samols, E. and Harrison, J. (1976). *Metabolism* (Suppl. 1) **25**, 1495–1497.

Samols, E. and Stagner, J. I. (1988). *Am. J. Med.* **85** (5A), 31–35.

Samols, E., Stagner, J., Ewart, R. B. and Marks, V. (1988). *J. Clin. Invest.* **82**, 350–354.

Sandler, S., Andersson, A. and Hellerström, C. (1987). *Endocrinology* **121**, 1424–1431.

Sarges, R. (1989). *Adv. Drug Res.* **18**, 140–175.

Sarges, R., Belletire, J. L. and Schnur, R. C. (1980). US Patent 4,210,667.

Sartor, G., Melander, A., Schersten, B. and Wahlin-Boll, E. (1980). *Eur. J. Clin. Pharmacol.* **17**, 285–293.

Satchithanandam, S., Vargofcak-Apker, M., Calvert, R. J., Leeds, A. R. and Cassidy, M. M. (1990). *J. Nutr.* **120**, 1179–1184.

Satoh, T., Nakafuku, M. and Kaziro, Y. (1992). *J. Biol. Chem.* **267**, 24149–24152.

Schade, D. S., Mitchell, W. J. and Griego, G. (1987) *J. Am. Med. Assoc.* **257**, 2441–2445.

Schäffer, L., Kjeldsen, T., Andersen, A. S., Wiberg, F. C. and Larsen, U. D. (1993). *J. Biol. Chem.* **268**, 3044–3047.

Schatz, H., Katsilambros, N., Nierle, C. and Pfeiffer, E. F. (1972). *Diabetologia* **8**, 402–407.

Schlessinger, J. (1988). *TIBS* **13**, 443–447.

Schlichtkrull, J. (1958). "Insulin Crystals." Ejnar Munksgaard Publisher, Copenhagen.

Schmid-Antomarchi, H., De Weille, J., Fosser, M. and Lazdunski, M. (1987). *J. Biol. Chem.* **262**, 15840–15844.

Schneider, J., Erren, T., Zofel, P. and Kaffarnik, H. (1990). *Atherosclerosis* **82**, 97–103.

Schöffling, F. K., Petzoldt, R., Hillebrand I., Schwedes, U. (1982). *In* "Genetic Environmental Interaction in Diabetes Mellitus" (J. S. Melish, ed.), pp. 339–343. Excerpta Medica, Amsterdam.

Schönborn, J., Heim, K., Rabast, U., Jaeger, H. and Ditschuneit, H. (1975). *Diabetologia* **11**, 375 (Abstr.).

Schrey, M. P. and Montague, W. (1983). *Biochem. J.* **216**, 433–441.

Schubart, U. K. (1982). *J. Biol. Chem.* **257**, 12231–12238.

Schuit, F. C. and Pipeleers, D. G. (1986). *Science* **232**, 875–877.

Schulz, E. (1968). *Arch. Klin. Med.* **214**, 135–162.

Schumann, F., Janssen, K., Aubell, R. and Christl, H. L. (1982). *In* "Proceedings of the First International Symposium on Acarbose" (W. Creutzfeld, ed.), pp. 367–372. Excerpta Medica, Amsterdam.

Schwartz, G. P., Burke, G. T. and Katsoyannis, P. G. (1989). *Proc. Natl Acad. Sci. USA* **86**, 458–461.

Schwartz, S. E., Levine, R. A., Singh, A., Scheidecker, J. R. and Track, N. S. (1982). *Gastroenterology* **83**, 812–817.

Schwedes, U., Pethold, R., Hillebrand, I., Schöffling, K. (1982). *In* "Proceedings of the First International Symposium on Acarbose" (W. Creutzfeld, ed.), pp. 275–281. Excerpta Medica, Amsterdam.

Sedoul, J. C., Pegron, J. F., Ballotti, R., Debant, A., Fehlmann, M. and Van Obberghen,

E. (1985). *Biochem. J.* **227**, 887–892.

Seino, S., Seino, M., Nishi, S. and Bell, G. I. (1989). *Proc. Natl Acad. Sci. USA* **86**, 114–118.

Selam, J. L., Slingenereyer, A., Saeidi, S., Mirouze, J., Richard, J. L. O., Rodies, M., Daynes, B. and Lapinski, H. (1985). *Diabetic Med.* **2**, 41–44.

Sellers, E. M. and Holloway, M. R. (1978). *Clin. Pharmacokinet.* **3**, 440–452.

Seltzer, H. S. (1979). *Compr. Ther.* **5**, 21–29.

Seltzer, H. S. (1989). *Endocrinol. Metab. Clin. North-Am.* **18**, 163–183.

Semba, K., Kamata, N., Toyoshima, K. and Yamamoto, T (1985). *Proc. Natl Acad. Sci. USA* **82**, 6497–6501.

Sener, A., Dufrane, S. P. and Malaisse, W. J. (1986). *Biochem. Pharmacol.* **35**, 3701–3708.

Sharp, G. W. G., Wiedenkeller, D. E., Kaelin, D., Siegel, E. G. and Wollheim, C. B. (1980). *Diabetes* **29**, 74–77.

Sharp, G. W. G., LeMarchaud-Brustel, Y., Yada, T., Russo, L. L., Bliss, C. R., Cormont, M., Monge, L. and Van Obberghen, E. (1989). *J. Biol. Chem.* **264**, 7302–7309.

Shaw, K. M., Bloom, A. and Bulpitt, C. J. (letter) (1977). *Br. Med. J.* **1**, 1415.

Shemer, J., Perrotti, N., Roth, J. and LeRoith, D. (1987). *J. Biol. Chem.* **262**, 3436–3439.

Shia, M. A. and Pilch, P. F. (1983). *Biochemistry* **22**, 717–721.

Shilo, S., Sotsky, M. and Shamoon, H. (1990). *J. Clin. Endocrinol. Metab.* **70**, 162–172.

Shima, K., Hirota, M. and Ohboshi, C. (1988). *Regul. Pept.* **22**, 245–252.

Shimazu, T. (1981). *Diabetologia* **20**, 343–356.

Shimizu, F., Shimizu, M. and Kamiyama, K. (1985). *Endocrinology* **117**, 2081–2084.

Shoelson, S. E., White, M. F. and Kahn, C. R. (1988). *J. Biol. Chem.* **263**, 4852–4860.

Shulman, G. I., Rothman, D. L., Jue, T., Stein, P. DeFronzo, R. A. and Shulman, R. G. (1990). *N. Engl. J. Med.* **322**, 223–228.

Shuster, L. T., Go, V. L., Rizza, R. A., O'Brien, P. C. and Service, F. J. (1988). *Diabetes* **37**, 200–203.

Siitonen, O., Huttunen, J. K., Järvinen, R., Palomäki, P., Aro, A., Juvonen, H., Korhonen, T. and Ritala, P. (1980). *Lancet* **i**, 217–223.

Silverstone, P. (1986). *Br. Med. J.* **292**, 933–934.

Sima, A. A., Lattimer, S. A., Yagihashi, S. and Greene, D. A. (1986). *J. Clin. Invest.* **77**, 474–484.

Sima, A. F., Bril, V., Nathaniel, V., McEwen, T. A., Brown, M. B., Lattimer, S. A. and Greene, D. A. (1988). *N. Engl. J. Med.* **319**, 548–555.

Simonson, D. C., Koivisto, V., Sherwin, R. S., Ferrannini, E., Hendler, R., Juhlin-Dannfeldt, A. and DeFronzo, R. A. (1984). *J. Clin. Invest.* **73**, 1648–1658.

Simonson, D. C., Delprato, S., Castellino P., Groop, L. and DeFronzo, R. A. (1987). *Diabetes* **36**, 136–146.

Simpson, H. C. R., Simpson, R. W., Lousley, S., Carter, R. D., Greckie, M., Hockaday, T. D. R. and Mann, J. (1981). *Lancet* **i**, 1–5.

Singh, S. K., Hatwal, A., Agrawal, J. K., Bajpai, H. S. and Singh, S. K. (1989). *Indian J. Pediatr.* **26**, 1007–1009.

Sirtori, C. R., Francheschini, G., Galli-Kienle, M., Cighetti, G., Galli, G., Bondioli, A. and Conti, F. (1978). *Clin. Pharmacol. Ther.* **24**, 683–693.

Sjöström, L. and William-Olsson, T. (1981). *Curr. Ther. Res.* **30**, 351–353.

Sjöstrom, L. and William-Olsson, T. (1982). *In Proc. Int. 1st Symp. Acarbose*, pp. 73–85. Exerpta Medica, Amsterdam.

Skolnik, E. Y., Batzer, A., Li, N., Lee, C.-H., Lowenstein, E., Mohammadi, M., Margolis, B. and Schlessinger, J. (1993a). *Science* **260**, 1953–1955.

Skolnik, E. Y., Lee, C.-H., Batzer, A., Vicentini, L. M., Zhou, M., Daly, R., Myers, M. J., Jr., Backer, J. M., Ullrich, A., White, M. F. and Schlessinger, J. (1993b). *EMBO J.* **12**, 1929–1936.

Smith, P. A., Rorsman, P. and Ashcroft, F.M. (1989). *Nature* **342**, 550–553.
Sodoyez, J. C. and Sodoyez-Goffaux, F. (1984). *Diabetologia* **27**, 143–145.
Somogyi, M. (1959). *Am. J. Med.* **26**, 169–191.
Sonnenberg, G. E., Kemmer, F. W., Cüppers, H. J. and Berger, M. (1983). *Diabetes Care* **6**, Suppl. 1, 35–39.
Soos, M. A. and Siddle, K. (1989). *Biochem. J.* **263**, 553–563.
Soos, M. A., Whittaker, J., Lammers, R., Ullrich, A. and Siddle, K. (1990). *Biochem. J.* **270**, 383–390.
Sorbinil Retinopathy Trial Research Group (1990). *Arch. Ophthalmol.* **108**, 1234–1244.
Sowers, J. R. (1991). *Am. Heart. J.* **122**, 932–935.
Spangler, R. (1990). *Diabetes Care* **13**, 911–922.
Spengler, M., Hänsel, G. and Boehme, K. (1992). *Horm. Metab. Res.* **26** (Suppl.), 50–51.
Speth, P. A. J., Jansen, J. B. M. J. and Lamers, C. B. H. W. (1983). *Gut* **24**, 798–802.
Stagner, J. I., Samols, E. and Bonner-Weir, S. (1988). *Diabetes* **37**, 1715–1721.
Stagner, J. I., Samols, E. and Marks, V. (1989). *Diabetologia* **32**, 203–206.
Standaert, M. L., Farese, R. V., Cooper, D. R. and Pollet, R. J. (1988). *J. Biol. Chem.* **263**, 8698–8705.
Steele-Perkins, G., Roth, R. A. (1990) *J. Biol. Chem.* **265**, 9458–9463.
Steinke, J., Patel, T. N., Ammon, H. P. T. (1972). *Metabolism* **21**, 465–470.
Stenman, S., Gropp, P. H., Saloranta, C., Totterman, K. J., Fyhrqvist, F. and Groop, L. (1988). *Diabetologia* **31**, 206–213.
Stewart, W. J., McSweeney, S. M., Kelett, M. A., Faxon, D. P. and Ryan, T. J. (1984). *Circulation* **70**, 788.
Stocks, A. E., Ma, A., Howlett, V. and Cameron, D. P. (1988). *Med. J. Aust.* **149**, 472–473.
Stowers, J. M. (1980). *The Royal Society of Medicine. International Congress and Symposium Series* **48**, 149–157.
Stribling, D. (1990). *Exp. Eye Res.* **50**, 621–624.
Stribling, D., Mirrlees, D. J. and Earl, D. C. N. (1983). *Diabetologia* **25**, 196 (Abstr. 362).
Strubbe, J. H. and Steffens, A. B. (1975). *Am. J. Physiol.* **229**, 1019–1022.
Stryjek-Kaminska, D., Pacula, P., Janeczko, E., Trusiewicz, D., Koneczna, A. and Dembe, K. (1989). *Diabetes Res. Clin. Pract.* **7**, 149–154.
Sturgess, N. C., Ashford, M. L. J., Cook, D. L. and Hales, C. N. (1985). *Lancet* **ii**, 474–475.
Sturm, M. (1992). *Wien. Klin. Wochenschr.* **104**, 329–336.
Sugden, M. C., Ashcroft, S. J. H. and Sugden, P. H. (1979). *Biochem. J.* **180**, 219–229.
Sun, X. J., Rothenberg, P., Kahn, C. R., Backer, J. M., Araki, E., Wilden, P. A., Cahill, D. A., Goldstein, B. J. and White, M. F. (1991). *Nature* **352**, 73–77.
Sun, X. J., Miralpeix, M., Myers, M. G., Jr., Glasheen, E. M., Backer, J. M., Kahn, C. R. and White, M. F. (1992). *J. Biol. Chem.* **267**, 22662–22672.
Sundkvist, G., Armstrong, F. M., Bradbury, J. E., Chaplin, C., Ellis, S. H., Owens, D. R., Rosen, I. and Sonksen, P. (1992). *J. Diabet. Complications* **6**, 123–130.
Sundler, F. and Böttcher, G. (1991). *In* "The Endocrine Pancreas" (E. Samols, ed.), pp. 29–51. Raven Press, New York.
Sussman, K. E., Crout, J. R. and Marble, A. (1963). *Diabetes* **12**, 38–45.
Suzuki, K. and Kono, T. (1980). *Proc. Natl Acad. Sci. USA* **77**, 2542–2545.
Suzuki, S., Oka, H., Yasuda, H., Ikeda, M., Cheng, P. Y. and Oda, T. (1983). *Endocrinology* **112**, 348–352.
Sweet, L. J., Morrison, B. D., Wilden, P. A. and Pessin, J. E. (1987). *J. Biol. Chem.* **262**, 16730–16738.
Sykes, S., Morgan, L. M., English, J. and Marks, V. (1980). *J. Endocrinol.* **85**, 201–207.
Syvälahti, E. K. G., Pihlajamaki, K. K. and Iisalo, E. J. (1974). *Lancet* **ii**, 232–233.

Szecowka, J., Grill, V., Sandberg, E. and Efendic, S. (1982). *Acta Endocrinol. (Copenh.)* **99**, 416–421.

Tadeo, T., Sathogi, S. and Masanori, K. (1982). European Patent 045,165 and 047,109.

Tagliaferro, V., Cassader, M., Bozzo, C., Pisu, E., Bruno, A., Marena, S., Cavallo-Perin, P., Cravero, L. and Pagano, G. (1985). *Diabete Metab.* **11**, 380–385.

Takayama, S., White, M. F., Lauris, V. and Kahn, C. R. (1984). *Proc. Natl. Acad. Sci. USA* **81**, 7797–7801.

Takayama, S., White, M. F. and Kahn, C. R. (1988). *J. Biol. Chem.* **263**, 3340–3447.

Täljedal, I.-B. (1982). In "Skandia International Symposion" (H. Boström and N. Ljungstedt, eds), p. 145. Almqvist & Wiksell, Stockholm.

Tamagawa, T., Niki, H. and Niki, A. (1985). *FEBS Lett.* **183**, 430–432.

Tanigawa, K., Kuzuya, H., Imura, H., Taniguchi, H., Baba, S., Takai, Y. and Nishizuka, Y. (1982). *FEBS Lett.* **138**, 183–186.

Tatemoto, K., Rökaeus, Å., Jörnvall, H., McDonald, T. J. and Mutt, V. (1983). *FEBS Lett.* **164**, 124–128.

Tattersall, R. (letter) (1992). *Brit. Med. J.* **305**, 831.

Tavare, J. M. and Denton, R. M. (1988). *Biochem. J.* **252**, 607–615.

Tavare, J. M., O'Brien, R. M., Siddle, K. and Denton, R. M. (1988). *Biochem. J.* **253**, 783–788.

Taylor, C. W. (1990a). *Biochem. J.* **272**, 1–13.

Taylor, R. H. (1990b). In "New Antidiabetic Drugs" (C. J. Bailey and P. R. Flatt, eds), pp. 119–132. Smith-Gordon, London.

Taylor, S. I., Kadowaki, T., Kadowaki, H. and Accili, D. (1990). *Diabetes Care* **13**, 257–279.

Tchoubroutsky, G. (1978). *Diabetologia* **15**, 143–152.

Teale, J. D. and Love, A. H. G. (1972). *Biochem. Pharmacol.* **21**, 1839–1848.

Thams, P., Capito, K. and Hedeskov, C. J. (1982). *Biochem. J.* **206**, 97–102.

Thoelke, H. and Ratzmann, K. P. (1989). *Dtsch. Med. Wochenschr.* **114**, 580–583.

Thomas, T. P., Ellis, T. R. and Pek, S. B. (1989). *Diabetes* **38**, 1371–1376.

Thorens, B., Sarkar, H. K., Kaback, H. R. and Lodish, H. F. (1988). *Cell* **55**, 281–290.

Tobe, K., Koshio, O., Tashiro-Hashimoto, Y., Takaku, F., Akanuma, Y. and Kasuga, M. (1990). *Diabetes* **39**, 528–533.

Todd, P. A., Benfield, P. and Goa, K. L. (1990). *Drugs* **39**, 917–928.

Toeller, M. (1990). *Diabetes Nutr. Metab.* **3** (Suppl. 1), 43–49.

Tornqvist, H. E. and Avruch, J. (1988). *J. Biol. Chem.* **263**, 4593–4601.

Tornqvist, H. E., Pierce, M. W., Frackelton, A. R., Nemenoff, R. A. and Avruch, J. (1987). *J. Biol. Chem.* **262**, 10212–10219.

Tornqvist, H. E., Gunsalus, J. R., Memenoff, R. A., Frackelton, A. R., Pierce, M. W. and Avruch, J. (1988b). *J. Biol. Chem.* **263**, 350–359.

Torsdottir, I., Alpsten, M., Andersson, H. and Einarsson, S. (1989). *J. Nutr.* **119**, 1925–1931.

Toyoda, N., Flanagan, J. E. and Kono, T. (1987). *J. Biol. Chem.* **262**, 2737–2745.

Travis, R. H. and Sayers, G. (1970). In "Goodman and Gilman's The Pharmacological Basis of Therapeutics" (A. Goodman, Gilman, T. W. Rall, A. S. Nies and P. Taylor, eds), 4th edn, pp. 1581–1603. Macmillan, New York.

Treherne, J. M. and Ashford, M. L. (1991). *Neuroscience* **40**, 523–531.

Trischitta, V., Gullo, D., Pezziano, V. and Vigneri, R. (1983). *J. Clin. Endocrinol. Metab.* **57**, 713–718.

Tromp, A., Hooymans, J. M., Barendsen, B. C. and van Doormaal, J. J. (1991). *Doc. Ophthalmol.* **78**, 153–159.

Tronier, B., Deigard, A., Andersen, T. and Madsbad, S. (1985) *Diabetes Res. Clin. Pract.* **1** (Supp. 1) S568.

Troy, S. M., Hicks, D. R., Kramal, M., Conrad, K. and Chiang, S. T. (1992). *Clin. Pharmacol. Ther.* **51**, 271–277.

Tucker, G. T., Casey, C., Phillips, P. J., Connor, H., Ward, J. D. and Woods, H. F. (1981). *Br. J. Clin. Pharmacol.* **12**, 235–246.

Turner, P. R., Tuomilehto, J., Happonen, P., La-Ville, A. E., Shaikh, M. and Lewis, B. (1990). Atherosclerosis **81**, 145–150.

Turner, R. C. and Holman, R. (1990). *Diabetes Care* **13**, 1011–1020.

Turner, R. C., Hosker, J. P. and Holman, R. R. (1987). *Medicographia* **9**, 42–45.

Ui, M. (1984). *Trends Biochem. Sci.* **7**, 277–279.

Ullrich, A., Bell, J. R., Chen, E. Y., Herrera, R., Petruzelli, L. M., Dull, T. J., Gray, A., Coussens, L., Liao, Y.-C., Tsubokawa, M., Mason, A., Seeburg, P. H., Grunfeld, C., Rosen, O. M. and Ramachandran, J. (1985). *Nature* **313**, 756–761.

Ullrich, A., Gray, A., Tam, A. W., Yang-Feng, T., Tsubokawa, M., Collins, C., Henzel, W., LeBon, T., Kathuria, S., Chen, E., Jacobs, S., Francke, U., Ramachandran, J. and Fujita-Yamaguchi, Y. (1986). *EMBO J.* **5**, 2503–2512.

University Group Diabetes Program (1970). *Diabetes* **19** (Suppl. 2), 785–830.

Uusitupa, M., Sodervik, H., Silvasti, M. and Karttunen, P. (1990). *Int. J. Clin. Pharmacol. Ther. Toxicol.* **28**, 153–157.

Uusitupa, M., Ebeling, T., Happonen, P., Voutilainen, E., Turtola, H., Parviainen, M. and Pyorala, K. (1991). *J. Cardiovasc. Pharmacol.* **18**, 496–503.

Vague, P., Juhan-Vague, I., Alessi, M. C., Badier, C. and Valadier, J. (1987). *Thromb. Haem.* **57**, 326–328.

Vallar, L., Biden, T. J. and Wollheim, C. B. (1987). *J. Biol. Chem.* **262**, 5049–5056.

Valverde, I., Vandermeers, A., Anjaneyulu, R. and Malaisse, W. J. (1979). *Science* **206**, 225–227.

Van Obberghen, E. and Kowalski, A. (1982). *FEBS Lett.* **143**, 179–192.

Van Obberghen, E., Rossi, B., Kowalski, A., Gazzano, H. and Ponzio, G. (1983). *Proc. Natl Acad. Sci. USA* **80**, 945–949.

Varticovski, L., Druker, B., Morrison, D., Cantley, L. and Roberts, T. (1989). *Nature* **342**, 699–702.

Velasco, J. M. (1987). *J. Physiol.* **398**, 15P.

Venkatesh, N., Lamp, S. T. and Weiss, J. N. (1991). *Circ. Res.* **69**, 623–637.

Verdy, M., Charbonneau, L., Verdy, I., Belanger, R., Bolte, E. and Chiasson, J. L. (1983). *Int. J. Obes.* **7**, 289–297.

Verspohl, E. J. and Ammon, H. P. T. (1980). *J. Clin. Invest.* **65**, 1230–1237.

Verspohl, E. J., Händel, M. and Ammon, H. P. T. (1979). *Endocrinology* **105**, 1269–1274.

Verspohl, E. J., Händel, M., Hagenloh, I. and Ammon, H. P. T. (1982). *Acta Diabetol. Lat.* **19**, 303–317.

Verspohl, E. J., Berger, U. and Ammon, H. P. T. (1986a). *Biochim. Biophys. Acta* **888**, 217–224.

Verspohl, E. J., Ammon, H. P. T., Williams, J. A. and Goldfine, I. D. (1986b). *Diabetes* **35**, 38–43.

Verspohl, E. J., Breuning, I., Ammon, H. P. T. and Mark, M. (1987). *Regulat. Pept.* **17**, 229–241.

Verspohl, E. J., Kaiser, P., Wahl, M. and Ammon, H. P. T. (1988). *Life Sci.* **43**, 209–219.

Verspohl, E. J., Breuning, I. and Ammon, H. P. T. (1989). *Am. J. Physiol.* **256** (*Endocrinol. Metab.* 19) E68–E73.

Verspohl, E. J., Ammon, H. P. T. and Klosa, M. (1990a). *Biochem. J.* **267**, 339–342.

Verspohl, E. J., Tacke, R., Mutschler, E., Lambrecht, G. (1990b). *Eur. J. Pharmacol.* **178**, 303–311.

Verspohl, E. J., Ammon, H. P. T. and Mark, M. (1990c). *J. Pharm. Pharmacol.* **42**, 230–255.

Vigneri, R. and Goldfine, I. (1987). *Diabetes Care* **10**, 118–122.

Vigneri, R., Gullo, D. and Pezzino, V. (1984). *Diabetes Care* **7** (Suppl. 1), 113–117.

Vincent, G. M., Janowski, M. and Menlove, R. (1991). *Cathet. Cardiovasc. Diagn.* **23**, 164–168.

Virsolvy-Vergine, A., Leray, H., Kuroki, S., Lupo, B., Dufour, M. and Bataille, D. (1992). *Proc. Natl. Acad. Sci. USA* **89**, 6629–6633.

Vogt, B., Mushack, J., Seffer, E. and Häring, H. U. (1990). *Biochem. Biophys. Res. Commun.* **168**, 1089–1094.

Vogt, B., Carrascosa, J. M., Ermel, B., Ullrich, A. and Häring, H. U. (1991a). *Biochem. Biophys. Res. Commun.* **177**, 1013–1018.

Vogt, B., Mushack, J., Seffer, E. and Häring, H. U. (1991b). *Biochem. J.* **275**, 597–600.

Vogt, B., Mühlbacher, C., Carrascosa, J. M., Obermaier-Kusser, B., Seffer, E., Mushack, J., Pongratz, D. and Häring, H. U. (1992). *Diabetologia* **35**, 456–463.

Vojtek, A. B., Hollenberg, S. M. and Cooper, J. A. (1993). *Cell* **74**, 205–214.

Von Kriegstein, E. (1985). *Ärtzl. Praxis* **37**, 302–304.

Vora, J. P. and Owens, D. R. (1991). *In* "Pharmacology of Diabetes" (C. E. Mogensen and E. Standl, eds) pp. 39–56 de Gruyter, Berlin, New York.

Vora, J. P., Owen, D. R. and Dolben, J. (1988). *Br. Med. J.* **297**, 1236–1239.

Wahl, M. A., Plehn, R. J., Landsbeck, E. A. and Ammon, H. P. T. (1991). *Endocrinology* **128**, 6, 3247–3252.

Wahl, M. A., Landsbeck, E. A., Ammon, H. P. T. and Verspohl, E. J. (1992). *Pancreas* **7**, 345–351.

Wahl, M. A., Straub, S. G., Ammon, H. P. T. (1993). *Diabetologia* **36**, 920–925.

Wåhlander, K., Ämmälä, C., Berggren, P.-O., Bokvist, K., Juntti-Berggren, L. and Rorsman, P. (1991). *In* "Wenner-Gren International Symposium Series" (T. Hökfelt, ed.).

Waldhäusl, W. (1987). *In* "Klinische Pharmacology" (H. P. Kuemmerle, G. Hitzenberger and K. H. Spitzy, eds), pp. 1–26. Ecomed Verlag, Landsberg, München.

Waldhäusl, W., Bratusch-Marrain, P., Breitenecker, F., Troch, I. and Komjati, M. (1984). *Diabetes* **33** (Suppl. 1A), 3.

Waldhäusl, W. K. (1986). *Diabetologia* **29**, 837–849.

Waldhäusl, W. K., Bratusch-Marrain, P., Kruse, V., Jensen, J., Nowotny, P. and Vierhapper, H. (1985). *Diabetes* **34**, 166–173.

Walker, A. R., Walker, B. F. and Richardson, B. D. (1970). *Lancet* **ii**, 51–52.

Walter-Sack, I., Ittner-Holland, A., Zöllner, N. and Wolfram, G. (1982). *In* "Proceedings of the First International Symposium on Acarbose" (W. Creutzfeld, ed.), pp. 223–224. Excerpta Medica, Amsterdam.

Walter-Sack, I. E., Wolfram, G. and Zollner, N. (1989). *Ann. Nutr. Metab.* **33**, 100–107.

Wang, J., Kwok, Y.-N., Baimbridge, K. G. and Brown, J. C. (1992). *Biochem. Biophys. Res. Commun.* **182**, 858–863.

Wang, J. L., Corbett, J. A., Marshall, C. A. and McDaniel, M. L. (1993). *J. Biol. Chem.* **268**, 7785–7791.

Ward, J. D. (1991). *In* "Textbook of Diabetes" (J. C. Pickup and G. Williams, eds), pp. 623–634. Blackwell Scientific Publications, Oxford.

Wardzala, L. J., Cushman, S. W. and Salans, L. B. (1978). *J. Biol. Chem.* **253**, 8002–8005.

Watkins, D. T. and Cooperstein, S. J. (1983). *Endocrinology* **112**, 766–771.

Weichert, W. and Breddin, H. K. (1988). *Diabéte Metab.* **14**, 540–543.

Weiss, M. E., Chatham, F., Kagey-Sobotka, A. and Adkinson, N. F., Jr. (1990). *Clin. Exp. Allergy*, **20**, 713–720.

Welsh, N. and Sandler, S. (1992). *Biochem. Biophys. Res. Commun.* **182**, 333–340.

White, M., Häring, H. U., Kasuga, M. and Kahn, C. R. (1984). *J. Biol. Chem.* **259**, 255–264.

White, N., Gingerich, R., Levandowski, L., Cryer, P. and Santiago, J. (1985a). *Diabetes* **34**, 870–875.

White, M. F., Maron, R. and Kahn, C. R. (1985b). *Nature* **163**, 76–80.

White, M. F., Takayama, Y. and Kahn, C. R. (1985c). *J. Biol. Chem.* **260**, 9470–9478.

White, M. F., Livingston, J. N., Backer, J. M., Lauris, V., Dull, T. J., Ullrich, A. and Kahn, C. R. (1988a). *Cell* **54**, 641–649.
White, M. F., Shoelson, B. E., Keutmann, H. and Kahn, C. R. (1988b). *J. Biol. Chem.* **68**, 2969–2980.
WHO Study Group (1985a). In "Technical Report Series: Diabetes Mellitus", 727, pp. 30–31. Geneva.
WHO Study Group (1985b). In "Technical Report Series: Diabetes Mellitus", 727, pp. 9–19. Geneva.
Wiholm, B. E. and Westerholm, B. (1984). *Acta. Med. Scand.* **683** (Suppl.), 107–117.
Wilden, P. A., Backer, J. M., Kahn, C. R., Cahill, D. A., Schroeder, G. J. and White, M. F. (1990). *Proc. Natl Acad. Sci. USA* **87**, 3358–3362.
Wiles, P. G., Guy, R., Watkins, S. M. and Reeves, W. G. (1983). *Br. Med. J.* **287**, 531.
Wiles, P. G., Hoskins, P., Leslie, R. D. and Pyke, D. A. (1984). *Br. Med. J.* **288**, 328–329.
Williams, D. R. F., James, W. P. T. and Evans, I. E. (1980). *Diabetologia* **18**, 379–383.
Williams, R. L., Blaschke, T. F., Meffin, P. J., Melmon, K. L. and Rowland, M. (1977). *Clin. Pharmacol. Ther.* **21**, 301–307.
Willms, B. and Sachse, G. (1982). *In Proc. 1st Int. Symp.* Acarbose, pp. 471–473. Excerpta Medica, Amsterdam.
Willms, B., Henrichs, H. R. and von Kriegstein, E. (1987). *Dt. Ärzteblatt* **84**, 203–204.
Wilson, D. E. (1983). *Ann. Intern. Med.* **98**, 219–227.
Wilson, D. P., Fesmire, J. D., Endres, R. K. and Blackett, P. R. (1985). *South. Med. J.* **78**, 636–638.
Wilson, J. A., Scott, M. M. and Gray, R. S. (1989). *Horm. Metab. Res.* **21**, 317–319.
Wing, L. M. H. and Miners, J. O. (1985). *Br. J. Clin. Pharmacol.* **20**, 482–485.
Wintermantel, C., Fischer, N., Muller, P. H., Velcovsky, H. G., Lischka, G. and Eggstein, M. (1988). *Dtsch. Med. Wochenschr.* **113**, 1142–1145.
Wogensen, L. D., Kolb-Bachofen, V., Christensen, P., Dinarello, C. A., Mandrup-Poulsen, T., Martin, S. and Nerup, J. (1990). *Diabetologia* **33**, 15–23.
Wolf, J., Wolf, E. and Hurter, P. (1987). *Monatsschr. Kinderheilk.* **135**, 770–774.
Wolfe, R. F., Nadel, E. R., Shaw, J. H. F., Stephenson, L. A. and Wolfe, M. H. (1986). *J. Clin. Invest.* **77**, 900–907.
Wollen, N. and Bailey, C. J. (1988a). *Diabete Metab.* **14**, 88–91.
Wollen, N. and Bailey, C. J. (1988b). *Biochem. Pharmacol.* **37**, 4353–4358.
Wollheim, C. B. and Biden, T. J. (1986). *J. Biol. Chem.* **261**, 8314–8319.
Wollheim, C. B., Dunne, M. J., Peter-Reisch, B., Bruzzone, R., Pozzan, T. and Petersen, O. H. (1988). *EMBO J.* **7**, 2443–2449.
Wolters, G. H. J., Wiegman, J. B. and Konijnendijk, W. (1982). *Diabetologia* **22**, 122–127.
Wright, A. D., Walsh, C. H., Fitzgerald, M. G. and Malins, J. M. (1979) *Br. Med. J.* **1**, 25–27.
Wright, K. S., Beck-Nielsen, H., Kolterman, O. G. and Mandarino, L. J. (1988). *Diabetes* **37**, 436–440.
Wu, M. S., Johnston, P., Sheu, E. H., Hollenbeck, C. B., Jeng, C. Y., Goldfine, I. D., Chen, Y. D. and Reaven, G. M. (1990). *Diabetes Care* **13**, 1–8.
Wyeth-Ayerst Int. Inc. (1989). "Alredase™." Franklin Scientific Projects Ltd., London, and Wyeth-Ayerst Int. Inc., Philadelphia.
Wymore, J. and Carter, J. E. (1982). *Arch. Intern. Med.* **142**, 381.
Yada, T., Russo, L. L. and Sharp, G. W. G. (1989). *J. Biol. Chem.* **264**, 2455–2462.
Yamada, K., Goncalves, E., Kahn, C. R. and Shoelson, S. E. (1992). *J. Biol. Chem.* **267**, 12452–12461.
Yamaguchi, Y., Flier, J. S., Yokota, A., Benecke, H., Backer, J. M. and Moller, D. E. (1991). *Endocrinology* **129**, 2058–2066.

Yamamoto, S., Ishii, M., Nakadate, T., Nakaki, T. and Kato, R. (1983). *J. Biol. Chem.* **258**, 12149–12152.

Yamatani, T., Chiba, T., Kadowaki, S., Hishikawai, R., Yamaguchi, A., Inui, T., Fujita, T. and Kawazu, S. (1988). *Endocrinology* **122**, 2826–2832.

Yanagawa, T., Yokoyana, A., Noya, K., Kasuga, Y., Takei, I., Maruyama, H., Kataoka, K., Saruta, T., Kawamura, S. and Toyama, K. (1990). *South. Med. J.* **83**, 1323–1326.

Yaney, G. C., Stafford, G. A., Henstenberg, J. D., Sharp, G. W. G. and Weiland, G. A. (1991). *J. Pharmacol. Exp. Ther.* **258**, 653–662.

Yang-Feng, T. L., Francke, U. and Ullrich, A. (1985). *Science* **228**, 728–731.

Yip, C. C., Hsu, H., Patel, R. G., Hawley, D. M., Maddux, B. A. and Goldfine, I. D. (1988). *Biochem. Biophys. Res. Comm.* **157**, 321–329.

Ylitalo, P., Oksala, H. and Pitkajarvi, T. (1985). *Arzneimittelforschung/Drug Res.* **35**, 1596–1599.

Yoon, J. W. and Ray, U. R. (1985). *Diabetes Care* **8** (Suppl. 1), 39–44.

Yoshimoto, A., Nakanishi, K., Anzai, T. and Komine, S. (1990). *Cell. Biochem. Funct.* **8**, 163–166.

Zaman, R., Kendall, M. J. and Biggs, P. I. (1982). *Br. J. Clin. Pharmacol.* **13**, 507–512.

Zawalich, W. S. and Diaz, V. A. (1986). *Diabetes* **35**, 1119–1123.

Zawalich, W. S., Diaz, V. A. and Zawalich, K. C. (1987). *Diabetes* **36**, 1420–1424.

Zawalich, W. S., Dierolf, B. and Zawalich, K. C. (1989a). *Endocrinology* **124**, 720–726.

Zawalich, W. S., Zawalich, K. C. and Rasmussen, H. (1989b). *Endocrinology* **125**, 2400–2406.

Zenobi, P. D. (1991). *Schweiz. Med. Wochenschr.* **121**, 475–481.

Zeuzem, S., Stahl, E., Jungmann, E., Zoltobrocki, M., Schöffling, K. and Caspary, W. F. (1990). *Diabetologia* **33**, 65–71.

Zick, Y., Sagi-Eisenberg, R., Pines, M., Gierschik, P. and Spiegel, A. M. (1986). *Proc. Natl Acad. Sci. USA* **83**, 9294–9297.

Ziegler, D., Mayer, P., Rathmann, W. and Gries, F. A. (1991). *Diabetes Res. Clin. Pract.* **14**, 63–73.

Zielmann, S., Schütte, G., Lenzen, S. and Panten, U. (1985). *Naunyn-Schmiedeberg's Arch. Pharmacol.* **329**, 299–304.

Zillikens, M. C., Swart, G. R., Van den Berg, J. W. and Wilson, J. H. P. (1989). *Aliment. Pharmacol. Ther.* **3**, 453–459.

Zinman, B. and Vranic, M. (1985). *Med. Clin. North Am.* **69**, 145–157.

Zinman, B., Vranic, M., Albisser, A. M., Hanna, A. K., Minuk, H. L. and Marliss, E. B. (letter) (1978). *N. Engl. J. Med.* **298**, 1202–1203.

Zuenkler, B. J., Trube, G. and Panten, U. (1989). *Naunyn-Schmiedeberg's Arch. Pharmacol.* **340**, 328–332.

# SUBJECT INDEX

## A

A-cells, 79, 100, 103, 104
$\beta$-adrenergic receptors, 101–102
insulin in regulation, 104
Acanthosis nigricans, 66
Acarbose, 75, 159–169, 179
actions, 159–160
administration, 161
chemistry, 159
clinical studies, 163–169
healthy volunteers, 163–165
type-I diabetes mellitus (IDDM), 165
type-II diabetes mellitus (NIDDM), 132, 165–169
drug interactions, 163
insulin therapy combination, 165, 168–169
lipid metabolism effects, 160–161, 164, 167
metformin combinations, 163
pharmacokinetics, 161–163
absorption, 161
distribution, 162
excretion, 162–163
half-life, 162
metabolism, 162
plasma levels, 162
side effects, 163
sulphonylureas combination, 161, 163, 168
uses, 161
Acetohexamide
pharmacokinetics, 119
side effects, 124
Acetylcholine, 101
Adenylate cyclase system
biguanide effects, 139
insulin secretion mechanism, 78, 92–93
sulphonylureas effects, 114–115
Adipose tissue
glucose transporter expression, 43, 44
glucose transporter function, 44–46
glucose uptake, 4, 45
insulin deficiency, 7

Adrenaline, insulin therapy interactions, 68
Adrenergic stimulation
glucose homoeostasis regulation, 5, 7
insulin secretion modulation, 100, 101–102
Adrenocorticotropic hormone (ACTH), 57
Age-associated factors
diabetes onset, 21
sulphonylureas pharmacokinetics, 120, 122
Alcohol
facial flushing response to sulphonylureas, 128–129
insulin therapy interactions, 68
Aldose reductase
biochemistry, 172–173
diabetic complications, 173
Aldose reductase inhibitors, 171–178
actions, 173–175
kidney, 174–175
neural tissue, 173–174
retina, 174
chemistry, 171–172
clinical trials, 177–178
drug interactions, 177
pharmacokinetics, 175–176
absorption, 175
distribution, 175
elimination, 176
half-life, 175
pathological changes, 176
plasma levels, 175
side effects, 176
structure, 172
toxic effects, 176
Alpha$_2$-adrenergic agonists, 102
Alpha-blockers, 67
Alrestatin, 172, 173
Anabolic steroids, 68
Anaphylactic reactions
insulin, 62–63
protamine, 68
Angiotensin-converting enzyme inhibitors, 67

type II diabetes mellitus
(NIDDM), 156–159
dosage, 153
drug interactions, 154
hydration rate, 152
lipid metabolism effects, 153,
158–159
pharmacokinetics, 153–154
side effects, 154
sulphonylureas interaction, 128
toxic effects, 154
uses, 152–153

**H**

Halofenate, 128
Hepatic glucose production (HGP), 3
insulin deficiency, 7
plasma glucose responsiveness, 14
stress response, 100
type II diabetes mellitus (NIDDM),
14
Hepatic impairment, 127
sulphonylureas pharmacokinetics,
120–121
Hepatomegaly, 68
HLA associations, 17
Honeymoon period, 19, 57, 64
Human insulin, 50, 51
absorption, 53
immunogenicity, 60, 64
lipoatrophy, 60
Hyperglycaemia
clinical symptoms, 18
insulin resistance, 66, 67
rebound see Somogyi phenomenon
Hyperlipidaemic states, 159, 161
Hypertension, 67
Hypoglycaemia, 21, 55–59
antibody-mediated insulin resistance,
66
continuous subcutaneous insulin
infusion (CSII), 72
drivers, 124
frequency, 57–58
hormonal changes, 56–57
insulin dosage adjustment, 56, 57
insulin secretion inhibition, 100
multiple daily injections (MDI), 72
sulphonylureas, 125–127
accumulation, 120

breast feeding, 125
clinical studies, 134–135
drug interactions, 127–128
neonatal effects, 124
overdosage, 121
symptoms, 55–56, 59, 121
treatment, 58–59, 121
unawareness, 56, 59
Hypothalamus, 6–7, 100

**I**

Incretin effect, 97, 98, 99
Indobufen, 128
Infectious aetiological factors, 18
Infectious complications, 19
Inositol phospho-oligosaccharides
(IPOs), 41, 42
Inositol triphosphate, insulin secretion
mechanism, 93, 94, 101
CCK$_8$ response, 99
Insulin
actions, 25–47
anabolic effects, 26
anticatabolic effects, 26
FFA mobilization inhibition, 6
glucose homoeostasis regulation,
3–7
growth-promoting effects, 26
islet A-cell/D-cell regulation, 103,
104
membrane transport processes, 26
protein biosynthesis regulation, 6, 9
bovine, 53, 55, 61, 64, 66
chemistry, 50
crystalline modifications, 50
physical exercise effect, 12
preparations, 50–52
absorption modification, 54–55
intermediate-acting, 50, 52
short/rapid-acting, 50, 51, 52
slow-acting/long-lasting, 51–52
pulsatile release, 4, 69
solubility, 50
structure, 50, 51
see also Bovine insulin; Human
insulin; Porcine insulin
Insulin allergy, 61–64
clinical manifestations, 62–63
anaphylaxis, 62–63
insulin resistance, 63

# CUMULATIVE INDEX OF AUTHORS

# CUMULATIVE INDEX OF TITLES